www.wadsworth.com

www.wadsworth.com is the World Wide Web site for Thomson Wadsworth and is your direct source to dozens of online resources.

At www.wadsworth.com you can find out about supplements, demonstration software, and student resources. You can also send email to many of our authors and preview new publications and exciting new technologies.

www.wadsworth.com

Changing the way the world learns®

Skills and Tools for Today's Counselors and Psychotherapists

From Natural Helping to Professional Counseling

Edward S. Neukrug
Old Dominion University

Alan M. Schwitzer
Old Dominion University

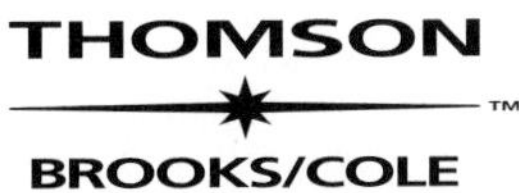

Australia • Canada • Mexico • Singapore • Spain
United Kingdom • United States

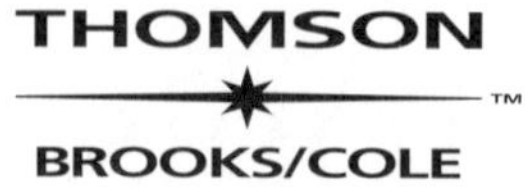

Skills and Tools for Today's Counselors and Psychotherapists: From Natural Helping to Professional Counseling, First Edition
Edward S. Neukrug and Alan M. Schwitzer

Executive Editor: Lisa Gebo
Assistant Editor: Alma Dea Michelena
Editorial Assistant: Sheila Walsh
Technology Project Manager: Barry Connolly
Executive Marketing Manager: Caroline Concilla
Senior Marketing Communications Manager: Tami Strang
Project Manager, Editorial Production: Rita Jaramillo
Art Director: Vernon Boes
Print Buyer: Rebecca Cross
Permissions Editor: Stephanie Lee
Production Service: Matrix Productions Inc.
Text Designer: John Edeen
Copy Editor: Frank Hubert
Cover Designer: Irene Morris
Cover Image: The Image Bank, Shaun Egan
Cover Printer: Webcom Limited
Compositor: Integra
Printer: Webcom Limited

Printed in Canada
1 2 3 4 5 6 7 09 08 07 06 05

Thomson Higher Education
10 Davis Drive
Belmont, CA 94002-3098
USA

Asia (including India)
Thomson Learning
5 Shenton Way
#01-01 UIC Building
Singapore 068808

Australia/New Zealand
Thomson Learning Australia
102 Dodds Street
Southbank, Victoria 3006
Australia

Canada
Thomson Nelson
1120 Birchmount Road
Toronto, Ontario M1K 5G4
Canada

UK/Europe/Middle East/Africa
Thomson Learning
High Holborn House
50/51 Bedford Row
London WC1R 4LR
United Kingdom

Library of Congress Control Number: 2004118287

ISBN 0-534-64490-2

To Kristina, Hannah, and Emma
You keep my feminine side alive and strong!
—E. S. N.

To my wife, Lisa, forever young
Laissez les bon temps rouler!
—A. M. S.

Contents

CHAPTER 2

CHAPTER 10

CHAPTER 11

Preface

Those who choose to become mental health professionals, such as counselors, psychotherapists, social workers, and psychologists, often describe themselves as "being the person who family and friends come to for help." In fact, people often choose the helping professions because they have been successful caregivers, mediators, or advisers in their personal lives. The qualities that others have seen in these *natural helpers*—qualities that have made them good listeners, calm responders, rational solution finders, or someone who asks the "right" questions—can often be fine-tuned and used in professional counseling and psychotherapy roles.

However, professional counseling and psychotherapy are about much more than being a natural helper. Professional practice requires

- an extensive academic knowledge base
- advanced mature self-development
- finely tuned professional helping and relationship skills
- the ability to rationally analyze the client's concerns and develop an effective plan for enabling the person to make changes and gains
- the knowledge and skill to implement a plan for change and make it work
- sound, ethical, and professional decision making

This book was written to introduce natural helpers to the knowledge and skills needed to become professional counselors. The text goes beyond the usual graduate skills textbook and presents critical issues graduate students will need to know if they are to be successful in today's highly complex world of professional counseling. As a result, we have divided the book into four parts that focus on eight core areas of knowledge and skills we believe are critical for the graduate student in training to master if he or she is to be an effective clinician. The eight core areas include (a) ethical, professional, and cross-cultural issues, (b) helper attitudes, (c) techniques, (d) diagnosis, (e) case conceptualization, (f) treatment planning, (g) case management, and (h) theory.

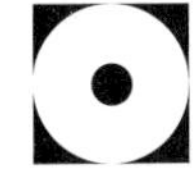

In addition to the text, the accompanying DVD offers brief explanations of the knowledge and skills presented in this text, provides demonstrations on how to use the skills most effectively, and reinforces much of what you will learn in your readings. As you read through the text, you will be periodically prompted to view the DVD that corresponds to your readings. At those points, we urge you to watch the DVD to augment what you have read.

Core Areas of Knowledge and Skills

The text has four parts: Part I: Understanding the Nature of the Helping Relationship, Part II: Clinical Skills: Attitudes and Techniques for Effective Counseling, Part III: Clinical Tools: Managing the Change Process, and Part IV: Professional Toolboxes. Seven of the eight core areas are fully covered in one or more chapters within these parts. The eighth area, theory, is discussed in various chapters throughout this text. However, because theory is so integral to the helping relationship, it should also be studied in a separate course. The parts, core areas, and the corresponding chapter(s) in which they are discussed are listed below.

PART I:
UNDERSTANDING THE NATURE OF THE HELPING RELATIONSHIP

All Core Areas:	Chapters 1 and 2
Core Area 1:	Ethical, Professional, and Cross-Cultural Issues (Chapter 3)

PART II:

CLINICAL SKILLS:	ATTITUDES AND TECHNIQUES FOR EFFECTIVE COUNSELING
Core Area 2:	Helper Attitudes (Chapter 4)
Core Area 3:	Techniques (Chapters 5–7)

PART III:

CLINICAL TOOLS:	MANAGING THE CHANGE PROCESS
Core Area 4:	Diagnosis (Chapter 8)
Core Area 5:	Case Conceptualization (Chapter 9)
Core Area 6:	Treatment Planning (Chapter 10)
Core Area 7:	Case Management (Chapter 11)
Core Area 8:	Theory (briefly mentioned in Chapters 9 and 10)

PART IV:
PROFESSIONAL TOOLBOXES
Provides a number of "tools" that can be used to expand the knowledge gained throughout the text and in the DVD. These include: Web sites for codes of ethics; additional material related to cross-cultural counseling; and examples of how to conceptualize cases, form diagnostic impressions, develop treatment plans, and write case reports.

The following presents a quick overview of the four parts in the text and the corresponding core areas that are covered in these parts.

Part I: Understanding the Nature of the Helping Relationship

Part I offers an overview of the helping relationship. Chapter 1 presents a synopsis of all the core areas that will be presented in the text, and Chapter 2 examines how these core areas are applied across the stages of the counseling relationship: the preinterview, rapport and trust building, problem identification, goal setting, work, closure, and the postrelationship. At the conclusion of Chapter 2, a table summarizes the core areas and presents an overview of what the reader will learn about in the text. Chapter 3 provides an examination of the first core area: ethical, professional, and cross-cultural issues.

Core Area 1: Ethical, Professional, and Cross-Cultural Issues (Chapter 3): For this core area, we define ethics and distinguish it from morality. We also present professional ethical codes and ethical hot spots and review some of today's critical ethical and legal issues, including breach of confidentiality, confidentiality of records, privileged communication, and confinement against one's will. Three models of ethical decision making are presented: decision-making models, moral models, and developmental models. Also, critical professional issues are discussed, including managed care, accountability, use of medication, and matching client problem with intervention strategy. Finally, there is an examination of cross-cultural counseling, and we raise the issue that counseling, as it is practiced today, does not always meet the needs of many people of color. Some models for cross-cultural counseling are presented.

Part II: Clinical Skills: Attitudes and Techniques for Effective Counseling

This part offers an in-depth examination of two critical core areas: attitudes and techniques needed when responding to the client.

Core Area 2. Helper Attitudes (Chapter 4): For this core area, we highlight the fact that some attitudes can negatively affect the helping relationship, and we discuss eight attitudes shown to be important to positive client outcomes. These include being empathic, genuine, accepting, and open-minded, and becoming increasingly cognitively complex, psychologically adjusted, good at relationship building, and competent. Four common concerns of beginning clinicians that sometimes affect their attitudes toward clients are also examined, including countertransference, dealing with difficult or resistant clients, the imposter phenomenon, and the white knight syndrome. Finally, we examine how attitudes toward clients from diverse backgrounds can affect our work with them.

Core Area 3. Techniques (Chapters 5–7): These chapters offer an in-depth examination of those skills that have been shown to be effective and demonstrate how the clinician can use them in the counseling and psychotherapeutic relationship. We offer information as well as suggestions for practicing the following skills: (a) the foundational skills of nonverbal behavior, silence and pause time, listening, paraphrasing, and empathy (Chapter 5); (b) information-gathering skills, including the use of questions, conducting a structured interview, and administering assessment procedures (Chapter 6); and (c) the commonly used relationship skills of affirmation giving; encouragement; modeling; self-disclosure; confrontation; solution-focused skills of offering alternatives, information giving, and advice giving; and collaboration (Chapter 7).

Part III: Clinical Tools: Managing the Change Process

This part identifies a number of core areas of knowledge and skills needed to manage the change process effectively. Often overlooked in counseling skills books and classes, we believe these tools are critical for the contemporary helper.

Core Area 4. Diagnosis (Chapter 8): To demonstrate this core area, we use the *DSM-IV-TR* as our guide as we explain the importance of diagnosis, present an overview of the *DSM-IV-TR*, show how to make a diagnosis, and suggest how the professional counselor can use this core area in treatment planning.

Core Area 5. Case Conceptualization (Chapter 9): For this core area, we show the process that allows the professional counselor to understand, through his or her unique theoretical perspective, a client's presenting problems and subsequently apply appropriate counseling skills and treatment strategies. One case conceptualization model, the inverted heuristic pyramid, is presented to help you understand the case conceptualization process.

Core Area 6. Treatment Planning (Chapter 10): For this core area, we focus on how to (a) select achievable goals, (b) determine treatment modes, and (c) document the attainment of goals. We also note that unlike natural helping, which is not planned, the treatment planning process allows the professional counselor to develop a deliberate, thoughtful method of providing counseling services.

Core Area 7. Case Management (Chapter 11): Being deliberate and accountable requires the professional counselor to practice a number of critical case management skills. Thus, for this core area, we highlight five important aspects of the case management process: (a) documentation, (b) consultation, supervision, and collaboration, (c) communication with stakeholders, (d) business-related activities, and (e) caseload management.

Another way of understanding the organization of this text is to list all the parts and chapters and show which of the eight core areas are covered in each. Table 1 provides such an overview.

Part IV: Professional Toolboxes

Part IV of the textbook provides developing counselors with a beginning set of tools to augment the learning that takes place in the book's 11 chapters and the various segments of the DVD.

Toolbox A is a listing of Web sites of Codes of Ethics for a number of mental health professional associations and thus provides you with a quick reference when making difficult ethical decisions.

Expanding on cross-cultural issues found in the text and DVD, Toolbox B provides a series of precise skills that might be helpful when counseling individuals from different cultural backgrounds, individuals from diverse religious

TABLE 1

Examining the Core Areas as a Function of Parts and Chapters of the Text

	CORE AREAS OF KNOWLEDGE AND SKILLS							
				CLINICAL TOOLS				
PARTS AND CHAPTERS	ETHICAL, PROFESSIONAL, CROSS-CULTURAL	ATTITUDES	SKILLS	DIAGNOSIS	CASE CONCEPTUALIZATION	TREATMENT PLANNING	CASE MANAGEMENT	THEORY*
Part I: Understanding the Nature of the Helping Relationship	X	X	X	X	X	X	X	X
Chapter 1: From Natural Helper to Professional Counselor	X	X	X	X	X	X	X	X
Chapter 2: The Stages of the Counseling Relationship	X	X	X	X	X	X	X	X
Chapter 3: Ethical, Professional, and Cross-Cultural Issues	X							
Part II: Clinical Skills: Attitudes and Techniques for Effective Counseling		X	X					
Chapter 4: Attitudes and Characteristics of the Effective Clinician		X						

TABLE 1 *(continued)*

CORE AREAS OF KNOWLEDGE AND SKILLS								
				CLINICAL TOOLS				
PARTS AND CHAPTERS	ETHICAL, PROFESSIONAL, CROSS-CULTURAL	ATTITUDES	SKILLS	DIAGNOSIS	CASE CONCEPTUALIZATION	TREATMENT PLANNING	CASE MANAGEMENT	THEORY*
Chapter 5: Foundational Skills			X					
Chapter 6: Information-Gathering			X					
Chapter 7: Commonly Used Skills			X					
Part III: Clinical Tools: Managing the Change Process				X	X	X	X	X
Chapter 8: Diagnosis				X				
Chapter 9: Case Conceptualization					X			X
Chapter 10: Treatment Planning						X		X
Chapter 11: Case Management						X		
Part IV: Professional Toolboxes	X	X	X	X	X	X	X	X

* Theory is critical to the helping relationship and also needs to be discussed in a separate course.

backgrounds, men and women clients, gay and lesbian clients, individuals who are HIV positive, homeless and poor people, older people, the mentally ill, and individuals with disabilities.

Toolbox C provides a sample report that shows a start-to-finish client case write-up, such as you might be required to prepare in a counseling agency or another professional setting. The sample clinical report is based on Sienna, whose case is discussed throughout the textbook and covers a wide range of areas one might address in a comprehensive report.

Toolbox D gives a description of the various diagnoses found in Axis I and Axis II of the DSM-IV-TR and thus expands on Chapter 8 of the textbook, which deals with developing DSM-IV-TR diagnostic skills.

Finaly, Toolbox E concerns the case of Alice, who we observe through an Intake Interview, Working Stage, and Closure Stage on the DVD. This Toolbox provides samples of case conceptualization, diagnosis, case notes, and treatment planning materials as applied to Alice and thus helps to expand the learning that takes place in chapters 8, 9, 10, and 11 of the text.

In summary, the text and DVD cover the eight core areas of knowledge and skills needed by the professional counselor to be effective in the helping relationship. Together, we hope that the text and DVD will start you on the path from being a natural helper to a professional counselor who has learned and can implement the eight identified core areas when working with clients.

Acknowledgments

Several people were instrumental in the development of this textbook and DVD. We owe our appreciation to Dr. Kyle Nicholas, Assistant Professor of Speech and Communication, for his insight and skill during the production of the DVD. We are indebted to the poet Tim Siebels for his role as DVD narrator. A special thanks goes to Phyllis, Anne, Charlie, and Dominique for all their valuable assistance and willingness to work long hours with us. We also would like to thank the production crew at Old Dominion University, who were always professional, cheerful, and ready to work! Debra Boyce, Patricia Cody, Angela Holman, and Jackie Stein provided valuable case material that helps bring the text alive. Of course, a sincere thanks goes to Lisa Gebo, Sheila Walsh, Rita Jaramillo, and Barry Connolly at Wadsworth, without whom this book and DVD could not have been successfully prepared and published. We would like to extend our gratitude to the following reviewers: Susan A. Adams, Delta State University; Michael Altekruse, University of North Texas; Joshua M. Gold, University of South Carolina–Columbia; Cindy Juntunen, University of North Dakota; P. Irene McIntosh, University of South Alabama; Rachelle Perusse, Plattsburgh State University of New York; and Kwamia N. Rawls, Seton Hall University. Thanks also to Aaron Downey at Matrix Productions, Frank Hubert, and Sally Scott for all of their hard work in completing the book. Finally, we appreciate our many students, whose collective journeys from natural helpers to professional counselors have informed our own work as educators.

PART ONE

Understanding the Nature of the Helping Relationship

The three chapters of Part I provide you with an overview of the text and offer you a sense of why the clinical skills and clinical tools that you will read and learn about in Parts II and III are so critical. In addition, you are introduced to the notion that being a professional counselor is a planned and deliberate process that entails the learning of a number of counseling skills and tools. This is contrasted with the qualities of the natural helper whose intentions are good but whose actions are not always conducive to a positive helping relationship.

Chapter 1 is entitled "From Natural Helper to Professional Counselor" and begins by reviewing the research on whether or not counseling and psychotherapy are effective. After establishing that counseling is effective, the chapter introduces you to the notion that clinical work with clients is a planned process and that you must learn a number of critical skills and tools to be effective at it. This leads into a discussion of eight core areas of knowledge and skills one should master to become a proficient, professional counselor, including (a) ethical, professional, and cross-cultural issues, (b) helper attitudes, (c) techniques, (d) diagnosis, (e) case conceptualization, (f) treatment planning, (g) case management, and (h) theory.

Chapter 2 introduces the relative importance of each of the core areas to the following stages of the counseling relationship: the preinterview, rapport and trust-building, problem identification, goal-setting, work, closure, and the postinterview. As we discuss the stages, we offer a case example to show how a client and a clinician work as they move through the stages of the counseling relationship, and we note that this case example (and others) will appear again in Part III of the text. The goals of the stages and how the core areas emerge as a function of the stages are summarized in the Chapter 2 Appendix, and these tables are also useful as a guide to the rest of the text. The chapter concludes with a discussion of the importance of continually trying to master the core areas throughout our careers and of remaining open to embracing changes in the core areas as we continue on our professional journey.

Chapter 3 is entitled "Ethical, Professional, and Cross-Cultural Issues." It starts by defining ethics and distinguishing between ethics and morality. Next, there is a discussion of the development and importance of professional ethical codes, and we highlight some codes of ethics and ethical hot spots in the helping professions. This is followed by a review of some critical ethical and legal issues, including breach of confidentiality, confidentiality of records, privileged communication, and confinement against one's will. As we continue, we offer three models of ethical decision making: decision-making models, moral models, and developmental models.

The next section of Chapter 3 examines a number of critical professional issues that impact the work of the clinician, including managed care, accountability, use of medication, and matching client problem with intervention strategy. The chapter continues with an examination of cross-cultural issues, where we specifically address the fact that counseling, as it is practiced today, often is not effective for many people of color. We next present some models of cross-cultural counseling and offer suggestions on how to work with a number of diverse groups. The chapter concludes by noting that improving our ability to work with cross-cultural clients, and indeed, with all clients, is a never-ending process; that is, we should always be fine-tuning our skills and learning how to be more effective with all of the clients with whom we work.

CHAPTER 1

From Natural Helper to Professional Counselor

Do counseling and psychotherapy work? That is the first critical question this chapter explores. And after presenting research that answers this question with a resounding "yes," we examine why counseling and therapy work and then distinguish what we call "natural helping" from professional counseling. This leads to a discussion of eight core areas of knowledge and skills needed if one is to become a professional counselor, including (a) ethical, professional, and cross-cultural issues, (b) helper attitudes, (c) techniques, (d) diagnosis, (e) case conceptualization, (f) treatment planning, (g) case management, and (h) theory. These essential core areas will be extensively discussed throughout this book. But let's start with the most basic question: Do counseling and psychotherapy work?

Do Counseling and Psychotherapy Work?

> *How well counselors perform, what they do, and what they will become is a complex interaction of credentialing requirements, expectations of the settings in which they are employed, personal characteristics, and the quality and content of their preparation as counselors.* (Herr, 1985, p. 33)

In 1952, Eysenck looked at 24 uncontrolled studies that examined the effectiveness of psychotherapy and found that "roughly two-thirds of a group of neurotic patients will recover or improve to a marked extent within about two years of the onset of their illness, *whether they are treated by means of psychotherapy or not*" (p. 322, italics added). Eysenck's research sent tremors through the professional community, and a debate ensued concerning the effectiveness of counseling. Although Eysenck's research was shown to be flawed, it did lead to debate concerning the effectiveness of counseling and resulted in hundreds of studies that examined counseling effectiveness. The results of this massive amount of research showed the following:

> *The evidence accumulated over the last 40 years is relatively clear: Counseling is a process from which most clients who remain involved for at least a few*

> *sessions benefit. When counseling effectiveness is calculated by determining the number of clients who improved, the results are amazingly similar across various studies. On the basis of both client and counselor ratings, approximately 22% of clients made significant gains, 43% made moderate changes, while 27% made some improvement. . . .* (Sexton, 1993, p. 82)

Sexton goes on to say that "counseling outcome research findings are so compelling that the debate regarding whether counseling is effective is no longer a major issue" (p. 84) (also see Sexton, 1999). Despite being assured that counseling works for a large majority of clients, questions concerning how it works and for whom it works best are still debated. For instance, a number of questions remained largely unanswered, including: Does counseling work for all types of problems? Does counseling work equally well for all cultural groups? Does counseling work equally well for all problems when conducted under all types of therapies? Are the effects of counseling long term? Does the personality style of the therapist have a differential effect on client outcomes? In an attempt to answer some of these questions, Lambert and Cattani-Thompson (1996) and Lambert and Ogles (2004) have reviewed the research on the effectiveness of counseling and found the following:

1. The vast majority of clients do better at the time of treatment termination.
2. For as many as 50% of clients, counseling can be effective in as few as 5 to 10 sessions.
3. Although 20% to 30% of clients will require treatment that is longer term, most of these will see improvements with counseling.
4. For the majority of clients, gains made in counseling seem to last long term.
5. As one might expect, less defensive, motivated clients who accept personal responsibility and do not have severe chronic problems do better in counseling.
6. Some techniques work better with specific problems, and clinicians should try to match techniques to problems.
7. Some clients will get worse in counseling, and clinicians should make every attempt to monitor client progress and make changes in technique or refer as quickly as possible.
8. The counselor–client relationship, or how the clinician brings himself or herself into the helping relationship, seems to be the best predictor of success in counseling.

As evidenced by the research, it is now clear that counseling is effective. It follows that clinicians should have the knowledge and skills that have been found to make it so. But how exactly does one gain such knowledge? That question is critical if we are to understand the nature of the effective counseling relationship.

Natural Helping Versus Professional Counseling

Have you ever listened to the radio talk-show host Dr. Laura or TV personality Dr. Phil? They certainly are heavy on the advice giving. It's not our style of doing counseling, and some have criticized them for being unprofessional, but they clearly are following their natural inclination to give advice. However, is following one's natural inclination or style the most effective way to do counseling? We would argue that it is not. In fact, the professional counseling relationship is quite different from the more familiar experience of natural everyday helping. Natural helpers, such as friends, relatives, and supportive others, rely on intuition, familiarity, natural responsiveness, and personal opinions as they spontaneously listen, support, encourage, challenge, analyze, make hopeful suggestions, and offer whatever advice they find most sensible. In contrast, the professional clinician attempts to purposely direct the counseling relationship by applying a broad range of critical skills in a systematic fashion.

HIGHLIGHT 1.1 **Counseling Does Work and Provides a Deliberate Mechanism to Help Clients**

In addition to the research that shows the efficacy of counseling, literally hundreds of publications have provided various mechanisms for how to do counseling. One manuscript by Daniels (2003) lists approximately 450 citations that speak to various skills important in the training of counseling.

Typically, we have found new students in clinical training describe themselves as natural "listeners," "analyzers," "problem solvers," or "challengers." And although such students have their hearts in the right place, they often have little knowledge of how to apply critical professional skills. For instance, those who define themselves as "natural listeners" tend to be caring, good listeners and focus on client self-expression and self-growth. These students might be heard saying the following:

1. "Counseling has to do with listening to another person's pain."
2. "I really want to show my clients I care about them—they are people!"
3. "I know I can help my client find out more about herself by listening intensely to her."

These new counselors are emphasizing active listening, empathic understanding, and rapport and trust building—skills that are most salient in the early stages of the counseling relationship. In their experience as natural helpers, they primarily have been "listening ears" who effectively offer support, help the person in need express himself or herself, and facilitate the client's understanding of his or her thoughts and feelings. However, they tend to be more reactive to clients, rarely guide or lead, and are usually less comfortable with case conceptualization, diagnosis, and treatment planning—skills that are critical in today's world. For them, the helping skills of listening, reflection, and empathic understanding, which we will study in Chapter 5, come naturally and will be strong assets early in their professional education and development.

In contrast to the listener, there are "analyzers," or students who mainly define counseling by assessing and analyzing client concerns and by focusing on gaining a better understanding of the issues. These students might be heard saying the following:

1. "I like to help people by analyzing and interpreting their problems for them."

2. "I love investigating the lives of clients—their past, present, and future. I think this helps clients understand the reasons for their feelings and problems and is a good basis for developing goals."
3. "Counseling is like a puzzle. I help the client put it together by probing and exploring parts of the client's psyche."

These new counselors are emphasizing case conceptualization, diagnosis, and treatment planning—skills that are most salient in the early to middle stages of the counseling relationship. In their experience as natural helpers, they primarily explore and probe and offer critical analyses of the problem's root causes and the factors that sustain or exacerbate the current situation. Usually, they are most comfortable deriving an intellectual understanding of client problems and less accustomed to soliciting expressions of emotion or listening empathically. They will enjoy learning about the skills of diagnosis, case conceptualization, and treatment planning (Chapters 8, 9, and 10) and will feel at home with the information-gathering skills we will discuss in Chapter 6. However, they might have a more difficult time with building relationships and using some of the foundational skills found in Chapter 5.

Then there are students who see themselves as "problem solvers." Here are some possible descriptions problem solvers might give of the counseling relationship:

1. "Counseling has to do with giving advice or direction."
2. "Why spend so much time analyzing or probing when you can get right down to the solution?"
3. "I love to offer guidance to a client. I think I can help a client, in a relatively short amount of time, solve his or her problem."

These students are emphasizing the work stage of the counseling relationship. In their experience as natural helpers, they primarily have been "problem solvers" and "action takers." They like to identify problems and tend to be more directive, attempting to mobilize the person in need to make decisions, take action, or decisively change behavior. Usually, they are most comfortable moving steadfastly toward problem resolution but are uncomfortable with listening, empathy, and case conceptualization. They tend to prefer the solution-focused skills of offering advice, offering alternatives, and giving feedback, which we will examine in Chapter 7, and they will also like the treatment-planning process described in Chapter 10. They may bring to the relationship an emphasis on brief counseling, solution-focused approaches, or guidance.

Finally, there are the "challengers." These students like to confront their clients, and you might find them saying the following about the counseling relationship:

1. "Why spend all that time listening to thoughts and feelings when you can directly ask a client why they feel a certain way?"
2. "Counseling has to do with pushing clients to understand how they created their current situation and challenging them to find ways of improving it."

PROFESSIONAL PERSPECTIVES 1.1

Pushing a Client Too Far

As a therapist at a mental health center, I (Ed Neukrug) worked with a psychiatrist who was the director of an inpatient unit. This psychiatrist was known for verbally confronting his clients in what some considered an abusive manner. Many a client (and therapist) were intimidated by him. One day, he chose the wrong client to confront, for as he berated this client for not following his treatment plan, the client lifted him in the air, held him against the wall, and told him, "Nobody tells me what to do." Many of the other clients (and quite a few therapists) could be heard quietly cheering on this client.

This example is an important reminder to the natural challenger that the manner in which a client is challenged is an artful skill that needs to be done carefully and appropriately and that other skills, such as listening, analysis, and problem solving, also need to be used if the natural challenger is to be effective.

3. "The counselor's role is to point out discrepancies between clients' actions, feelings, and behaviors."

The challenger likes to confront the manner in which the client views the world. This student cares little for understanding the stages of the helping relationship and has little patience for the natural rhythm of the helping relationship—concepts we examine in Chapter 2. In fact, this student often thinks that he or she can quickly push the client into seeing the world in a different manner and will often confront clients through the use of questions, particularly "why" questions, as we will discuss in Chapter 6. This student is not particularly comfortable with empathy, as he or she believes there is no reason to take a lot of time indirectly getting to the problem when you can ask the client directly what's going on. Similarly, case conceptualization is not seen as a particularly important skill by these students because it relies on having a complex cognitive understanding of the client's predicament and on understanding theory and is not, on the surface, goal oriented. However, he or she may feel comfortable challenging a client and telling the client his or her diagnosis while assisting the client in creating a treatment plan—concepts we will examine in Chapters 7 and 10, respectively (see Professional Perspectives 1.1).

As suggested in the examples given, each new trainee has a natural inclination toward a style of being with a client. And it should be stressed that each style has a unique and important perspective to offer to the counseling relationship. However, often trainees know little about how to apply their style in the most effective manner, how to apply their style in a timely fashion, or how knowledge and skills in other core areas will increase the probability that he or she will work effectively with clients. Although you might find that you have more of an affinity for one style of helping over the others (see Exercise 1.1), we believe that if you are to be an effective clinician, you must be well-rounded and deliberate; that is, you will need to learn a wide range of core knowledge and skills and be able to apply them in a manner that can be most helpful to the client. Thus, one purpose of this text is to move you from your natural helping style toward a professional counseling approach in which you have at your disposal a large repertoire of knowledge and skills.

EXERCISE 1.1 **Natural Styles of Helping**

Using the scale shown, give yourself a rating for each style of natural helping listed. Then, rank order the style and write its corresponding score. See the example below. As you read through the text, identify those skills that most coincide with your natural style. These are the skills you will likely be particularly good at, and you probably will have a more difficult time learning the skills associated with your secondary styles.

1	2	3	4	5	6	7	8	9	10
Not at All Important Possibly Harmful				Moderately Important			Critically Important Probably Very Helpful		

STYLE

___ Listener: Likes to understand another's point of view by listening and showing empathy. Has feelings for another.

___ Analytical: Likes to explore, probe, and offer a critical analysis of a situation. Involved in the intellectual process of understanding a client's predicament.

___ Problem Solver: Likes to define the problem, set goals, and take action to reach a solution.

___ Challenger: Likes to push and confront a client into viewing the world differently.

EXAMPLE *Rank*	*Score*	YOUR SCORE AND RANK *Rank*	*Score*
1. Listener	10	1. ____________	____
2. Analyzer	8	2. ____________	____
3. Problem Solver	3	4. ____________	____
4. Challenger	2	5. ____________	____

Core Areas of Knowledge and Skills

As noted earlier, becoming a professional counselor means that you have mastered the knowledge and skills in a number of core areas, such as the eight that we have identified. In this text, each core area, with the exception of theory, has one or more chapters dedicated to it. Theory is mentioned briefly throughout the text, and you will likely have a separate course devoted to it.

PART I:
UNDERSTANDING THE NATURE OF THE HELPING RELATIONSHIP
All Core Areas: Chapter 1
All Core Areas: Chapter 2
Core Area 1: Ethical, Professional, and Cross-Cultural Issues (Chapter 3)

PART II:
CLINICAL SKILLS: ATTITUDES AND TECHNIQUES FOR EFFECTIVE COUNSELING
Core Area 2: Helper Attitudes (Chapter 4)
Core Area 3: Techniques (Chapters 4–7)

PART III:
CLINICAL TOOLS: MANAGING THE CHANGE PROCESS
Core Area 4: Diagnosis (Chapter 8)
Core Area 5: Case Conceptualization (Chapter 9)
Core Area 6: Treatment Planning (Chapter 10)
Core Area 7: Case Management (Chapter 11)
Core Area 8: Theory (briefly mentioned in Chapters 1, 2, 9, and 10)

PART IV:
PROFESSIONAL TOOLBOXES
Expands on core areas of knowledge and skills presented in text and DVD.

What follows are brief descriptions of these core areas. As you read through the text, you will have an opportunity to delve further into each of them.

Ethical, Professional, and Cross-Cultural Issues

The natural helper has not learned, and likely has little interest in learning, the broad array of professional and ethical issues that can impact on a helping relationship. These issues are critical to the relationship because they affect the manner in which the clinician works with his or her client. For instance, understanding the limits of our ability as a therapist, how we describe our work to our clients (e.g., professional disclosure statements), knowing the limits of confidentiality, assuring that we have the necessary knowledge of cross-cultural differences in our application of helping skills, understanding the importance of the boundaries of the helping relationship, knowing what to do when a client is in danger of harming himself or herself or another, and knowing when to refer a client to another therapist are just a few of the myriad ethical concerns that might be faced by the professional counselor and are addressed in ethical codes (see Toolbox A for Web sites of the ethical codes of select mental health professional associations). Ethical, professional, and cross-cultural issues will be discussed at length in Chapter 3 and highlighted at other times throughout the text.

Helper Attitudes

The natural helper relies on his or her intuitive sense of what attitudes and behaviors should be applied in the informal helping relationship. In contrast, the professional counselor has adopted personality characteristics that have been theoretically or empirically shown to be critical to the effective helping relationship. It is essential that the professional counselor learns how to let go of behaviors and attitudes that would be detrimental to the helping relationship and purposefully and actively adopt new behaviors and attitudes that will facilitate client growth. Research on effectiveness of counseling has pinpointed some attitudes that seem to be more critical than others. Some of these include being empathic, genuine, accepting, and open-minded. Others include cognitive complexity, being adjusted psychologically, being able to build a relationship with your client, and being competent (see Neukrug, 2003, 2004). These characteristics will be examined in Chapter 4.

Techniques

Natural helpers tend to randomly apply a hodgepodge of techniques when helping an individual. Unfortunately, their techniques have often been shown not to be theoretically or empirically sound. Professional counselors, on the other hand, have at their disposal a wide range of helping skills that have been shown to be effective in assisting clients through the stages of the helping relationship. A number of chapters in this text are dedicated to understanding these skills, including Chapter 5, which covers the foundational skills of silence and pause time, listening, paraphrasing, and empathy; Chapter 6, which examines the information-gathering skills of asking questions, conducting a structured interview, and administering assessment procedures; and Chapter 7, which examines the commonly used skills of affirmation-giving, encouragement, modeling, self-disclosure, collaboration, and confrontation, as well as the commonly used solution-focused skills of offering alternatives, information-giving, and advice-giving.

Diagnosis

Studies have shown that a large percentage of Americans have or will experience an emotional disorder (Hersen & Van Hasselt, 2001). Thus, regardless of where a counselor is employed, he or she will be working with clients who have serious emotional problems, and often, these clients will be given a diagnosis based on their symptoms (see Davison & Neale, 2004). Whereas the natural helper will not apply a formal diagnosis, he or she may come up with a nonresearched diagnosis from popular literature. On the other hand, the professional counselor will rely on a systematic mechanism of making a diagnosis that relies on professional sources, such as the *Diagnostics and Statistical Manual-IV, Text Revision* (American Psychiatric Association, 2000). Making an accurate diagnosis is critical for treatment planning because it helps determine the kinds of goals and techniques to be used. Recognizing this, most training programs now include in their curriculum a focus on psychopathology and diagnosis (Hinkle, 1994a; Hohenshil, 1993, 1994).

Controversy still exists about the use of diagnosis and includes such issues as (a) Is diagnosis a social construction? (b) Why are minorities misdiagnosed at higher rates than Whites? and (c) Is associating a person with a diagnostic "label" in the long run harmful to how the client views himself or herself and how others view the client? Despite this controversy, it is clear that all clinicians today must be familiar with how to make a diagnosis and with the purposes diagnoses serve (Fong, 1995; Hinkle, 1994a, 1994b; Hohenshil, 1994). Thus, how to diagnosis clients' symptoms will be discussed in detail in Chapter 8.

Case Conceptualization

Case conceptualization, the next logical step after making a preliminary diagnosis, is the process that allows the clinician to understand, through his or her unique theoretical perspective, a client's presenting problems and subsequently apply appropriate counseling skills and treatment strategies. Whereas experienced counselors develop their own systematic method of conceptualizing client problems, natural helpers do not have a mechanism for understanding clients. If not given a method for case conceptualization, beginning counselors and therapists, who are often still struggling with their theoretical orientation, will have a difficult time conceptualizing client problems. This leaves students floundering, often relying on their intuition, falling back on basic counseling skills, and, much like natural helpers, randomly attempting a hodgepodge of techniques (Martin, Slemon, Hiebert, Hallberg, & Cummings, 1989). Thus, we believe it is critical that every student have a model of case conceptualization. One model of case conceptualization that we will discuss in this text is Schwitzer's (1996, 1997) inverted pyramid heuristic (IPH). How to conceptualize client problems will be discussed in detail in Chapter 9.

Treatment Planning

Whereas natural helpers rarely, if ever, develop a planned mechanism for working with clients, the professional counselor and therapist has the knowledge and professional responsibility to provide a client with a treatment plan that will address presenting issues. A treatment plan is based on one's conceptualization of client problems and on the diagnosis of the client. It establishes the process that will be used to address identified problems and can include such elements as the length of treatment, intervention skills, and possible medication that might be used. Treatment planning is critical in the accountability process because it defines a method of treatment that can later be used to evaluate progress. Treatment planning will be addressed in Chapter 10.

Case Management

Case management has been viewed as the overall process involved in maintaining the optimal functioning of clients (Sullivan, Wolk, & Hartmann, 1992; Woodside & McClam, 2003). Thus, case management involves a broad array of activities including (a) documentation, (b) consultation, supervision, and collaboration, (c) communicating with stakeholders, (d) business-related activities, and (e) caseload management. Whereas the natural helper has rarely even considered the vast majority of the case management issues just listed, the professional counselor sees case management as a critical piece of his or her work with the client. And with a greater emphasis on accountability in the mental health professions, these issues have become increasingly important. Thus, case management will be examined in detail in Chapter 11.

Theory

Generally, natural helpers have not thought through their understanding of human nature, which is basic to one's theoretical orientation. In contrast, professional counselors should be able to clearly identify their view of human nature and the subsequent theory of change that is derived from it. Theories, and the view of human nature that they are based on, typically take into account the effects of biology, genetics, and environment (e.g., family, neighborhood, social situation) on the personality development of the individual. Theories are heuristic; that is, they are researchable and testable and ultimately allow us to discard those aspects shown to be ineffective. Having a counseling theory is the clinician's template for conceptualizing client problems, applying techniques, and predicting change (Brammer & MacDonald, 2003; Brammer, Shostrom, & Abrego, 1993). To "function without theory is to operate without placing events in some order and thus to function meaninglessly" (Hansen, Rossberg, & Cramer, 1994, p. 9). Today, there are dozens of counseling theories, although only a handful are practiced by the majority of clinicians (Neukrug, Milliken, & Shoemaker, 2001; Neukrug & Williams, 1993). Although it is not the purview of this text to focus in depth on theory, theory is mentioned throughout the text and is critical to understanding the case conceptualization process described in Chapter 9.

LEARNING TO BE A COUNSELOR: An Ongoing Process

You are about to take the journey from natural helper to professional counselor. However, whether you have never been a counselor, have 50 years of counseling experience and are first obtaining your degree, or are a master therapist recognized around the world, you have something in common—you still have a lot to learn. During that learning process, we hope you spend time examining and delving deeper into each of the core areas identified in this book.

As you continue on your journey, and as years pass, you will find that the core knowledge and skills identified in this book will evolve. As they transform, we believe that each of us has the responsibility to remain knowledgeable about how the core areas have changed and how other new core areas may arise. Stay informed, keep practicing, and remember that the best clinicians are those who have a solid foundation but also recognize advances in the field and are willing to judiciously change with the times.

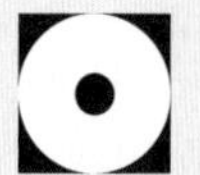

At this point, we recommend that you pause reading the text, turn to the DVD, and view the section entitled:

Introduction

Chapter Summary

This chapter began by examining the research on the effectiveness of counseling and psychotherapy. We first presented Eysenck's (1952) study, which suggested that professional counseling might not be effective. However, due to the furor this study created, and the fact that the study was found to have serious methodological flaws, a vast amount of follow-up research was conducted that showed the efficacy of counseling and psychotherapy. We concluded that the vast majority of clients do better as a result of counseling, with most of them making gains within 10 sessions. We also noted that the reason counseling works seems to be a mixture of counselor attitudes and the techniques used.

As the chapter continued, we distinguished the natural helper from the professional counselor. We suggested that many beginning counselors enter training with one of four natural orientations to working with clients: listeners, analyzers, problem solvers, or challengers. We also suggested that each of these styles works best at different stages of the helping relationship and that the effective helper is well-rounded and deliberate; that is, he or she has learned a wide range of core knowledge and skills and can apply them in a manner that can be most helpful to the client. Thus, we proposed that the purpose of this text is to move you from your natural helping style toward a professional counseling approach in which you have at your disposal a large repertoire of knowledge and skills.

Based on the literature, we next went on to identify eight core areas of knowledge and skills we deemed critical if one is to be an effective clinician, including: (a) ethical, professional, and cross-cultural issues, (b) helper attitudes, (c) techniques, (d) diagnosis, (e) case conceptualization, (f) treatment planning, (g) case management, and (h) theory. We noted that each core area cited, with the exception of theory, has one or more chapters dedicated to it.

The chapter concluded with a discussion of the importance of continually trying to master the core areas of knowledge and skills throughout our careers and the importance of remaining open to embracing changes in the core areas and, ultimately, in the skills and tools we use.

CHAPTER 2

The Stages of the Counseling Relationship

In contrast to natural helpers, who do not tend to view the helping relationship as a process, professional counselors understand that the relationship has a natural progression that begins with the building of a therapeutic alliance, leads toward the identification of problems, moves forward toward working on those problems, and has a clear ending based on the attainment of goals. Each stage in this helping relationship is seen as an important building block in the overall helping process and carries with it a unique primary goal. In this chapter, we identify the primary goal of each stage of the helping relationship. Then, we show how each of the core areas of knowledge and skills identified in Chapter 1 are critical in varying ways during every stage of the counseling relationship. The chapter concludes with three tables that summarize the stages and the critical knowledge and skills areas that are needed in each stage.

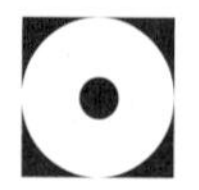

If you have not done so already, we recommend that you pause reading the text, turn to the DVD, and view the section entitled:

Introduction

Understanding the Stages of the Counseling Relationship

If clinicians are to be successful, they must understand the natural unfolding progression of the helping relationship and how to apply the core areas of knowledge and skills, identified in Chapter 1, at an opportune moment. Thus, this chapter describes the stages of the helping relationship, notes the primary goal of the stage, and then details which core areas of knowledge and skills are associated with each stage. The core areas of knowledge and skills are described under three general headings: Clinical Skills, where attitudes and techniques are discussed; Clinical Tools, where diagnosis, case conceptualization, treatment planning, case management, and theory are covered; and Ethical, Professional, and Cross-Cultural Issues. Each of these core areas are covered in the subsequent chapters of this text. The stages include the preinterview, rapport and trust building, problem identification, goal setting, work, closure, and the postrelationship (Neukrug, 2002).

The Preinterview (Preparatory) Stage

The preinterview process consist of the counselor's preparation for the first meeting as well as the client's experiences prior to that meeting, including making the decision to seek help and taking the first steps inside the agency walls. The primary goal at the preinterview stage is to prepare for an optimal first professional encounter with the client (see Chapter 2 Appendix for a summary of this stage).

Clinical Skill

ATTITUDES During the preinterview stage, it is the clinician's responsibility to take a self-inventory of his or her attitudes to assure that he or she is psychologically ready to work with clients throughout all of the stages. Although each attitude is critical throughout all of the stages, some emerge as more important than others as a function of stage. *Being open-minded and accepting, being psychologically adjusted,* and *cognitive complexity* deserve special mention at the preparatory stage. Although at times it is natural for clinicians to have difficulty being nonjudgmental, it is critical to begin each new counseling relationship with an open-minded, accepting attitude and an inviting manner. Also, because clients come to counseling for a myriad of reasons, the counselor must have the psychological preparedness to handle whatever emotionally charged or value-laden issues the client presents. In addition, the clinician must have the cognitive complexity to understand that any information obtained in the early stages likely gives only a glimpse of the whole client picture. Thus, the clinician should not try to jump to premature conclusions about the client, and the clinician should be psychologically able to deal with whatever issues the client brings to therapy.

Clinical Tool

CASE MANAGEMENT If the relationship is to begin on a positive note, good case management is needed even before meeting the client for the first time (Neukrug, 2002, 2004). For instance, the counselor should assure an appointment time is made and be punctual for the interview. Also, he or she should assure that all related paperwork and agency files are in order and review any advance information such as reports from previous clinicians, assessment results, or other clinical material. Preparatory case management also requires that the counselor and administrative staff handle all preinterview phone contacts, scheduling matters, waiting room situations, and so forth in a professional and courteous manner that gives a positive impression to the soon-to-be client.

Ethical, Professional, and Cross-Cultural Issues

COMPETENCE AND PROFESSIONAL LIMITATIONS Prior to the helping relationship beginning, the clinician should determine if the client's concerns and dynamics are within the counselor's range of competencies and whether the agency or setting is appropriate for the presenting problem. Knowing one's professional limits is important if the clinician is to make thoughtful and wise decisions about whether to counsel the client, seek consultation and/or supervision, or refer the client to another professional.

OFFICE DECOR Professional counselors are intentional about the image they want their office to convey. In general, professional items and neutral decor are preferable, although some personal items like family photos are acceptable. Although items reflecting personal values, such as political flyers and religious books, are usually avoided, this is not always the case. For instance, the clinician who works in a religiously based counseling center or one who works in a counseling center for gays and lesbians might be more apt to have materials that are biased toward the values of his or her clients. Ultimately, the clinician should make purposeful, wise decisions about office decor, taking into account its impact on clients.

KNOWLEDGE OF AND SKILLS TO USE WITH DIVERSE CLIENTS As the ethnic/cultural background of the client is determined, the clinician needs to consider whether he or she has the knowledge and skills necessary to be effective with the client. If not, the clinician should do the preparatory work to gain the needed knowledge and skills or refer the client to someone who is more familiar with the client's culture.

ATTITUDES TOWARD DIVERSE CLIENTS Prior to meeting with the client, the clinician needs to take a self-inventory to assure that he or she does not hold biases toward the client's culture. Because biases can be unconscious, such a self-inventory must be taken very seriously.

CASE ILLUSTRATION 2.1 Preinterview (Preparatory) Stage

The following case example is provided in installments throughout this chapter to highlight the clinical responsibilities associated with each stage of the counseling relationship. (Please note that we will return to this case in Part III of the text.)

> Sienna, a 23 year old, African American, second-year college female, calls the student counseling center presenting moderate, persistent depression. Sienna comes from an intact family, now lives on campus with an assigned roommate, and is involved with a White male college student.

PREINTERVIEW CLIENT DYNAMICS

Sienna's self-referred main concerns were low mood and feelings of depression lasting for several months. Prior to seeking counseling, Sienna had tried to cope by using an old coping mechanism of "just trying to be happy," distracting herself with social activities, working out, and concentrating on school. When her problems continued, she tried new ways of coping, including discussing her problems with her resident assistant and seeking support from her best friend and from her boyfriend. Finally, when none of these helped change her mood, she began downsliding—that is, feeling worse, having less energy, performing poorly academically, and having growing, distressing self-doubts about her ability to handle adult life.

PREINTERVIEW CLINICAL DYNAMICS

When she contacted the center, basic information was gathered from Sienna and she was given an initial appointment (case management). The counselor was a clinician experienced with college student mood problems but also was prepared to refer Sienna to a consulting psychiatrist to evaluate her for medication or hospitalization if needed (competence). Based on the limited information the counselor had received about the client prior to intake, she prepared herself for tearfulness, presentations of sadness, and perhaps pessimistic thoughts of leaving school or even suicide but also tried to remain open to whatever issues may arise (openness). She also made a mental note of the importance of being accepting and nonjudgmental regarding Sienna's problem and the fact that the limited amount of information that she had might not be a full indication of the extent of Sienna's problem (cognitive complexity). In addition, the counselor, who is White, completed a self-inventory to assure she was not holding biases and reflected on the literature she had read concerning working with female, African American young adults.

EXERCISE 2.1 **Reflections on the Preinterview**

In small groups, consider the following issues that clinicians often face during the preinterview stage of the counseling relationship.

1. RESOLVING ISSUES AND EXPECTATIONS OF COUNSELING: Think of a time when you were confronted with the emergence of a new stressor, longstanding unresolved developmental concern, or growing entrenched problem in your own life. How did you resolve the concern? How might you have felt seeking counseling for the first time about your problem? What expectations would you have about the counselor?
2. MAINTAINING A NONJUDGMENTAL ATTITUDE: It is natural for clinicians to face difficulties being nonjudgmental at times. Which clients, or what counseling issues, do you believe will be most challenging for you as you attempt to remain nonjudgmental? How will you manage this when confronted by a new client with the characteristics or issues you identified?

Stage 1: Rapport and Trust Building

Stage 1 begins with the actual interview, and the primary goal of this stage is to gather initial information about the client and establish a trusting, facilitative therapeutic alliance. Although Stage 1 begins with the first interview, it can last from one to many sessions depending on the client and the nature of the problem (see Chapter 2 Appendix for a summary of this stage).

Clinical Skills

ATTITUDES Having *empathy* and showing *acceptance* are two attitudes that assist in building a strong alliance early in the clinical relationship. These attitudes help the client feel safe, encourage self-disclosure, and set the tone for the helping relationship. Unlike natural helpers who are often uncomfortable with the strong emotions of helpees, as client self-disclosure occurs, the professional counselor has the ability to listen and be accepting of the expression of deep emotions, such as sobs of depression, rage, or feelings of guilt and shame. This ability is the result of the clinician's work on his or her own psychological adjustment.

The beginning of the helping relationship is critical to successful outcomes, and clinicians must have embraced the notion that if they do not have the *competence* to work with a particular client, they will seek consultation or supervision, or refer the client to a clinician who can be effective with the client.

TECHNIQUES The major goal of this stage is to build trust and rapport, and the foundational skills of *silence* and *pause time, listening, paraphrasing,* and *empathic understanding* are critical to this process. *Information gathering* is important at this early stage because it helps the clinician understand the totality of the client's situation. In addition, in this age of accountability, information is needed quickly to form diagnostic impressions and to develop treatment plans, which often are required by funding sources and insurance companies. Thus, *conducting a structured interview* and gently probing and *asking questions* are often used during this early part of the helping relationship and continued in Stage 2. One of the challenges faced by the counselor during this stage is to build a strong therapeutic alliance through the use of foundational skills and also to conduct the information gathering that needs to take place, which often requires skills that are not as conducive to relationship building. As the clinician readies to move on to the next stage, *collaboration* is important because the clinician wants to assure that his or her expectations match those of the client.

Clinical Tools

CASE CONCEPTUALIZATION Although the case conceptualization process has barely begun in this stage, clinicians do begin to make some tentative hypotheses about client issues and possible ancillary concerns that will be used later in the case conceptualization process.

DIAGNOSIS As the client begins to identify issues, the clinician will very tentatively consider diagnoses. However, it is critical that the clinician wait until more information is gathered in Stage 2 before making a firm diagnosis of symptoms.

CASE MANAGEMENT Extensive case management early in the helping relationship is usually needed to ensure that all related paperwork and intake assessment materials are completed, billing and other business matters are attended to, necessary correspondence with other professionals is conducted, and agency records have been addressed.

Ethical, Professional, and Cross-Cultural Issues

PROFESSIONAL COMPETENCE During Stage 1, the clinician should confirm that the client's concerns and dynamics are within the counselor's range of competencies and that the agency or setting is appropriate for the presenting problem. Thus, the clinician should make thoughtful decisions about whether counseling can be productive for the client's presenting problem, whether to make an effective referral, or whether to consult with another professional.

CROSS-CULTURAL COMPETENCE As the clinician gets to know the client, he or she should become acutely aware of gaps in knowledge and skills that exist relative to the client's ethnic/cultural background (Arredondo, 1999). In addition, competent cross-cultural clinicians should be cognizant of any biased attitudes they might have toward a client. When gaps in knowledge or skills cannot be appropriately dealt with to assure positive client outcomes, or when counselors have biased attitudes that cannot be overcome, the client should be referred to another clinician.

COUNSELOR SELF-DISCLOSURE Professional counselors are planful about self-disclosure, and they make purposeful decisions concerning what, if any, personal information will be shared with clients. Self-disclosure should only be done when it is expected to benefit the client. Some clinicians share very little personal information to keep the focus squarely on the client, but other counselors use more self-disclosure. Regardless of how much sharing the clinician believes will be helpful, a general rule during Stage 1 is to focus almost completely on the client and then to gradually allow more counselor self-disclosure later in the process.

ESTABLISHING BOUNDARIES Another way professional counseling is different from natural helping is that the relationship has built-in limits. During Stage 1, clients should obtain a clear picture of how often and for how long sessions will take place, what they can expect and should not expect from the counselor during the relationship, and how to reach the counselor for emergency as well as nonemergency matters (e.g., suicidal thoughts, billing, cancellations, rescheduling, etc.).

ASSESSING FOR HARM TO SELF OR OTHERS Although more formally done in Stage Two (see the subsection on Assessing for Psychopathology and Breaking Confidentiality), it is critical that clinicians are aware of any signs that the client might be potentially harmful to self or others. Clinicians should know how to ask questions to assess for such lethality and when it is ethically and legally critical to break confidentiality.

PROFESSIONAL DISCLOSURE STATEMENT AND INFORMED CONSENT To help orient clients and to assure there are no misunderstandings, it is often wise for the helper to provide a verbal or written professional disclosure statement that describes such counseling-related issues as the helper's theoretical orientation, credentials held, the purpose of the interview, relevant agency rules, limits to confidentiality, legal issues, fees for service, and so forth (American Mental Health Counselors Association [AMHCA], 1987; Corey, Corey, & Callanan, 2003). After reviewing the professional disclosure statement, the helper should obtain the client's informed consent for the helping process to proceed. Such consent involves the client giving his or her verbal or written permission to participate in the helping interview. (Professional disclosure statements and informed consent will be discussed in more detail in Chapter 6.)

CASE ILLUSTRATION 2.2 Stage 1: Rapport and Trust Building

During Sienna's initial interview, she starts to sob profusely and states that she does not understand why she is so depressed. She reports having fleeting thoughts of wanting to kill herself, but states that she does not have a plan and believes that suicide would be an "easy way out." She quickly identifies a number of issues in her life that seem important, but she is not sure that they are particularly "causing" her current state of depression. The issues in her life include being sad about moving away from home, being confused about dating a person who is from a different culture, finding school more work than she had imagined, and having difficulties with her roommate. She notes that she has felt depressed in the past, " but these feelings are much more intense," and she is concerned that she will not be able to concentrate on her schoolwork.

CLIENT DYNAMICS

As with most clients, making it to the first session took some amount of courage. Although nervous about meeting with her counselor for their first time, Sienna was also relieved, and the counselor quickly helped her feel more at ease by allowing her a few moments to look around the office. Sienna also felt more comfortable after the counselor offered her a professional disclosure statement that highlighted the nature of the counseling relationship and the limits of confidentiality. Sienna was now relatively comfortable sharing her thoughts about what brought her to the session and responding to the counselor's inquiries. Sienna was only vaguely aware of the counselor's mix of inquiry and empathic listening skills.

CLINICAL ISSUES

The counselor realized the importance of sharing the professional disclosure statement and explaining the limits of confidentiality, although it was a little awkward taking care of these issues prior to Sienna talking about why she had come to the counseling center. After signing the informed consent statement, the counselor asked Sienna to discuss what brought her to the interview. This was followed by the counselor gathering information. At the same time, the counselor tried to make sure she listened empathically to Sienna in an effort to understand the client at deeper levels and to assist in building rapport. This balance between inquiry and empathy at times felt awkward to the counselor. However, to gather information so as to understand the full context of the client's difficulties, and in an effort to build rapport, both were deemed important skills during this first session.

Although the counselor had experienced some moderate depression herself a few years back, she chose not to self-disclose at all during the session because it would seem to give the wrong message as to the nature of the counseling relationship and the kinds of boundaries that would exist. During the session, the counselor had little difficulty handling Sienna's sometimes strong affect and did not attempt to "rescue" her from these strong feelings. Although she was supportive of Sienna, she also knew it was important to set boundaries by explaining the center's appointment schedule and emergency on-call contacts. Due to the level of depression Sienna was exhibiting and her inability to concentrate on school, the counselor also considered a referral for Sienna to be evaluated for possible antidepressant medication. In addition, a second appointment later in the week was set up for Sienna to see the counselor.

EXERCISE 2.2 **Reflections on Rapport and Trust Building**

In small groups, consider the following questions that clinicians often face during the rapport and trust building stage of the counseling relationship.

1. OFFICE DECOR: Describe what you believe is appropriate decor in a counseling office, how you might prepare the physical environment of your own office, and what messages you would want to convey by your selections.
2. SELF-DISCLOSURE: When, if ever, do you believe it would be appropriate or necessary to self-disclose in a helping relationship?
3. CLIENT AFFECT: Which client emotions do you believe will be most challenging for you when working with a client? How might you respond when confronted by a client expressing the feelings you described?
4. BUILDING THE RELATIONSHIP AND GATHERING INFORMATION: How comfortable might you feel trying to balance the foundational skills needed to build a relationship (e.g., empathic understanding) with the information-gathering skills needed to gain a deeper understanding of the client (e.g., questions, structured interview)?

Stage 2: Problem Identification

The primary goal of Stage 2 is to identify, describe, and understand the client's concerns (Schwitzer, 1996, 1997). Although problems begin to emerge in Stage 1, they are fully identified in Stage 2, and the stage is set to establish goals in Stage 3. This often takes a few sessions (see Chapter 2 Appendix for a summary of this stage).

Clinical Skills

ATTITUDES Whereas natural helpers tend to jump into problem solving prior to fully understanding an individual's concerns, professional counselors methodically collect and make sense of all the key information and then design a careful plan for change. Such a methodical, planful process requires *cognitive complexity* (Duys & Hedstrom, 2000). Thus, it is not surprising that new counselors tend to experience more ambiguity, more confusion, and less confidence, and they delay treatment planning more than seasoned practitioners (Hill & Ridley, 2001; Ladany, Marotta, & Muse-Burke, 2001; Martin, Slemon, Hiebert, Hallberg, & Cummings, 1989). Of course, *competence,* or having a thirst for continually seeking the most effective ways of working with a client, is critical at this stage.

TECHNIQUES During this stage, the clinician uses his or her *foundational skills* to follow the client's story and to gently guide the storytelling so that all the important information is covered. In addition, *empathic understanding* can allow the client to delve deeper into a problem and is critical if rapport and trust are to be maintained. During this stage, clinicians must also be skilled at in-depth *information gathering* to identify client needs and issues (Seligman, 2004). Information gathering, begun in Stage 1, assures that enough information can be collected to make a good decision about the treatment that will follow. To facilitate the gathering of information, a number of techniques are used, including *asking questions* and the use of a *structured interview.* Other kinds of information-gathering tools include having clients complete intake forms, problem checklists, informal rating scales, and personality measures. As clinicians leave this stage and get ready for goal setting and treatment planning, they use *collaboration* to assure that they are in sync with the client regarding what issues are to be addressed.

Clinical Tools

CASE CONCEPTUALIZATION In Stage 2, the case conceptualization process begins by identifying client needs from among the presenting concerns. The clinician then examines whether associated features, or additional concerns that accompany the client's central reason for seeking counseling, are present. Next, the clinician explores whether unrecognized or undetected problems might also be present. Finally, the clinician attempts to identify etiological factors, which are the roots, origins, or causes of the client's difficulties, and sustaining factors, which are the circumstances or forces currently keeping the problem going. Ultimately, the clinician's theoretical orientation will influence how the clinician views the information gathered and how those problems will be addressed (Stage 3).

DIAGNOSIS Although very tentatively begun in Stage 1, a diagnosis is formally made during this stage. Professional counselors and psychotherapists must be skilled using the *DSM-IV-TR* (American Psychiatric Association [APA], 2000) to make clinical diagnoses (Seligman, 1998, 2004). Diagnoses are used to describe client problems, lend direction in treatment planning, and communicate about client concerns with other clinicians.

CASE MANAGEMENT During this stage, the clinician should take accurate case notes, check on business-related issues, and attend to any progress reports that may be required for supervisors, insurance companies, and funding agencies.

Ethical and Professional Issues

ASSESSING FOR PSYCHOPATHOLOGY AND BREAKING CONFIDENTIALITY Today's professional counselor encounters a wide range of client functioning (Seligman, 2004). As the clinician delves further into the client's issues, significant clinical concerns may arise. For instance, the therapist may be faced with a client who is suicidal, shows potential for harming others, or is evidencing other signs of psychopathology. It is the clinician's responsibility to know when to break confidentiality due to an assessment of probable client harm toward self or others. If psychopathology is missed or not diagnosed accurately, the clinician may be working on inappropriate goals, inadvertently damaging the client, or be responsible for harm caused to others by not acting quickly enough.

REFERRAL As problems are identified during this stage, referrals to other resources are sometimes needed. Thus, clinicians must recognize when to refer a client (a) for a physical examination to rule out a medical problem, (b) for testing to better identify a diagnosis, (c) for a psychiatric evaluation for medication, or (d) to another counselor because the identified problem appears beyond one's area of competence.

CONSULTATION AND SUPERVISION As clients reveal deeper parts of themselves, they will sometimes present issues with which the clinician has little experience or will tap into unfinished issues in the clinician's life. Thus, it is always prudent for a clinician to have a supervisor with whom he or she can consult. Supervision allows the clinician to understand how his or her issues may interfere with effective treatment, offers different perspectives on understanding client problems, and is a mentoring process that can gradually assist the clinician in improving his or her skills (Bernard & Goodyear, 2004).

CASE ILLUSTRATION 2.3 Stage 2: Problem Identification

After Sienna's first session, she was asked and readily agreed to complete a number of assessment instruments to help fully understand some of the issues underlying her presenting problem. During the next session, she finds herself feeling increasingly comfortable in the helping relationship and begins to identify additional issues important to her, including feelings of enmeshment with her parents, dependence on her boyfriend, and lack of clarity about her values. She also realizes that many of her symptoms, such as problems sleeping, lack of concentration, lethargy, and poor appetite, are related to her depression.

CLIENT DYNAMICS

As Sienna continues in counseling, she begins to feel more trusting of her counselor. She soon feels comfortable sharing additional information about herself and even finds that she gets in touch with issues of which she was not aware. In addition, she now feels comfortable when the clinician gently probes into her life and feels safe enough to answer her probes as fully as possible. She is realizing that sharing the deepest parts of herself will eventually lead to her feeling better, and ideally, to having a more fulfilling life.

Through counseling, Sienna comes to understand that she was experiencing many unrecognized associated features of depression, such as lethargy, trouble getting up in the morning for classes, trouble sleeping, poor appetite, and trouble concentrating on schoolwork. Sienna also recognizes an undetected concern that seems to be both an etiological and sustaining factor—her emotional dependence on her parents before going to college and on her boyfriend and others since coming to college.

Sienna soon sees a connection between her depression and feelings of enmeshment with her parents. She notes that her parents had always tried to keep her "close to home," and now that she is at college, she feels a freedom that had never existed before. However, her new found freedom is connected to feelings of

(continued)

(continued)

guilt and shame. On the one hand, she tries to be free from her parents, and on the other hand, she experiences guilt and shame about behaving in a manner in which her parents would not approve. She also realizes that although she feels a strong sense of love for her boyfriend, she is increasingly feeling dependent on him. She begins to wonder if she always needs to be emotionally tied to someone—first her parents, now her boyfriend. Despite her sense of caring for him, she also wonders if seeing someone from another culture could be an act of rebellion toward her parents. She soon realizes that despite her freedom from her parents, she finds that she espouses many of her parents' values and is beginning to wonder if these values are ones she would want as her own. She is increasingly gaining clarity on the many issues she has to work on.

CLINICAL ISSUES

Although the clinician initially accepts the presenting problems as potential issues for Sienna to work on, she also realizes that there may be other underlying concerns. Although she does not initially share these thoughts with Sienna, through the building of trust and later through probing, Sienna eventually comes to realize this also. In addition, the interpretation of assessment instruments helps the client gain new insights about herself.

Sienna had described depression as one reason for coming to the counseling center, and her test results were consistent with moderate depression and emotional dependence. However, as the clinician uses foundational skills to build rapport, and as the clinician also gathers additional information, a number of potential issues to work on come to the forefront, including (a) depression, which is sometimes debilitating, (b) problems with her roommate, (c) inability to concentrate and study, (d) emotional dependence on others, and (e) confusion about her values.

As the clinician works with Sienna and gets to know her on deeper levels, she begins to formulate a possible diagnosis for Sienna's problems. Such a diagnosis will assist in treatment planning and in any possible referrals that may need to be made. In this case, the clinician tentatively diagnoses Sienna as having an adjustment disorder with depressed mood and, for now, rules out diagnoses of dysthymia or a major depressive disorder.

EXERCISE 2.3 **Reflections on Problem Identification**

In small groups, consider the following questions that clinicians often face during the problem identification stage of the counseling relationship.

1. IDENTIFYING CLIENT CONCERNS AND MAINTAINING SUPPORT: With the main goal of Stage 2 being to identify, describe, and understand the client's concerns, describe how you might balance the continual probing that is critical in this stage with the need to maintain a supportive trusting relationship.
2. POTENTIAL FOR HARM: What might your response be to a client who presents with suicidal thoughts; self-harm, such as cutting oneself; threats of harm to someone else; or severe psychopathology, such as delusions or hallucinations?

Stage 3: Goal Setting and Treatment Planning

The primary goal of Stage 3 is to specify expected outcomes of the counseling process. At this stage, goals that will lead to a plan of therapeutic action are determined (Jongsma & Peterson, 2003) (see Chapter 2 Appendix for a summary of this stage).

Clinical Skills

ATTITUDES In contrast to natural helpers, professional counselors and psychotherapists collaborate with their clients to set specific goals for change. Based on these goals, treatment plans are devised that can vary according to the client's interests and needs, the counselor's theoretical orientation, and the counseling agency's mission. The development of a treatment plan requires *cognitive complexity* and clinical *competence* because it is an involved process that requires clinicians to consider alternative ways of reaching goals and necessitates that the clinician has a repertoire of clinical skills.

TECHNIQUES Professional counselors must be skilled at setting reasonable, measurable goals. Treatment plans focused on such goals can prevent the onset of problems, improve normal psychosocial development and adjustment, and/or therapeutically resolve more distressing, disruptive problems that are firmly entrenched (Drum & Lawler, 1988). A number of skills can assist in setting goals and treatment plans that are achievable. For instance, *offering alternatives* and *giving information* can offer new directions for the client when setting goals, and, if done carefully, *advice giving* can be critical in helping to reach one's goals. Whichever techniques are used, it is imperative that goals and treatment plans are developed *collaboratively* so that the client feels a sense of ownership and empowerment in his or her own therapeutic process.

Clinical Tools

CASE CONCEPTUALIZATION The case conceptualization process, which began in Stage 2, continues in Stage 3 as goals are developed and a treatment plan is put in place. The treatment plan is based on the clinician's unique view of the world, which is a function of his or her theoretical orientation.

DIAGNOSIS Although already made, the competent and reflective clinician always reconsiders the accuracy of the original diagnosis and is open to changing it if necessary.

TREATMENT PLANNING The goals, which are an outgrowth of case conceptualization, become a critical element in the treatment planning process. Treatment plans are individualized to meet client needs and include measurable milestones for charting the client's progress (Jongsma & Peterson, 2003). A good treatment plan requires a clinician who has extensive knowledge of intervention skills that can be matched to the goals that have been set. Skillful treatment planning is a road map that sets the stage for the work to follow.

CASE MANAGEMENT During goal setting and treatment planning, the clinician should take accurate case notes, check on business-related issues, and attend to any progress reports that may be required for supervisors, insurance companies, and funding agencies.

Ethical, Professional, and Cross-Cultural Issues

LIMITATIONS OF THE SETTING In recent years, an increasing number of constraints have been placed on the counseling relationship, including limitations on the number of sessions, the amount of reimbursement for clients from healthcare agencies, and time restraints due to large caseloads (Ackley, 1997; Seligman, 2004). With such constraints, clinicians have a professional responsibility to set goals that are reasonable for the number of contacts, amount of time the client is seen, and professional attention the clinician is able to devote to the client. When client needs cannot be met due to existing constraints, the clinician is obligated to help the client find a more amenable setting in which to achieve his or her counseling goals.

CASE ILLUSTRATION 2.4 Stage 3: Goal Setting

Sienna has identified a number of important issues in her life and now voices some concern over what to do next. As she does so, the clinician assures her that the two of them will work collaboratively on identified goals based on the issues noted earlier. Realizing that it is now the end of the third session, and the center only allows for twelve sessions, Sienna is faced with some important decisions about which issues to focus on. With the help of her counselor, she develops a hierarchy of the problems she would like to tackle. Based on this hierarchy, Sienna decides to do the following:

1. Seek psychiatric consultation for possible medication to address her depressive symptoms. Medication, if taken, could also help with a number of the associated symptoms such as lack of appetite, sleep disturbance, and inability to concentrate.
2. Hold off on dealing with her roommate problems. Sienna sees this as the least of her concerns and hopes that once she is feeling better, the problem will dissipate and/or she will have the strength to talk with her roommate directly.
3. Learn study skills and design a time management log with her counselor to help her study.
4. Spend the rest of her sessions discussing her feelings of emotional dependence and her confusion over her values. Sienna hopes this will help her understand herself more clearly and lead to greater decision-making skills.
5. Reevaluate her goals after eight sessions to see if they are realistic.

CLIENT DYNAMICS

Sienna feels a sense of accomplishment related to her ability to identify issues and delve more deeply into herself. She also has an underlying sense that she must soon work on identified problems. She begins to seek direction from her counselor, who helps her identify which problems to focus on. She is beginning to feel a sense of collaboration—almost teamwork—as the two of them begin to develop a treatment plan. She is both apprehensive and excited about working on her issues.

CLINICAL ISSUES

The counselor felt good about progress made during the session. She was able to help Sienna identify a broader range of issues than she had originally come in with and has now offered her a mechanism to work on these issues. The main service constraint for Sienna and the counselor was a 12-session-per-school-year limit employed by the counseling center. In consultation with the counselor, Sienna had come up with what the counselor thought was a reasonable treatment plan for the limited number of sessions. It was critical that the counselor have a good referral base for possible medication, and her diagnosis of adjustment disorder with depression will be helpful to the psychiatrist to whom she refers. To work with Sienna, the counselor must be well read about effective treatments of depression and its related symptoms. In addition, the counselor should know how to teach study skills or refer to others who can do so, and the counselor should be able to develop a time management log. Finally, the counselor should understand the developmental issues that many late adolescents and young adults face—autonomy and value identification.

EXERCISE 2.4 **Reflections on Goal Setting and Treatment Planning**

In small groups, consider the following questions that clinicians often face during the goal setting and treatment planning stage of the counseling relationship.

1. SERVICE LIMITATIONS: What are your attitudes about the following service limitations: (a) session limits, (b) client ability to pay, (c) caseload size? Discuss how you might raise and discuss these topics with a client. Role-play these issues with a fellow student.
2. GOALS AND FOCUS: Consider how the goals of counseling will change as a function of whether one is focusing on prevention, normal developmental issues, or in-depth psychotherapy work. What professional settings are a good match for the type of counseling goals with which you would prefer to work?
3. CASE MANAGEMENT: In this age of accountability, case management issues have become paramount. What case management concerns would you have at this stage in the counseling relationship and how comfortable do you feel spending a fair amount of time doing the necessary paperwork?

Stage 4: Work

Perhaps it is misleading to wait until the fourth stage to say that "work" has begun, since in many ways work starts the moment the client contacts the counseling setting. However, it is during Stage 4 that the "work" of facilitating progress toward specified treatment goals formally begins (see Chapter 2 Appendix for a summary of this stage).

Clinical Skills

ATTITUDES In Stage 4, both the client and counselor work. The counselor works by applying his or her advanced skills and intervention strategies. Thus, the counselor shows *competence* and mastery of a number of skills that will assist the client toward reaching his or her goals. Becoming a competent clinician begins with mastery of the skills covered in this textbook, is reinforced and strengthened with advanced coursework and extensive supervised practical experience, and continues after one's professional training is completed by keeping up with the literature and being involved with professional workshops and conferences. Competence is more than just learning the skills—it is a desire and thirst for knowledge. It is an attitude that says, "learning never ends."

TECHNIQUES Some universal helping skills are commonly used during the work stage. For instance, it is not unusual during this stage to find clinicians using *affirmation giving,* as the client reaches goals; modeling of new behaviors by the counselor for the client; selective *self-disclosure* on the part of the counselor as an example of ways to reach goals and to affirm the client in his or her goal-seeking behavior; and *confronting* the client in an effort to encourage new ways of understanding the problem while encouraging change.

Also during the work stage, the clinician must be skilled in applying theory to practice in an effort to reach identified goals set in the previous stage. Sometimes called *theory-driven skills,* today's professional counselors employ one of three different approaches to clinical work: (a) a purist adherence to a single theoretical orientation, (b) eclecticism, or (c) an integrative approach. Purists consistently use the same formal model of doing therapy (e.g., person-centered, cognitive-behavioral, psychodynamic, reality therapy, existential, gender-aware approach, family systems, or another approach). Eclectic counselors form different treatment combinations for each client on the basis of their clinical experience, counseling knowledge base, or other professional preferences. Clinicians with an integrative framework use one dominant model as their main basis for viewing clinical work and also planfully borrow techniques and concepts into their main model to tailor fit the approach to client needs. Although this text will not go into depth about the various theoretical orientations to which one could adhere, effective clinicians should be able to apply their theoretical approach to a wide range of client goals.

Clinical Tools

CASE CONCEPTUALIZATION AND TREATMENT PLANNING The issues the client works on is an outgrowth of the case conceptualization process that started during the problem identification stage, continued into the goal setting and treatment planning stage, and is now focused on in the work stage. It therefore makes sense that one's treatment plan will be based on the case conceptualization process; that is, the course of treatment is based on which problems were identified, the goals set, and how the counselor's theory will be used to reach those goals. In essence, a road map is formed earlier in the relationship that guides the use of advanced skills and theory-driven skills during the work stage. For instance, Sienna's goal of working on her dependence needs were identified earlier in the helping relationship and led toward a treatment plan. How this goal is now attained, during the work stage, may differ quite a bit depending on the clinician's theoretical orientation.

DIAGNOSIS AND TREATMENT PLAN RECYCLING As the client begins to work on his or her issues, it may become evident that the goals chosen and the treatment plan devised may not be meeting the client's needs and therefore should be revised. Clinicians should be open to revising the goals and treatment plans based on progress made during this stage.

CASE MANAGEMENT During the work stage, the clinician should continue to take accurate case notes, check on business-related issues, and attend to any required progress reports that may be required for supervisors, insurance companies, and funding agencies.

Ethical and Professional Issues

PROFESSIONAL COMPETENCE Whereas natural helpers offer temporary support, professionals take on the ethical and legal responsibility for assisting the client in need. Thus, throughout the counseling relationship, the clinician must keep an eye on whether the client's concerns and dynamics are within the counselor's range of competencies. During the work stage, the clinician must adequately apply his or her theoretical orientation to client goals; modify goals and treatment plans when necessary; suggest additional assessment; seek peer consultation or clinical supervision; make decisions about alternative treatment modes, such as group or family counseling or inpatient hospitalization; and know when to help the client move on to a clinician with different competencies better suited to the client's needs. Being competent, then, is a professional responsibility and carries with it an attitude that assumes vigilance on the part of the clinician to assure that the best clinical work is being practiced.

CASE ILLUSTRATION 2.5 Stage 4: Work

Sienna enters the work stage of the counseling relationship realizing that change is within reach and that she must actively work on her goals to make this happen. She focuses on each of the identified issues and begins to tackle them one at a time. She is given a referral to a psychiatrist, who defers prescribing antidepressant medication until it is seen whether counseling can produce enough improvement in mood. She also receives a referral to a study skills group. In addition, the counselor helps Sienna create a log for managing her time. Finally, Sienna begins to discuss her relationship with her parents and the kinds of values that were instilled in her. She begins to sort through the values that seem most important to her.

(*continued*)

(continued)

CLIENT DYNAMICS

Now that goals have been agreed on, Sienna realizes that she has work to do in the helping relationship. Although she seeks guidance from the clinician, she realizes that much of the work is in her hands; that is, she must actively take steps to change her life. She feels both apprehensive and eager about the work she has to do. With some well-appreciated help from her therapist, she finds a psychiatrist with whom to consult about medication, finds a study skills groups, and develops a time management log. Now she feels ready to work on what she perceives to be the most difficult part of counseling—her relationship with her parents and how that defines who she is.

CLINICAL ISSUES

The counselor employs an integrative approach in her work with Sienna. Although her main grounding was humanistic, she has incorporated into her approach a number of techniques from other theories, including brief counseling, psychodynamic theory, systems theory, developmental theory, and cognitive/behaviorism. As she works with Sienna, she (a) sets goals to be reached in a limited number of sessions (brief), (b) develops a time management log and reinforces Sienna's adherence to it (behavioral), (c) refers to a study skills group to learn about new behaviors (behavioral), (d) discusses family issues from a systemic and psychodynamic perspective, and (e) explains life stage developmental issues to Sienna (psychoeducational).

EXERCISE 2.5 **Reflections on Work**

In small groups, consider the following questions that clinicians often face during the work stage of the counseling relationship.

1. APPROACHES TO CLINICAL WORK: What do you think are the advantages and disadvantages of the purist, eclectic, and integrative approaches to professional counseling? At this point in your development, which one of these seems the best fit for you?
2. BRIEF OR LONG-TERM TREATMENT: At this point in your development, which seems the best fit with your own natural helping style: (a) a brief approach that deals directly with symptom relief or (b) a longer term, indirect approach that focuses on underlying causes?
3. COMPETENCE THROUGHOUT ONE'S CAREER: In what ways can you challenge yourself to broaden your theoretical viewpoint through future learning and practice?

Stage 5: Closure

Stage 5, the closure stage, is sometimes referred to as the termination phase of treatment, and its primary goals are to summarize, review, and make the transition out of counseling as smooth as possible (see Chapter 2 Appendix for a summary of this stage).

Clinical Skills

ATTITUDES During the closure stage, the therapist helps the client review and summarize the changes achieved and goals attained; outlines areas for the client to continue working on after termination; and discusses the experience of the counseling relationship, particularly feelings about the relationship coming to an end. Within professional boundaries, the clinician may share some of his or her experiences of the relationship and feelings about termination.

Helping clients process their thoughts and feelings during this stage facilitates movement from the dependence they often feel during the relationship to the independence needed once counseling ends. *Empathy* and *acceptance* are two key attitudes that help the client review progress made and deal with current feelings about closure and autonomy, while *genuineness* is critical if the clinician is to be real regarding his or her feelings about the relationship coming to an end.

As the relationship closes, clinicians are often faced with a wide range of feelings, some of which may be uncomfortable to acknowledge. For instance, they may feel a sense of accomplishment; they might second-guess the work done; and they can grow alert to feelings toward the client they developed in earlier stages but did not act on, such as need for approval, frustration, anger, or sexual attraction. Most often, these are common, passing feelings. However, to remain helpful to the client during closure, the clinician must manage his or her own reactions to termination. Dealing with these reactions is a part of the professional's work duties, and developing the emotional capacity to handle them requires the counselor to be *adjusted psychologically*.

TECHNIQUES During closure, the clinician must be skilled at bringing the relationship to a productive conclusion. The foundational skills associated with *listening* and *empathy*, and the commonly used skills of *affirmation giving*, *modeling*, and *self-disclosure*, are used to help the client discuss his or her thoughts and feeling about the relationship and to assist in saying good-bye. For instance, effective clinicians can listen and understand the strong feelings some clients have about ending. Good clinicians are able to model genuineness by self-disclosing appropriate feelings when saying good-bye. Seasoned professionals can affirm client progress and the positive changes that have been made, while also *challenging* the client to continue to move on in his or her life. At the end of this stage, the clinician *collaborates* with the client to assure that expectations about follow-up are similar and to make sure that there is no unfinished business.

Clinical Tools

CASE MANAGEMENT Extensive case management usually is needed at the end of the counseling relationship to ensure that all related paperwork and billing issues are up-to-date, correspondence with other professionals is handled, and any after-planning and follow-up have been arranged.

Ethical and Professional Issues

AFTER-PLANNING At closure, it is the clinician's responsibility to help the client plan for needs following termination. For instance, when necessary, concrete arrangements should be made for follow-up visits, referral to another professional such as a psychiatrist or school counselor, or transition to another treatment mode, like group or family counseling. Specific suggestions for self-guided after-work should be made when needed, such as reading assignments or a self-help program for continued behavior change. Overall, the client should leave with a good sense of how to keep up the progress already made, a mechanism to continue to work independently toward unreached goals, and a road map to tackle any challenges or obstacles that might be encountered.

CASE ILLUSTRATION 2.6 Stage 5: Closure

Although told at the beginning of the helping relationship that there was a maximum of twelve sessions at the counseling center, Sienna is somewhat surprised when the counselor notes, during the tenth session, that there are only two sessions left. Although initially feeling apprehensive, Sienna begins to mentally review what she has done in counseling. She is relieved when the counselor also begins to review the course of the helping relationship and summarizes the gains that have been made. In addition, the counselor begins to focus on how Sienna will follow up with the psychiatrist to reevaluate whether to prescribe a low dose of an antidepressant, maintain her time management log, continue with her study skills group, and integrate the knowledge she has gained about herself relative to her family and developmental stage. Sienna is also relieved when the counselor suggests that she join an 8-week self-esteem group for college students. Although a little apprehensive, when the last session ends, Sienna thanks her counselor and feels ready to move on.

CLIENT DYNAMICS

Sienna is actually a little panic stricken when she realizes that the counseling relationship will be ending. However, she does not show the full extent of her panic to the counselor and realizes that one of her issues has been emotional dependence on others. Sienna begins to think that she can function on her own and be healthy without the counselor, and she decides to discuss this notion with her counselor during the sessions that are left. She sees this as a large step for herself. Sienna also realizes that she is in charge of her life and that she is capable of continuing the changes she has made. She is going to miss her counselor a lot but knows that she can contact her if there is an emergency. She is also looking forward to her new group experience.

CLINICAL ISSUES

Due to Sienna's dependence issues, the counselor is prepared for a negative reaction from Sienna when she tells Sienna that they have only two sessions left. She knows that it will be important to structure the next couple of sessions in a manner that will relieve anxiety as they move out of the helping relationship. In the eleventh and final twelfth sessions, the counselor structures the discussion to help Sienna summarize the changes she has experienced, talk out loud about how the counseling experience had been for her, and talk about continuing work on her own. They also discuss how she will maintain contact with the psychiatrist, continue her time management log, and continue with her study skills group. She also purposefully tells Sienna about the self-esteem counseling group in an effort to ease her out of the individual counseling relationship. She believes the group will be a good transition from individual counseling to independent functioning.

During the last session, the counselor and Sienna discuss how Sienna would handle things if she felt herself "losing ground" or if some of her mood problems reemerged every now and then. In addition, the counselor expresses her positive feelings and admiration for the work Sienna has accomplished. Finally, the counselor feels it is especially important to reach a clear termination so Sienna can practice her newly developing emotional independence with a successful closure rather than allowing the sessions to continue too long.

EXERCISE 2.6 **Reflections on Closure**

In small groups, consider the following questions that clinicians often face during the closure stage of the counseling relationship.

1. COUNSELOR'S REACTIONS: People differ in how they experience relationship endings and in how they go about saying good-bye. What have your experiences been with relationship endings? What are your attitudes regarding counseling as a temporary relationship that will ultimately come to an end?
2. CHANGES IN FOCUS AND OVEREXTENDED COUNSELING: The counseling relationship may extend beyond the predetermined closure point because important new issues arise that must be addressed due to client dependence or as a result of counselor ambivalence about termination. When you find a counseling relationship continuing past expectations, how will you decide the cause? How will you determine what is appropriate? How might you deal with an overextended counseling relationship?

Stage 6: Postinterview

We believe that patients [and clients] can and should return as needed.
(Budman & Gurman, 1988, p. 20)

Closure of the relationship may not be the ultimate conclusion of the counselor's contact with the client, and it is not unusual for some clients to return to the same counselor or seek another professional sometime in the future (Neukrug, Milliken, & Shoemaker, 2001; Neukrug & Williams, 1993). Clients may need to revisit old concerns, return with new problems, or come back during life transitions to explore adjustment and development. Thus, the primary goal of the postinterview is to maintain appropriate availability (see Chapter 2 Appendix for a summary of this stage).

Clinical Skills

ATTITUDES Clinicians should continue to maintain a professional stance in their relationships with clients, even after counseling has ended. This allows the client to foster his or her independence yet leaves the door open for the client to seek the same clinician again for counseling. The *competent* clinician has the desire to follow up with clients and has the ability, due to his or her own *psychological adjustment,* to maintain appropriate boundaries despite the end of the clinical relationship.

Clinical Tools

CASE MANAGEMENT Case management continues beyond the end of the counseling relationship. At the postinterview stage, case management is needed to store and protect files and records, conduct any needed monitoring or follow-up contacts, conduct follow-up assessment when it is used, finalize any billing or business matters, and respond to requests for information from referral resources and possible future clinicians the clients might see.

Ethical and Professional Issues

MAINTAINING BOUNDARIES Clinicians should continue to maintain a professional stance in their relationships with clients even after counseling has ended, and ethical codes support this view (see American Counseling Association [ACA],1995; National Association of Social Workers [NASW], 1999; also see list of ethical code Web sites in Toolbox A), Thus, most clinicians try to avoid any close relationships with clients after termination. This includes dating and romantic relationships, friendships, positions of power like clinical supervisor or dissertation adviser, and other relationships that are too familiar.

ETHICS OF FOLLOW-UP ASSESSMENT Follow-up contacts such as letters, surveys, questionnaires, and phone calls can help measure client satisfaction and goal attainment. This type of information helps the counselor evaluate which approaches have been most successful (Hutchins & Cole, 1997; Kleinke, 1994) and provides a brief chance to reinforce the client's progress (Neukrug, 2002, 2004). It is also an opportunity for the client to request additional counseling if needed. Although many clients appreciate and benefit from follow-up, others prefer no interaction once closure is reached. Therefore, clinicians should be sensitive to these differing reactions when conducting follow-up. One or two attempts can be made, usually within a few weeks to 6 months after closure, but a clinician should avoid multiple, relentless attempts to contact clients.

CASE ILLUSTRATION 2.7 Stage 6: The Postinterview

At termination, Sienna was asked to complete closure paperwork and measures of change. Her assessment instruments showed significant improvement in most areas, and she reported substantial goal accomplishment.

After counseling had ended, Sienna followed up with her group counseling experience and her appointment with the psychiatrist, who felt that progress had been made and no further appointments would be necessary. Over time, she stopped using her time management log but continued with her study skills group until it had ended. After 2 months, as agreed on during the last session, the counselor made a follow-up phone call to Sienna. Sienna noted that she was doing well, despite some moments of depression. She stated that she had broken up with her boyfriend but at times missed him terribly. She noted that her relationship with her parents was more distant than in the past but that it seemed to have a new, "healthier" quality. She stated that she was happy to hear from the counselor and no longer felt counseling to be necessary. The counselor noted that she had sent a client satisfaction survey and encouraged Sienna to complete it fully and honestly. She noted that she would not see the survey directly but that her supervisor reviewed all of the returned surveys and, once a year, gave her feedback while maintaining the anonymity of clients.

CLIENT DYNAMICS

Sienna feels good when counseling ends and, despite some momentary setbacks, continues with progress in all areas of her life. She reflects back on her counseling experience with a sense of accomplishment and satisfaction. Although not wanting to go back into counseling, she is not opposed to it should other significant issues develop in her life. In quiet, alone moments, she realizes that her view of herself and of life in general has significantly changed.

CLINICAL ISSUES

Results from counseling are often longlasting, although clients sometimes lose track of how much has changed for them. Sienna's case is an example of how change is self-perpetuating. She now sees herself differently, understands her relationship with her parents in a new way, and has a new outlook on her future. The clinician can feel a sense of accomplishment with the progress Sienna made but should also reflect on other ways she could have assisted Sienna with her goals.

Exercise 2.7 **Reflections on the Postinterview**

In small groups, consider the following questions that often face clinicians during the postinterview stage of the counseling relationship.

1. PROFESSIONAL BOUNDARIES: Over the years, the kinds of boundaries a counselor should have relative to his or her relationship with former clients have been debated. What are your beliefs about this? For example, should the counselor have any personal-social contact after termination of counseling? Would it make a difference if the client initiated the contact? Are friendships allowable after a specified amount of time? What about intimate or romantic relationships? What about professional relationships such as instructor, clinical supervisor, or colleague?
2. ETHICAL GUIDELINES AND PROFESSIONAL BOUNDARIES: What do the most common professional ethical guidelines, such as those of the ACA, APA, and NASW, say about postcounseling relationships between clinicians and counselors? Find out and discuss. (See list of Web sites of code of ethics of professional associations in Toolbox A.)

LEARNING TO BE A COUNSELOR: An Ongoing Process

Understanding the natural progression of the counseling relationship is critical to your success at being a clinician. But understanding it isn't enough. One has to live it. And as you live it, you realize that each counseling relationship has a rhythm of its own that unravels naturally if we allow it to. This means that each of us has to have patience to allow for the unfolding of this relationship: patience so we don't push our clients too fast; patience so we can enjoy our work and "go with the flow" of this critical relationship; and patience so we can give our "patients" time to heal from whatever pain they have to deal with in life—and then move on.

Sometimes having patience will not be easy, especially when you are beginning this journey and want so badly to watch your clients get better quickly. However, if you can allow yourself the freedom to let clients heal in their own time, your clients will get better more quickly than if you tried to push them along, and you will enjoy the journey more.

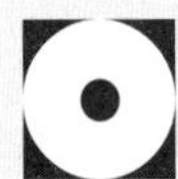

If you like, you can skip ahead in the DVD and view the sections entitled:

Clinical Tools and Intake Interview Introduction

Intake Interview

Working Stage Interview

and

Termination Interview

You will also be prompted to view these sections of the DVD later in the text.

Chapter Summary

This chapter identified seven stages of the helping relationship, which included: (a) the preinterview stage, (b) the rapport and trust building stage, (c) the problem identification stage, (d) the goal setting stage, (e) the work stage, (f) the closure stage, and (g) the postrelationship stage. For each of these stages, we identified its primary goal and discussed how each of the eight core areas of knowledge and skills emerge as a function of stage. These goals and the core areas of knowledge and skills are summarized in the Chapter 2 Appendix. As we discussed the stages, we offered a case example, Sienna, to show how a client and a clinician work as they move through the stages of counseling, and we noted that this example (and others) will be discussed again in Part III of the text.

The chapter concluded with a discussion concerning the importance of clinicians allowing the progression of the helping relationship to unravel naturally. It was suggested that patience is a critical factor in this process and that sometimes such patience comes with experience.

Summarizing the Stages

As you can see throughout the chapter, there are a myriad of counseling skills, clinical tools, and professional and ethical issues to which a clinician must attend throughout the counseling relationship. The following tables in the Chapter 2 Appendix help summarize the stages and the important core areas associated with them.

CHAPTER 2 APPENDIX: Stages and Associated Core Areas of Knowledge and Skills

TABLE 2.1
Attitudes and Skills throughout the Helping Relationship

STAGE	GOAL	CRITICAL ATTITUDES	CRITICAL TECHNIQUES
Preinterview	Preparation for optimal first encounter	• Acceptance: Ready self to accept client's issues and feelings. • Open-Mindedness: Ready self to not jump to conclusions about client. • Cognitive Complexity: Information gained is just one small piece of whole. • Psychological Adjustment: Take self-inventory to assure emotional readiness to work with client and to deal with any issue the client might touch upon.	• None. Client hasn't met with clinician.
Stage 1: Rapport and Trust Building	Establish a trusting, facilitative, therapeutic relationship	• Empathy: So client will feel heard, to build the alliance, and to encourage client self-disclosure. • Acceptance: So client will feel welcomed and safe. • Relationship Building: Most critical factor to successful client outcomes. Make sure one builds an alliance. • Psychological Adjustment: Being able to handle client's emotions and emotions of self toward client. • Competence: If clinician does not have competence to work with client, he or she will seek consultation, supervision, or refer client.	• Foundational Skills: Silence and pause time, listening, paraphrasing, and empathic understanding to build relationship and understand client fully. • Information Gathering: Asking questions and use of structured interview to probe and gather information to understand extent of client situation and to begin the process of developing a diagnosis and forming a treatment plan. • Commonly Used Skill: Collaboration to assure client and counselor expectations regarding treatment match.

Stage 2: Problem Identification	Identification, description, and understanding of client concerns	• Cognitive Complexity: Important for making sense of client situation after gathering information. • Being Competent: Is facile at using necessary skills to build relationship and gather information to identify client needs.	• Foundational Skills: To follow and guide story and maintain rapport. In particular, empathic understanding for delving deeper into problems and obtaining broader view of client's situation. • Information Gathering: To identify needs to develop goals in next stage. Use of questions, structured interview, intake forms, checklists, ratings scales, personality tests. • Commonly Used Skill: Collaboration to assure client and counselor identification of problem areas match.
Stage 3: Goal Setting and Treatment Planning	Specification of expected outcomes	• Cognitive Complexity: Clinician should have alternative ways of reaching goals that are based on client's expressed needs. • Being Competent: Clinician should be able to accurately identify problems and set achievable goals and treatment plan by having a repertoire of skills.	• Goal Setting Skills: Giving advice, offering alternatives, and giving information can all be critical when collaboratively setting goals. • Commonly Used Skill: Collaboration when setting goals and developing treatment plans to assure that goals and intervention strategies match.
Stage 4: Work	Facilitate progress toward specified outcomes	• Being Competent: Competence and mastery of a number of skills that will assist the client toward reaching his or her goals. "Learning never ends."	• Theory-Driven Skills: Used to work on goals from clinician's theoretical orientation (e.g., single orientation, eclecticism, integrative). • Commonly Used Skills: Affirmations, encouragement modeling, self-disclosure, confronting client to view problem in new ways while encouraging change.

(*continued*)

TABLE 2.1 *(continued)*

STAGE	GOAL	CRITICAL ATTITUDES	CRITICAL TECHNIQUES
Stage 5: Closure	Summarize, review, and resolve client experience	• Being Empathic, Accepting, and Genuine: Helpful in understanding and accepting client's feelings and thoughts about the ending of the therapeutic relationship. • Psychological Adjustment: Important for counselor's sometimes ambivalent feelings about closure and feelings toward client.	• Foundational Skills: Listening and being empathic are used to summarize progress, hear client's feelings about ending, and highlight significance of relationship. • Commonly Used Skills: Affirmation giving to affirm client progress. Modeling to show client how to say good-bye. Self-disclosure to express clinician's feelings concerning end of helping relationship. Collaboration to assure no unfinished business, to assist in saying good-bye, and to assure similar expectations regarding follow-up.
Stage 6: Postinterview	Maintain appropriate availability	• Competence: Assures for proper follow-up. • Psychological Adjustment: Important for maintenance of postrelationship boundaries.	None: Client no longer in therapeutic relationship.

TABLE 2.2
Clinical Tools throughout the Helping Relationship

STAGE	PRIMARY GOAL	CASE CONCEPTUALIZATION	DIAGNOSIS	TREATMENT PLANNING	CASE MANAGEMENT
Preinterview	Preparation for optimal first encounter	None: Haven't yet met client.	None: Haven't yet met client.	None: Haven't yet met client.	• Attend to appointment times, paperwork, files, advance information (e.g., previous reports, assessment results), preinterview contacts, etc.
Stage 1: Rapport and Trust Building	Establish a trusting, facilitative, therapeutic relationship	• Very early hypotheses made about client concerns and ancillary issues.	• Very tentative diagnosis may begin, but clinician is open to changing diagnosis in Stage 2.	None: Too early in relationship.	• Attend to paperwork, intake issues, billing, business matters, correspondence with other professionals, and agency records.
Stage 2: Problem Identification	Identification, description, and understanding of client concerns	• Begins with problem identification and examines possible undetected features, associated features, etiological factors, and sustaining factors.	• Diagnosis is formally made. Used to describe client problems, communicate client concerns with other professionals, and in treatment planning.	None: Too early in relationship.	• Write case notes, check on business-related issues, attend to required progress reports for supervisors, insurance companies, and funding agencies.
Stage 3: Goal Setting and Treatment Planning	Specification of expected outcomes	• Process continues as clinician develops goals and treatment plans. Conceptualization and resulting treatment plan are based on clinician's theoretical orientation.	• Competent and reflective clinician always reconsiders accuracy of original diagnosis and is open to changing it if necessary.	• Based on previously identified goals. Outgrowth of case conceptualization. Road map for work stage.	• Write case notes, check on business-related issues, attend to required progress reports for supervisors, insurance companies, and funding agencies.

(*continued*)

TABLE 2.2 *(continued)*

STAGE	PRIMARY GOAL	CASE CONCEPTUALIZATION	DIAGNOSIS	TREATMENT PLANNING	CASE MANAGEMENT
Stage 4: Work	Facilitate progress toward specified outcomes	• Client's work is an outgrowth of case conceptualization process.	• Recycling: Revisit diagnosis if client is not meeting goals.	• Treatment plan is an outgrowth of case conceptualization process that tentatively started in Stage 2, continued into the Stage 3, and is now focused on in this stage. • Recycling: Revisit treatment plan if client is not meeting goals.	• Write case notes, check on business-related issues, attend to required progress reports for supervisors, insurance companies, and funding agencies.
Stage 5: Closure	Summarize, review, and resolve client experience	None: Counseling coming to an end.	None: Counseling coming to an end.	None: Counseling coming to an end.	• Extensive near end of helping relationship: ending paperwork, billing issues, correspondence with other professionals, after-planning.
Stage 6: Postinterview	Maintain appropriate availability	None: Counseling is finished.	None: Counseling is finished.	None: Counseling is finished.	• Protect files and records, conduct monitoring, conduct follow-up contact and assessment, finalize business matters, respond to requests from referral sources.

TABLE 2.3
Ethical and Professional Issues throughout the Helping Relationship

STAGE	PRIMARY GOAL	ETHICAL, PROFESSIONAL, AND CROSS-CULTURAL ISSUES
Preinterview	Preparation for optimal first encounter	• Competence and Professional Limitations: Client's concerns should be within counselor's competencies. Make thoughtful and wise decisions about whether one needs to consult, seek supervision, and refer. • Office Decor: Consider what might be offensive to clients. Be intentional about how you decorate your office. • Knowledge of, and Skills to Use with, Diverse Clients: Assure you have the knowledge and skills. • Attitudes toward Diverse Clients: Take a self-inventory to assure no biases.
Stage 1: Rapport and Trust Building	Establish a trusting, facilitative, therapeutic relationship	• Professional Competence: Assure client's concerns within range of competence. • Assess for Cultural Competence: Assure that you are aware of the knowledge, skills, and attitudes necessary to work effectively with clients from diverse backgrounds. • Self-Disclosure: Should be planful, purposeful, and limited during this stage. • Establishing Boundaries: Client should understand the boundaries of a counseling relationship (e.g., length of sessions, expectations of relationship, emergency and nonemergency ways of contacting clinic). • Assessing for Harm to Self or Others: Know what questions to ask and when it is ethically and legally important to break confidentiality. • Professional Disclosure Statement: Given to client. • Informed Consent: Received from client.
Stage 2: Problem Identification	Identification, description, and understanding of client concerns	• Assessing Potential for Harm and Psychopathology: As client issues emerge, clinician should know how to assess for psychopathology and when to break confidentiality. • Referral: Know when to refer for physical problems, testing, evaluation for medication, or referral to another clinician. • Consultation and Supervision: Disclosure of deeper issues by client may tap into clinician's unfinished business. Be open to consultation and supervision to work through these issues.

(*continued*)

TABLE 2.3 *(continued)*

STAGE	PRIMARY GOAL	PROFESSIONAL, ETHICAL, AND CROSS-CULTURAL ISSUES
Stage 3: Goal Setting and Treatment Planning	Specification of expected outcomes	• Limitations of Setting: Take into account limits settings place on number of sessions, client's ability to pay, size of caseload, and other factors.
Stage 4: Work	Facilitate progress toward specified outcomes	• Professional Competence: Myriad issues face the competent professional during the work stage, including adequately applying theory, modifying goals when necessary, seeking consultation and supervision, deciding on alternative treatment modes, referring to another clinician. Be up on best practices in field.
Stage 5: Closure	Summarize, review, and resolve client experience	• After-Planning: When necessary, arrange for follow-up, referrals to others, transition to other treatment modes, specific suggestions for self-guided after-work, etc.
Stage 6: Postinterview	Maintain appropriate availability	• Maintaining Boundaries: Avoid nonprofessional contact after relationship. • Ethics of Follow-Up: Evaluate self by measuring client satisfaction and goal attainment. Follow-up can also reinforce progress by client. Offer opportunity to seek counseling again if needed. Avoid relentless contacts for clients not interested in follow-up.

Ethical, Professional, and Cross-Cultural Issues

Whereas natural helpers generally have a healthy sense of what is "right and wrong," professional counselors have a refined sense of their ethical and professional responsibilities. Thus, it is important that the professional counselor be able to address ethical questions that may arise, professional concerns that can impact the helping relationship, and cross-cultural issues when working with people of color. This chapter addresses these important areas.

The chapter starts by defining ethics and distinguishing between ethics and morality. Next, we discuss the development of and need for an ethical code that guides the clinician's behavior. Then, we highlight some codes of ethics and ethical hot spots, and this is followed by a review of some critical ethical and legal issues, including breach of confidentiality, confidentiality of records, privileged communication, and confinement against one's will. As we continue, we offer three models of ethical decision making: decision-making models, moral models, and developmental models.

As the chapter moves along, we examine a number of critical professional issues that impact the work of the clinician, including managed care, accountability, use of medication, and matching client problem with intervention strategy. The chapter concludes with an examination of cross-cultural issues, at which point we specifically address the fact that counseling does not work for many people of color and examine some models for cross-cultural counseling.

Ethical Issues

Ethics has become a critical area of importance for clinicians because it affects almost every aspect of their work. Thus, in this section, we define ethics and contrast it with morality, discuss the development of and need for ethical codes, highlight some codes of ethics and ethical hot spots, examine some critical ethical and legal issues, and offer three models of ethical decision making.

Defining Ethics

Within the mental health professions, concern regarding the impact of client behavior on self and others has gained increased notoriety and often drives the kinds of clinical decisions made. Whereas natural helpers deal with such questions from an individual moral perspective, professional counselors respond from an ethical stance. But what exactly is the difference between decision making based on morals and decision making based on ethics?

Morality is generally concerned with how an individual conducts oneself and is often the reflection of values of a group, such as an individual's family, religious sect, culture, or nationality. In contrast, ethics generally describes the collectively agreed on "correct" behaviors within the context of a professional group (Barry, 1982; Gladding, Remley, & Huber, 2001; Mowrer, 1967; Sieber, 1992; Swenson, 1997). Therefore, what might be immoral behavior for a minister might be ethical behavior for a counselor. For instance, relying on his or her sect's religious writings, a minister might oppose abortion. On the other hand, relying on ethical guidelines that assert a client's right to self-determination, a clinician might support a client's decision to have an abortion. Sometimes an individual's moral beliefs will conflict with his or her professional ethics (e.g., when a clinician's religious beliefs concerning abortion are in contrast to his or her ethical obligation regarding self-determination). Clearly, trying to make sense of one's values, what is right and wrong, and professional ethics can at times be quite an undertaking. And to make things even more confounding, sometimes the law will contradict one's values, sense of morality, and even professional ethics (Swenson, 1997).

EXERCISE 3.1 **Ethical versus Moral Beliefs**

In the space provided on the left, write down a strong moral belief that you hold. Then, describe a professional situation in which you might find yourself responding in a manner opposed to your personal moral beliefs (see example). Next, discuss in small groups how you might handle such a situation. You might want to examine one of the professional ethical codes as you do this exercise (see Web sites for professional ethical codes in Toolbox A).

MORAL BELIEF	PROFESSIONAL ETHICS THAT MIGHT CONTRAST WITH MORAL BELIEFS
1. I'm against the death penalty.	If I was counseling a client who had a loved one who was murdered, I might have to listen attentively to the client's desire to see the murderer receive the death penalty. And I would be obligated to be nonjudgmental with the client regarding his or her belief.
2.	
3.	
4.	

The Development of and Need for Ethical Codes

The establishment of ethical guidelines is relatively new to the helping professions. For instance, the American Psychological Association (APA) first published its code of ethics in 1953, the National Association of Social Workers (NASW) established its guidelines in 1960, and the American Counseling Association (ACA) developed its ethical guidelines in 1961. Because ethical standards are to some degree a mirror of changes in society, the associations' guidelines have undergone a number of major revisions over the years to reflect society's ever-changing values (see ACA, 1995; APA, 2003; NASW, 1999).

Despite some differences, it is interesting to note that the ethical guidelines of the helping professions of counseling, psychology, and social work all share similar values while serving a number of other general purposes (Corey, Corey, & Callanan, 2003; Loewenberg & Dolgoff, 2005; Mabe & Rollin, 1986; VanZandt, 1990):

1. They protect consumers and further the professional standing of the organization.
2. They are a statement about the maturity and professional identity of a profession.
3. They guide professionals toward certain types of behaviors that reflect the underlying values considered desirable in the profession.
4. They offer a framework in the sometimes difficult ethical decision-making process.
5. They can be offered as one measure of defense if the professional is sued for malpractice.

Although ethical guidelines can be of considerable assistance in a professional's ethical decision-making process, there are also limitations to the use of such a code (Mabe & Rollin, 1986):

1. There are many issues that cannot be handled in the context of a code.
2. There are some difficulties with enforcing the code, or at least the public may believe that enforcement committees are not tough enough on their peers.
3. There is often no way to bring the interests of the client, patient, or research participant systematically into the code construction process.
4. There are parallel forums in which the issues in the code may be addressed, with the results sometimes at odds with the findings of the code (e.g., in the courts).
5. There are possible conflicts associated with codes: between two codes, between the practitioner's values and code requirements, between the code and ordinary morality, between the code and institutional practice, and between requirements within a single code.
6. There is a limited range of topics covered in the code, and because a code approach is usually reactive to issues already developed elsewhere, the requirement of consensus prevents the code from addressing new issues and problems at the cutting edge (pp. 294–295).

Although there are positive and negative aspects to the use of ethical guidelines, the professional associations all clearly feel the development of such codes has been crucial to the professionalization of the mental health fields.

EXERCISE 3.2 **Developing Ethical Guidelines**

In groups of approximately six students, develop five to ten ethical guidelines you think would be critical to include in a professional ethics code. When you have finished, share these with the class, and as a class, come up with a final list of as many guidelines you would like to include. Compare this list with the existing ethical code of one or more of the helping professions (see Toolbox A).

Codes of Ethics and Ethical "Hot Spots"

Today, all of the major mental health professional associations have ethical codes that guide the practice of mental health professionals. Thus, we find ethical guidelines for counselors (ACA, 1995), psychologists (APA, 2003), social workers (NASW, 1999), marriage and family therapists (American Association of Marriage and Family Therapy [AAMFT], 2001), psychiatrists (American Psychiatric Association [APA], 2001), human service professionals (National Organization of Human Service Education [NOHSE], 1995), and others (see Toolbox A). Although there is much in common among the various ethical standards, differences do exist, and a conscientious professional will have some knowledge of the varying ethical guidelines. Although all ethical codes cover dozens of potential ethical problem areas, some issues that have gained prominence in the literature in recent years include the following: confidentiality, competence, dual relationships and conflicts of interest, inappropriate fee assessment, informed consent, misrepresentation of credentials, and sexual relationships with clients (APA, 2002; Neukrug, Milliken, & Walden, 2001) (Table 3.1).

Critical Ethical and Legal Issues

> *The study of ethics provides guidance for professionals, aids in stating professionals' responsibilities to society, provides society with reassurance, and helps professionals maintain their integrity and freedom from outside regulation. When legislatures pass laws requiring conduct incompatible with ethical codes, professional associations first try to change the laws. If that fails they modify the ethical codes to fit the new laws.* (Swenson, 1997, p. 58)

Literature in the mental health professions cites a number of important ethical concerns that have significantly impacted on the work of the clinician. Often, these are associated with important legal issues. The following sections highlight some of these critical issues, including breach of confidentiality, confidentiality of records, privileged communication, confinement against one's will, and the importance of malpractice insurance when doing counseling.

Breach of Confidentiality

Probably, the most discussed area of ethical behavior has to do with permissibility to break confidentiality. This was highlighted by the much-publicized *Tarasoff* case,

TABLE 3.1
Comparison of How Ethical Codes Address Ethical Hot Spots

ETHICAL HOT SPOT	ACA ETHICAL STANDARDS	NASW ETHICAL STANDARDS	APA ETHICAL STANDARDS
Confidentiality and Breach of Confidentiality	*Section B.1.: Confidentiality: Right to Privacy: a. Respect for Privacy.* Counselors respect their clients' right to privacy and avoid illegal and unwarranted disclosures of confidential information . . . *c.Exceptions.* . . . does not apply when disclosure is required to prevent clear and imminent danger to the client or to others or when legal requirements demand that confidential information be revealed.	*Section 1.07: Social Workers' Ethical Responsibilities to Clients: Privacy and Confidentiality:* *(c)* Social workers should protect the confidentiality of all information obtained in the course of professional services, except for compelling reasons. . . . does not apply when disclosure is necessary to prevent serious, foreseeable, and imminent harm to a client or other identifiable person.	*Section 4: Privacy and Confidentiality: 4:05: Disclosures:* *(b)* Psychologists disclose confidential information without the consent of the individual only as mandated by law, or where permitted by law for a valid purpose such as to (1) provide needed professional services; (2) obtain appropriate professional consultations; (3) protect the client/patient, psychologist, or others from harm; . . .
Competence	*Section C.2.: Professional Competence: a. Boundaries of Competence.* Counselors practice only within the boundaries of their competence, based on their education, training, supervised experience, state and national professional credentials, appropriate professional experience. Counselors will demonstrate a commitment to gain knowledge . . .	*Section 4.01: Social Workers' Ethical Responsibilities as Professionals: Competence: (a)* Social workers should accept responsibility or employment only on the basis of existing competence or the intention to acquire the necessary competence. *(b)* Social workers should strive to become and remain proficient in professional practice . . .	*Section 2: Competence: 2.01 Boundaries of Competence:* *(e)* . . . [psychologists] take reasonable steps to ensure the competence of their work and to protect clients/patients, students, supervisees, research participants, organizational clients, and others from harm. *2.03 Maintaining Competence:* Psychologists undertake ongoing efforts to develop and maintain their competence.
Dual Relationships and Conflicts of Interest	*Section A.6.: The Counseling Relationship: Dual Relationships: a. Avoid When Possible.* Counselors . . . avoid exploiting the trust and dependency of clients. Counselors make every effort to avoid dual relationships that could impair	*Section 1.06: Social Workers' Ethical Responsibilities to Clients: Conflicts of Interest: (a)* . . . Social workers should inform clients when a real or potential conflict of interest arises and take reasonable steps to resolve the issue in a manner that makes the	*Section 3.06: Human Relations: Conflict of Interest:* Psychologists refrain from taking on a professional role when personal, scientific, professional, legal, financial, or other interests or relationships could reasonably be

(continued)

TABLE 3.1 *(continued)*

ETHICAL HOT SPOT	ACA ETHICAL STANDARDS	NASW ETHICAL STANDARDS	APA ETHICAL STANDARDS
	professional judgement or increase the risk of harm to clients . . .	clients' interests primary and protects clients' interests to the greatest extent possible . . .	expected to (1) impair their objectivity, competence, or effectiveness . . .
Inappropriate Fee Assessment	*Section A.10.a.: The Counseling Relationship: Fees and Bartering a. Advance Understanding.* Counselors clearly explain to clients . . . all financial arrangements related to professional services . . . *b. Establishing Fees.* In establishing fees . . . counselors consider the financial status of clients . . .	*Section 1.13: Social Workers' Ethical Responsibilities to Clients: Payment for Services: (a)* When setting fees, social workers should ensure that the fees are fair, reasonable, and commensurate with the services performed. Consideration should be given to clients' ability to pay.	*Section 6.04: Record Keeping and Fees: Fees and Financial Arrangements: (a)* As early as is feasible . . . psychologists and recipients of psychological services reach an agreement specifying compensation and billing arrangements. *(b)* Psychologists' fee practices are consistent with law. *(c)* Psychologists do not misrepresent their fees.
Informed Consent	*Section A.3.a.: The Counseling Relationship: Client Rights a. Disclosure to Clients.* . . . throughout the counseling process as necessary, counselors inform clients of the purposes, goals, techniques, procedures, limitations, potential risks and benefits of services to be performed . . .	*Section 1.03: Social Workers' Ethical Responsibilities to Clients: Informed Consent: (a)* . . . Social workers . . . inform clients of the purpose of the services, risks related to the services, limits to services because of the requirements of a third-party payer, relevant costs, reasonable alternatives, clients' right to refuse or withdraw consent . . .	*Section 10.01: Therapy: Informed Consent to Therapy: (a)* . . . psychologists inform clients . . . about the nature and anticipated course of therapy, fees, involvement of third parties, and limits of confidentiality and provide sufficient opportunity for the client/patient to ask questions and receive answers . . . .
Misrepresentation of Qualifications	*Section C.4.: Professional Responsibility:Credentials: a. Credentials Claimed.* Counselors claim or imply only professional credentials possessed and are responsible for correcting any known misrepresentations of their credentials by others . . .	*Section 4.01: Social Workers' Ethical Responsibilities as Professionals: Misrepresentation: (c)* Social workers should ensure that their representation to clients, agencies, and the public of professional qualifications, credentials, education, competence, affiliations, services provided, or results achieved are accurate . . .	*Section 2.01: Competence: Boundaries of Competence: (a)* Psychologists provide services, teach, and conduct research with populations and in areas only within the boundaries of their competence, based on their education, training, supervised experience, consultation, study, or professional experience.

Sexual Relationship with Client	*Section A.7.: The Counseling Relationship: Sexual Intimacies with Clients: a. Current Clients.* Counselors do not have any type of sexual intimacies with clients and do not counsel persons with whom they have had a sexual relationship. *b. FormerClients.* Counselors do not engage in sexual intimacies with former clients within a minimum of two years after terminating . . .	*Section 1.09: Social Workers' Ethical Responsibilities to Clients: Sexual Relationships: (a)* Social workers should under no circumstances engage in sexual activities or sexual contact with current clients, whether such contact is consensual or forced. *(c)* Social workers should not engage in sexual activities or sexual contact with former clients. . . .	*Section 10: Therapy: 10.05 Sexual Intimacies With Current Therapy Clients/Patients:* Psychologists do not engage in sexual intimacies with current therapy clients/patients.*10.08: Sexual Intimacies With Former Therapy Clients/Patients: (a)* Psychologists do not engage in sexual intimacies with former clients/patients for at least two years . . .

Source: American Counseling Association (ACA), *Code of Ethics and Standards of Practice*, 1995; reprinted by permission. National Association of Social Workers (NASW), *Code of Ethics of the National Association of Social Workers*, 1999; reprinted by permission. American Psychological Association (APA), *Ethical Principles of Psychologists and Code of Conduct*, 2003; reprinted by permission.

in which a clinician and others were successfully sued for not warning a client's former girlfriend of potential harm that the client posed to her. This case involved a client named Prosenjit Poddar who was being seen at the counseling center at the University of California at Berkeley. Poddar told his psychologist that as a result of his girlfriend's recent threats to break up with him and date other men, he intended to kill her. As a result, his psychologist informed his supervisor and the campus police of his client's threat, at which point the campus police detained Poddar. The supervisor reprimanded the psychologist for breaking confidentiality, and finding no reason to further detain Poddar, the campus police released him. Two months later, he killed his girlfriend, Tatiana Tarasoff. Tatiana's parents sued the university, the therapist, the supervisor, and the police and won their suit against all but the police. The decision, which was seen as a model for "duty to warn," was interpreted by courts to mean that a therapist must make all efforts to prevent danger to another or to self. It is also interesting to note that the police won their lawsuit because in detaining the client, and subsequently assessing him using the most recognized and substantiated means, they came to the decision that he was not in danger of harming Tarasoff. Thus, even if your decision making results in unfortunate circumstances, if you do follow the best practice of your profession, you have a much greater likelihood of having the court on your side.

As a result of cases like *Tarasoff*, it is now assumed that clients have a right to expect that their conversations with counselors are private, except:

- when a client is in danger of harming himself or herself or someone else; this is known as "duty to warn"
- when a child is a minor and the law states that parents have a right to information about their child
- when a client asks the helper to break confidentiality (e.g., your testimony is needed in court)
- when a helper is bound by the law to break confidentiality (e.g., most states have mandatory reporting of child abuse and some have mandatory reporting of elder abuse)
- when revealing information about a client to the helper's supervisor to benefit the client
- when a helper has a written agreement from his or her client to reveal information to specified sources (e.g., other social service agencies that are working with the same client)
- when a clinician or the clinician's records are subpoenaed by the court and the clinician is not protected by a privileged communication statute (see the next section)

Privileged Communication

Privileged communication is a conversation conducted with someone that state or federal law identifies as a person with whom conversations may be privileged—that is, legally kept confidential (i.e., attorney–client, doctor–patient, therapist–patient, clergy–penitent, husband–wife, etc.). In the case of clinicians, the goal of the law is to encourage the client to engage in conversations without fear that the clinician

PROFESSIONAL PERSPECTIVES 3.1
Jaffee v. Redmond

"Mary Lu Redmond, a police officer in a village near Chicago, responded to a 'fight in progress' call at an apartment complex on June 27, 1991. At the scene, she shot and killed a man she believed was about to stab another man he was chasing. The family of the man she had killed sued Redmond, the police department, and the village, alleging that Officer Redmond had used excessive force in violation of the deceased's civil rights. When the plaintiff's lawyers learned that Redmond had sought and received counseling from a licensed social worker employed by the village, they sought to compel the social worker to turn over her case notes and records and testify at the trial.

Redmond and the social worker claimed that their communications were privileged under an Illinois statute. They both refused to reveal the substance of their counseling sessions even though the trial judge rejected their argument that the communications were privileged. The judge then instructed jurors that they could assume that the information withheld would have been unfavorable to the police-woman, and the jury awarded the plaintiffs $545,000 (Remley et al., 1997, p. 214).

After a series of appeals, the Supreme Court heard the case on February 26, 1996. The Court decided that the licensed therapist did indeed hold privilege and that the judge's instruction to the jury was therefore unwarranted.

will reveal the contents of the conversation (e.g., in a court of law), thus ensuring the privacy and efficacy of the counseling relationship. The privilege belongs to the client and can be asserted or waived only by the client (Attorney C. Borstein, personal communication, September 21, 2004; Swenson, 1997, p. 464). Privileged communication should not be confused with confidentiality, which is the *ethical* (not legal) obligation of the counselor to keep conversations confidential (Glosoff, Herlihy, & Spence, 2000).

A 1996 ruling upheld the right to privileged communication (*Jaffee v. Redmond*, 1996; see Professional Perspectives 3.1). In this case, the Supreme Court held the right of a licensed social worker to keep her case records confidential. Describing the social worker as a "therapist" and "psychotherapist," the ruling will likely protect all licensed therapists in federal courts and may affect all licensed therapists who have privileged communication (Remley, Herlihy, & Herlihy, 1997).

Confidentiality of Records

Although it is a gray area, clients probably have a legal right to view their counseling records, and increasingly, they have been exercising these rights in schools and agencies (Swenson, 1997). In fact, most ethical codes state that clients should be provided access to their records if the client is competent and the material is not misleading or detrimental. Relative to children, although ethical guidelines usually support a child's right to confidential counseling, it has generally been assumed that parents have the right to view records of their children (Attorney C. Borstein, personal communication, September 21, 2004; Davis & Mickelson, 1994; Hubert, 1996; Swenson, 1997). Of course, specific local and state laws may vary, and counselors should make themselves aware of how local laws apply.

In terms of federal law, the Freedom of Information Act of 1974 allows individuals access to any records maintained by a federal agency that contain personal information about the individual, and every state has followed along with similar laws governing state agencies (Public Citizen, 2002). Similarly, the Buckley Amendment of 1974, otherwise known as the Family Education Rights and Privacy Act (FERPA), assures parents the right to access their minor children's educational records (Committee on Government Operations, 1991).

More recently, the passage of the Health Insurance Portability and Accountability Act (HIPAA) assures the privacy of client records and the sharing of such information (Zuckerman, 2003). In general, HIPAA restricts the amount of information that can be shared without client consent and allows for clients to have access to their records, except for process notes used in counseling (U.S. Department of Health and Human Services, 2003). In fact, HIPAA requires agencies to show how they have complied with this act. As a result of HIPAA, mental health professionals will generally have to do the following:

- "Provide information to patients about their privacy rights and how that information can be used.
- Adopt clear privacy procedures for their practices.
- Train employees so that they understand the privacy procedures.
- Designate an individual to be responsible for seeing that privacy procedures are adopted and followed.
- Secure patient records." (American Psychological Association Practice Organization, 2002, p. 2)

Confinement Against One's Will

In 1975, Kenneth Donaldson, who had been committed to a state mental hospital in Florida and confined against his will for 15 years, sued Dr. J. B. O'Connor, the hospital superintendent, and his staff for intentionally and maliciously depriving him of his constitutional right to liberty (see *Donaldson v. O'Connor,* 1975). Donaldson, who had been hospitalized for paranoid schizophrenia, said he was not mentally ill and, even if he was, stated that the hospital had not provided him with adequate treatment. Over the 15 years of confinement, Donaldson, who was not in danger of harming himself or others, had frequently asked for his release and had relatives who stated they would attend to him if he was released. Despite this, the hospital refused to release him, stating that he was still mentally ill. The Supreme Court unanimously upheld lower court decisions stating that the hospital could not hold him against his will if he was not in danger of harming himself or others (Swenson, 1997).

This decision led to drastic changes in the mental health delivery system around the country. No longer would state mental hospitals be the dumping grounds for individuals with mental illness or emotional problems. Today, every state in the country prohibits a clinician from long-term confinement of an individual against his or her will unless there is a clear indication that the person is a danger to self or others. And even in this case, a court hearing to show cause is generally necessary.

Best Practices

> *Regardless of how careful counselors are . . . malpractice lawsuits can still occur.* (Gladding, 2000, p. 69)

As you can see from the previous discussion of ethical hot spots and the sometimes resulting lawsuits, making ethical decisions can be an arduous and potentially career threatening process. It is therefore essential that clinicians are equipped with the clinical knowledge and tools necessary to make the best decisions when working with clients. Showing a court that you have followed best practices in your profession can be critical in winning a lawsuit. Although ethical guidelines are not legal documents, following one's professional association's code of ethics can be an important piece of evidence in showing best practices have been followed. Gerald Corey and his colleagues give an extensive list of ways in which clinicians can assure that they have been following best practices (Corey & Corey, 2003; Corey et al., 2003). For instance, they note that clinicians should:

- have a clear definition of fees and know about billing regulations
- keep good records
- preserve appropriate confidentiality
- avoid searches of students by school counselors
- avoid dual relationships, especially having sex with a client
- consult with colleagues when need be
- whenever possible, obtain permission from a client to consult with others
- use informed-consent procedures
- have a sound theoretical approach and a clear understanding of why one uses certain techniques
- know how to assess clients who are a danger to themselves and others and what to do if one is in danger
- have a contract with their place of employment regarding the legal liability for professional training
- assess progress to client goals and teach clients how to assess their own progress
- maintain their competence
- have clear, well-documented treatment plans
- report suspected abuse as required by law
- consider bartering for services as generally unwise and maybe unethical
- not abandon their client (e.g., avoid long absences)
- refer and transfer clients wisely
- be aware of potential legal problems when discussing abortion and birth control
- treat their clients with respect
- avoid power relationships with clients
- maintain malpractice insurance

EXERCISE 3.3 **Ethical Dilemmas**

On your own, consider what you might do if faced with the following scenarios. Then, share your responses in small groups or in the class. You may want to review one or more of the professional ethical codes when making your responses (see Toolbox A).

1. *Breach of Confidentiality:* A client of yours, who has attempted suicide a number of times, states that you are not helping her and suddenly bolts out of your office and says, "I don't know what I'm going to do now." What should you do?
2. *Breach of Confidentiality:* You are working with a 14 year old who is sexually active and refuses to use protection. What should you do?
3. *Privileged Communication:* You are a licensed therapist and you receive a subpoena from the spouse of one of your clients asking you to testify in court about the parenting of your client. What should you do?
4. *Privileged Communication:* You have not yet obtained your license and your client reveals to you that she has committed a serious crime. The police come to you, asking to see your counseling records. What should you do?
5. *Confidentiality of Records:* A client of yours asks to see all of your case notes. Does the client have the legal right to do so? Do the ethical guidelines of your professional association support the client's right to see the records? What should you do?
6. *Confidentiality of Records:* You are seeing an 8-year-old client who reveals that her parents verbally, but not physically, abuse her. They constantly yell at her and talk to her in a derogatory tone. One day, they come to you wanting to see their daughter's records. What should you do?
7. *Confinement Against One's Will:* A client of yours has an acute schizophrenic episode and is not able to physically take care of himself (does not dress properly for the weather and does not eat properly). Can you have your client confined to an inpatient hospital? What should you do?
8. *Confinement Against One's Will:* A new client of yours suddenly tells you he is suicidal and is intending to go home and shoot himself. What should you do?

Resolving Ethical Dilemmas

In view of the practical limitations of ethical guidelines noted earlier, and in search of a more flexible and comprehensive approach to resolving ethical dilemmas, models of ethical decision making have been devised (Cottone & Claus, 2000; Welfel, 2002). This section of the chapter offers three such models: decision-making models, moral models, and developmental models. These models are not mutually exclusive; that is, they can be used simultaneously.

Decision-Making Models

Decision-making models provide the clinician with a step-by-step approach to making ethical decisions. They are practical, hands-on approaches that are particularly useful for the beginning clinician. One such approach, developed by Corey et al. (2003), is a seven-step practical, problem-solving model that consists of (a) identifying the problem, (b) identifying the potential issues involved, (c) reviewing the relevant ethical guidelines, (d) obtaining consultation, (e) considering possible and probable courses of action, (f) enumerating the consequences of various decisions, and (g) deciding on the best course of action. Corey's and other similar models can be a great aid to the clinician in the sometimes thorny ethical decision-making process.

Moral Models

Whereas Corey's model emphasizes pragmatism, other models stress the role of moral principles in this ethical decision making. For instance, Kitchener (1984, 1986) describes the role of five moral principles in making ethical decisions that include promoting the *autonomy* of the client (e.g., independence, self-determination, freedom of choice); the *beneficence* of society (promoting the good of others); the *nonmaleficence* of people (avoidance of harm toward others); *justice* or fairness to all (providing equal and fair treatment to all people); and *fidelity* of the counseling relationship (loyalty, commitment, and faithfulness). The clinician who employs this model will not necessarily decline the use of codes but will refer to them while using these moral principles in his or her decision-making process.

Another moral model by Rest (1984) suggests following a critical decision-making path that includes making an interpretation about the situation, gauging and selecting the moral principles that underlie the decision to be made (e.g., a person should not murder), and acting on the basis of the selected moral principle(s). At each stage in the model, Rest (1984) has pinpointed potential counselor difficulties in employing this way of making ethical decisions: (a) The counselor may misinterpret or fail to see the need for moral action; (b) the counselor may be incapable of making a principled moral judgment in the face of a complex dilemma; (c) the counselor may be unable to plan a course of action; and (d) the counselor may lack the will to act.

Developmental Models

Professional helpers are confronted routinely by stressful, ambiguous, and complex ethical dilemmas (Corey et al., 2003; May & Sowa, 1992; Welfel & Lipsitz, 1983). For guidance, helpers can turn to ethical codes and to the decision-making and moral models already discussed. However, as helpful as codes and these models may be, evidence suggests that the ability to make wise ethical decisions may be influenced by the counselor's level of ethical, moral, and cognitive development (Hayes, 1994; Magolda & Porterfield, 1988; Neukrug, Lovell, & Parker,1996; Neukrug & McAuliffe, 1993; Van Hoose & Paradise, 1979; Welfel & Lipsitz, 1983).

In most developmental models, lower level thought characteristically tends toward black-and-white thinking, concreteness, rigidity, oversimplification, stereotyping, self-protectiveness, and authoritarianism, while higher level thinking is more flexible, complex, nondogmatic, and more sensitive to the context in which a decision is being made (cognitive complexity) (Cottone, 2001; Kohlberg, 1984; McAuliffe, Eriksen, et al., 2000; Pascarella & Terenzini, 1991). Although few adults (or clinicians) reach the higher levels of this development (Lovell, 1999), these models suggest that if afforded the right opportunities, most adults can. Interestingly, this development seems to be universal across cultures (Snarey, 1985).

Clinicians at the lower levels are rigid and dualistic about ethical decision making, often "want the answer," and are likely to adhere rigidly to a clearly written ethical code. These clinicians might regard ethical codes as the singular authority, with any further soul searching deemed a needless exercise in overcomplicating matters. On the other hand, clinicians at higher levels of development, although fully aware of their ethical guidelines, may adhere less rigidly to guidelines and are more apt to use codes as a tool in a deeply reflective decision-making process (Neukrug et al., 1996). Although both types of clinicians may use decision-making models, given the same ethical dilemma, the manner in which they employ them could be strikingly different. Considering how two different counselors, Jaime, who is a "dualist," and Dale, who is a "relativist," might respond to the ethical dilemma posed in the case of John.

> *John, a 55-year-old gay man, is seriously depressed and feels that he has no reason to continue living. Although he has been seeing you, his counselor, for several months, his outlook on life has not changed, and he is determined to end what he considers an "empty existence" before death overtakes him. John's partner of 15 years, Jim, died of AIDS 2 years ago after suffering prolonged pain and anguish. Although John himself has lived with HIV for more than 10 years, he has recently been diagnosed with AIDS, and the new medications he has been taking to treat the disease have become increasingly less effective. He believes that the reality of his own mortality has become apparent. John, whose parents died when he was 6, has no surviving relatives or any close friends. He and Jim had isolated themselves from others and, to safeguard their privacy, severed all social ties years ago. As a self-employed writer who has chosen a solitary lifestyle, John has no support system and is not interested in trying to develop one now. He tells you that he has lived long enough and has accomplished most of what he wished to do in life. He is now ready to die and wants only to get it over with as quickly and painlessly as possible. He asks you to help him decide on the most efficient means of achieving this goal. As his counselor, what should you do?*

Although both clinicians are convinced that John has both the motivation and means to end his life, the processes they employ in coming to their conclusion, and in this case, the eventual decisions they arrive at, differ markedly. For instance, perceiving the severity of the situation, Jaime refers to the ethical guidelines of her professional association and decides that she must intervene to save her client's life. She knows that not to do so would be in violation of the ethical codes because the guidelines state that it is her responsibility to "prevent clear and imminent danger to the client or others." In addition, she recognizes that legal action could be taken against her if a suicide occurred. Besides, examining Kitchener's (1984) decision-making model, she knows that for the good of society (beneficence), John must not kill himself because he would not be following the law, and society would fall apart if everyone was lawless; that it is important that she does all she can to prevent him from emotionally harming others as would occur if he were to commit suicide (nonmaleficence); that he must be in a better state of mind to make a rational decision (autonomy); that many people in life have to undergo very difficult ordeals, and why should he be an exception (fairness); and that she has been committed to the counseling relationship, and to his life, and so should he (fidelity). Jaime therefore concludes that she has no choice. Against his wishes, she has John committed to a psychiatric facility.

Dale also understands the seriousness of John's condition but resolves the dilemma differently. She reviews the ethical guidelines and is quickly reminded that the code advises a clinician to take action when clients endanger themselves or others and that they equally emphasize the need to respect the privacy of the client and the client's freedom to choose his or her goals in counseling (see ACA, 1995; APA, 1999; NASW, 2003). She ponders the apparently conflicting advice found in the guidelines. She reflects and considers Kitchener's (1984) model. Knowing that John does not want to live, maybe she should allow him to choose death (autonomy). However, she wonders whether John is capable of making such a decision in his deteriorated physical and mental state. She then considers whether killing oneself is in best the interest of society (beneficence). She also considers who would be emotionally harmed if he did choose suicide and who would be harmed if he were prevented from killing himself (nonmaleficence). In a quandary, she thinks more and reflects on her sessions with him. She wonders what is fair and just in this situation (fairness). She considers how loyal he has been to the counseling relationship and how committed she has been to helping him (fidelity). She consults with others, particularly those who might have views differing from hers. Finally, after reflecting on a variety of different scenarios, Dale makes her decision. She hopes she has made the best decision.

Jaime's decision making exemplifies dualistic thinking that relies on external authority to distinguish between right and wrong. She reflects little, comes to decisions quickly, and does not value consultation and differing opinions. In contrast, Dale's relativistic ethical reasoning is characterized by introspection, a willingness to fully consider a variety of variables, and the determination that after deliberate and exhaustive review, she will have to come up with some decision on this complex situation.

It is important to highlight the fact that clinicians who are at varying stages developmentally could come to the same decisions. This model assumes that what decision is made is not as crucial as how the individual made that decision (this is why Dale's decision is not identified). Jaime's decision is based on little reflection, a rigid adherence to rules and regulations, little understanding of the contextual world of the client, and a reliance on outside authority (the code). Dale's decision is made with introspection, openness, reflection, a deep understanding of the client, and a desire to examine opposing points of view. In many ways, Dale has a more difficult time in the decision-making process because she has examined varying viewpoints and may always have some doubt about her decision. Jaime, on the other hand, is so convinced that her decision is correct that she may never question herself.

Final Thoughts on Resolving Ethical Dilemmas

Developmental theory suggests that the clinician's general skill at making ethical decisions tends to increase over time (Pelsma & Borgers, 1986; Tennyson & Strom, 1986; Van Hoose, 1980), and in this process, it is likely that the clinician will include some kind of decision making and moral model. Ideally, as you continue down your career path in the helping professions, over time, you will not need to have "the answer" but instead will make reflective ethical decisions that show self-understanding, a grasp of your ethical guidelines, and an understanding of ethical decision-making models. Although you may not always be confident that you have made the best decision, you will be secure in the fact that you have made a deeply reasoned decision.

EXERCISE 3.4 **Resolving Ethical Dilemmas**

Review the ethical dilemmas in Exercise 3.3. Use the decision-making model, moral models, and the guidelines described by the higher developmental level clinician to discuss how you might respond to one or more of the dilemmas.

Professional Issues

A number of issues affect the manner in which clinicians do their work. This section examines a few of the more critical ones, including managed care, accountability, use of medication, and matching client problem with intervention strategy.

Managed Care

> *the discussion ranges over lawyers and legal liability, advertising brochures and corporate logos, data bases and form letters, niche marketing and high-tech, multi-feature phone systems. Unhappy about their experience with managed care companies—the intrusive micromanagement of their work, rigid time limits, endless paperwork and the struggle to get reimbursed—they [seven therapists] have decided, like thousands of other therapists in America, to pool their talents and find a way to do together what is increasingly hard to do independently, practice their profession with a reasonable degree of freedom, autonomy and integrity—and still make a living.* (Wylie, 1995, pp. 20–21)

The cost of healthcare, particularly mental health services, skyrocketed in the second part of the 20th century and apparently will continue to do so in this century (Janesick, & Goldsmith, 2000; Smith, 1999). As a result, health insurance companies offer fewer services for mental health treatment, demand stricter documentation of the services they do provide, want evidence that treatment is progressing, and have an expectation that most treatment will be brief (Granello & Witmer, 1998).

In an effort to decrease the cost of healthcare, many businesses have opted to join managed care organizations such as HMOs (health maintenance organizations) or PPOs (professional provider organizations). These organizations limit the choices individuals have in selecting their providers (e.g., physicians and therapists), limit the number of counseling sessions, usually have an accountability process whereby clinicians must show that what they are doing is working within a reasonable amount of time, and require large amounts of paperwork in an effort to control the healthcare system and lower costs. Despite the fact that most mental health providers have negative feelings about managed care, evidence seems to say this change is here to stay (Danzinger & Welfel, 2001).

It is clear that as changes in our healthcare system continue, our usual ways of offering counseling will change. Clinicians are faced with a dilemma. They can continue to offer traditional counseling services knowing that insurance companies are likely to limit the number of counseling sessions, resulting in clinicians (a) offering services for free, (b) offering services at a reduced fee, or (c) terminating services in the middle of treatment. Or they can become knowledgeable about brief treatment approaches and the skills that accompany them. These approaches, until recently, have been rarely taught in traditional training programs (Daniels, 2001).

Changes in the delivery of mental healthcare services will affect how we conceptualize our clients' problems as we increasingly are asked to view our clients through the brief treatment prism. These changes will also affect the kinds of helping skills used by clinicians and have brought a whole new realm of ethical and professional issues to the forefront. For instance, do brief treatment approaches show the same efficacy as the more traditional approaches, and can a clinician end therapy because the managed care organization will no longer pay for treatment?

Accountability

> *Demands for accountability have focused not just on cost control but also on enhancing the quality of care.* (Eisen, Clarridge, Stringfellow, Shaul, & Cleary, 2001, p. 115)

Managed care, increased government regulations in the schools, and the oversight of agency funding sources have all led to the increased importance of accountability in the delivery of mental health services (Borders, 2002; Manderscheid, Henderson, & Brown, 2001). In fact, some have suggested that issues related to accountability have become more important than one's theoretical alignment (Sexton, 1999). Ideally, this increased focus will lead to better clinical services.

As agencies and educational settings examine what kinds of interventions work best, they will ask their clinicians to adopt the counseling theories and methods that show the most efficacy. Although some clinicians will do this readily, it will raise the ire of others. Ponder how you might react if approached by a supervisor and asked to change your counseling style because another has been shown more effective than the one you are using. Finally, the age of accountability has raised a myriad of new professional and ethical issues such as: "Do I practice what I was taught, or do I practice what my supervisor tells me to do in an effort to show the HMO that I am practicing a method shown more efficacious for the problem at hand?" And, "If torn between two diagnoses, do I write down the one that will be more amenable to the organization to which I am accountable (e.g., more apt to pay)?"

Use of Medication

Although modern-day psychotropic medications have been used for more than 50 years, recent advances in brain research and the subsequent development of even better medications will greatly affect the mental health professions. Today, there are promising new medications that can be beneficial in the treatment of psychoses, depression, anxiety, attention deficit disorder, dementia, and other related illnesses (Schatzberg & Nemeroff, 2001). With increasing evidence that some emotional disorders are genetically linked (Neukrug, 2001), and with research now suggesting that the treatment of some problems, such as depression, may be best facilitated through a combination of therapy and psychotropic medication, it is becoming evident that the use of medications as an adjunct to counseling is critical today (Conte, Plutchik, Wild, & Karasu, 1986; Ingersoll, 2000; Norden, 1996).

As the use of medication becomes increasingly widespread, and as advances in psychotropic medication continue, the role of the clinician in the development of a treatment plan that includes medication will increase, and the manner in which the clinician responds to the client will change. For instance, medication forces the clinician to:

1. use helping skills early in the relationship that will assess the client's need for medication (e.g., structured interviews, questions, probing)
2. use helping skills that will allow us to broach the topic of medication in a manner that will not offend the client
3. change the kinds of helping skills being applied as the client changes his or her outlook toward life as a result of medication
4. develop a process to continue to monitor the use of medication if the client ends counseling prior to the discontinuation of medication.

Whether or not medication should be used as an adjunct to counseling, and how one broaches this possibly delicate topic with clients, has become increasingly important. In fact, today, the clinician who does not consider a medication referral for some clients is open to possible malpractice suits because, in some cases, avoidance of the use medication may be viewed as practicing incompetent therapy (Ingersoll, 2000; Sarwer-Foner, 1993).

Matching Client Problem with Intervention Strategy

Increasingly, research has shown the importance of pairing a specific intervention technique with an identified client problem. For instance, Seligman (2004) suggests that clinicians use treatment plans specifically designed for certain disorders, including disorders in children and adolescents, situational disorders, mood disorders, anxiety disorders, behavior and impulse control disorders, disorders that have both a physical and psychological component, personality disorders, and psychotic and dissociative disorders. These treatment plans provide a number of recommendations for addressing each disorder. As you reads these various plans, it quickly becomes evident that clinicians must be facile with a wide range of intervention techniques if they are to work adequately with a wide range of clients. Thus, texts must increasingly provide the student with the basis for learning a number of critical skills necessary to work with a variety of disorders.

Whereas clinicians traditionally have tended to practice one style of counseling, today's competent clinician typically no longer relies on one theoretical orientation when working with a range of client problems. In fact, the ethical guidelines of psychologists, counselors, and social workers all address the importance of gaining training, supervision, and consultation while learning up-to-date skills.

> *Psychologists planning to provide services, teach, or conduct research involving populations, areas, techniques, or technologies new to them undertake relevant education, training, supervised experience, consultation, or study.* (APA, 2003, Standard 2.01.c)

and

> *Social workers should provide services in substantive areas or use intervention techniques or approaches that are new to them only after engaging in appropriate study, training, consultation, and supervision from people who are competent in those interventions or techniques.* (NASW, 1999, Standard 1.04.b)

and

> *Counselors practice in specialty areas new to them only after appropriate education, training, and supervised experience. While developing skills in new specialty areas, counselors take steps to ensure the competence of their work and to protect others from possible harm.* (ACA, 1995, Standard C2.b)

EXERCISE 3.5 **Discussing Issues**

In small groups, discuss how managed care, accountability, use of medication, and matching client problem with intervention strategy will affect the ways in which clinicians do their work in the future.

Cross-Cultural Issues

> *Every person is like all persons, like some persons, and like no other person.* (paraphrased from Kluckhohn & Murray; in Speight, Myers, Cox, & Highlen, 1991, p. 32)

Although it is a critical professional issue like the other professional issues just highlighted, cross-cultural counseling deserves special notice because it has gained an importance in the field that few other issues have in the relatively short history of the mental health professions. The relatively recent focus on cross-cultural issues is at least partly due to the fact that counseling does not work for many people of color and that new models of cross-cultural counseling have arisen.

Counseling Does Not Work for Many People of Color

The rise to prominence of cross-cultural counseling is due to the fact that, unfortunately, counseling does not work for many clients from diverse backgrounds. In fact, a large body of evidence shows that minority clients are frequently misunderstood, often misdiagnosed, and, relative to White clients, find therapy less helpful, attend therapy at lower rates, and terminate therapy more quickly (Garretson, 1993; Gonzales et al., 1997; Good, 1997; Lee & Mixson, 1995; McKenzie, 1999; Morrow & Deidan, 1992; Poston, Craine, & Atkinson, 1991; Solomon, 1992; Wilson & Stith, 1991). In addition, clients with cultural backgrounds different from their helper may experience the helping relationship more negatively than when the helper is of the same culture (Atkinson, 1985; Atkinson, Poston, Furlong, & Mercado, 1989; Phelps,

PROFESSIONAL PERSPECTIVES 3.2

Lack of Awareness of Own Biases and Prejudices

Robertiello and Schoenewolf (1987) note a number of mistakes that were made by helpers due to their lack of awareness of their own biases.

1. The liberal White therapist who refuses to deal with a Black client's mistrustful and suspicious dreams of him due to the helper's denial of the tension in the relationship.
2. The feminist helper who blindly encourages her client to leave her husband because he is a batterer. The client leaves her husband but ends up in another battering situation because the helper did not examine what part the woman was playing in picking abusive men.
3. The helper who reassures her client that her homosexual feelings do not mean she is a lesbian. The helper does this out of fear of dealing with the client's sexuality and instead tries to ignore the subject. The client may or may not be homosexual, but reassuring her that she is not does not allow the client to explore her sexuality.
4. The helper who refuses to hear her client's atheistic views because they are contrary to her religious beliefs. This has the effect of cutting off meaningful conversations in other areas because the client lost trust in the helper.

Taylor, & Gerard, 2001). Thus, it is understandable that today we find minority clients underrepresented at mental health centers (Sue & Sue, 2002). Clinicians must learn the attitudes and skills that will best fit the unique needs of minority clients and be able to interpret client statements without biases and prejudice (see Chapter 4 for a discussion of attitudes that can deleteriously affect clients of color).

Clinical Work with People of Color

If clinicians are to ameliorate the problems that seem inherent to their work with minority clients, they must have (a) an ever-increasing awareness of their own assumptions, values, and biases, (b) an understanding of the worldview of the culturally different client, and (c) the ability to apply adequate intervention strategies when working with culturally different clients (Arredondo, 1999; Kim & Lyons, 2003; Pedersen, Draguns, Lonner, & Trimble, 2002) (see Professional Perspectives 3.2).

Our work with diverse clients can be understood through a model presented by Speight et al. (1991). Coming from an existential perspective, they note that in trying to understand individuals, we need to be aware of their uniqueness (Eigenwelt), their common experiences held in groups and cultures (Mitwelt), and their shared universal experiences (Umwelt) (Binswanger, 1962, 1963) (Figure 3.1). Although this model can be used with any client, it reminds us of the uniqueness of each client, the tendency for all clients to have experiences unique to their cultural group, and the fact that all of us share universal experiences (e.g., sadness from losing a loved one).

In this text, you will learn the basic techniques necessary to be an effective clinician. These techniques should be effective with most clients much of the time. However, due to a client's affinity with his or her unique cultural group

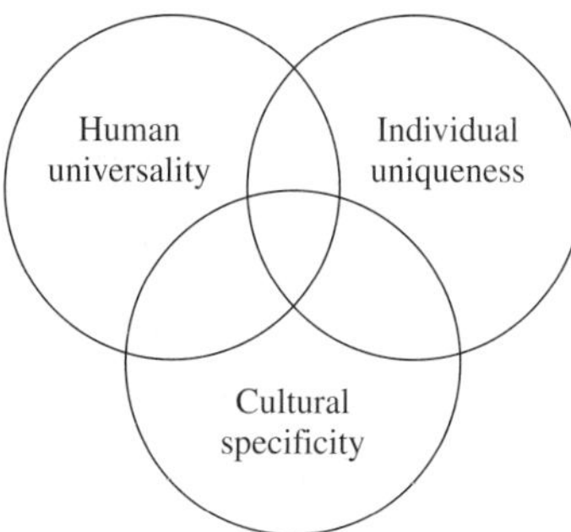

Figure 3.1 Each Sphere Represents a Unique Aspect of the Individual. The intersection where the spheres overlap suggests that we can only understand the totality of our clients' situation if we can understand the uniqueness of these three components.

Source: From "A Redefinition of Multicultural Counseling," by S. L. Speight, J. Myers, C.F. Fox, and P. S. Highlen, 1991, *Journal of Counseling and Development, 70*, 29–36. Copyright 1991. American Counseling Association. Reprinted by permission.

(Mitwelt), some techniques may be more conducive to work with specific minority clients at certain times. In Toolbox B, you will find some general guidelines for how to counsel individuals from different ethnic and racial groups, individuals from diverse religious backgrounds, women and men, gay men and lesbian women, individuals who are HIV positive, the homeless and the poor, older persons, the mentally ill, and individuals with disabilities. However, you will also want to gain a deeper understanding of specific cultural groups and be able to apply appropriate techniques to those groups (Nwachuku & Ivey, 1992). This might be gained in a counseling theories class, a class on multicultural counseling, immersing yourself in cultures different from your own, or working with a clinical supervisor who is from a culture different from yours.

LEARNING TO BE A COUNSELOR: An Ongoing Process

Sue and Sue (2002) note that working with culturally different clients should be viewed as a constantly changing process. In this context, they state that the helping relationship "is an active process, that it is ongoing, and that it is a process that never reaches an end point. Implicit is recognition of the complexity and diversity of the client and client populations, and acknowledgment of our own personal limitations and the need to always improve" (p. 227). Our view, however, is that working with *all* clients is a constantly changing process that involves actively taking steps to keep in touch with the ever-changing ethical, professional, and cross-cultural issues that are affecting one's profession. Clinicians are responsible for continually assuring themselves that they keep up-to-date. This is accomplished by being an active member in one's professional associations, attending workshops and continuing education opportunities, and being open to consultation and supervision. This active participation in the profession is an important way that professional counselors distinguish themselves from natural helpers.

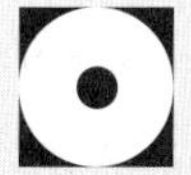

At this point, we recommend that you pause reading the text, turn to the DVD, and view the section entitled:

Introduction

Chapter Summary

This chapter examined ethical, professional, and cross-cultural issues related to the counseling relationship. First, we defined ethics, noting that in the context of the helping professions, it has to do with the consensus viewpoint of one's professional association and contrasted it with a person's individual morality. We then noted that the development of ethical guidelines is relatively new for the helping professions, starting in the 1950s. Next, we highlighted a number of reasons ethical codes are needed and some problems with ethical guidelines. We examined some ethical hot spots, including confidentiality, competence, dual relationships and conflicts of interest, inappropriate fee assessment, informed consent, misrepresentation of credentials, and sexual relationship with clients. We also showed how each of these hot spots is addressed by the ACA, APA, and NASW ethical guidelines. This section next reviewed some critical ethical and legal issues, including breach of confidentiality, confidentiality of records, privileged communication, and confinement against one's will, and described a number of best practices when doing counseling. The section ended with a discussion about ways of resolving ethical dilemmas and presented the decision-making, moral, and developmental models of ethical decision making.

The next section examined four important professional concerns that impact the nature of the helping relationship. First, we discussed managed care, noting how it has affected the number and kind of sessions available to clients and thus the way that treatment is offered. Then, we discussed accountability and its importance in helping clinicians look at which techniques can be most useful. Next, we noted how the widespread use of medication has changed the way treatment is offered. Finally, we suggested that clinicians have to increasingly rely on the efficacy of the match between the client's problem and the technique used and less on their own theoretical orientation.

The last section examined cross-cultural issues in counseling, and we noted that, unfortunately, minority clients are frequently misunderstood, often misdiagnosed, find therapy less helpful than their majority counterparts, attend therapy at lower rates than majority clients, tend to terminate therapy more quickly than majority clients, experience therapy as less helpful, and find clinicians less helpful if they are from a different culture.

As the discussion of cross-cultural counseling continued, we examined steps that must be taken if clinicians are to be effective with clients of color, including (a) having an ever-increasing awareness of one's assumptions, values, and biases, (b) having an understanding of the worldview of the culturally different client, and (c) being able to apply adequate intervention strategies when working with culturally different clients. Then, we offered an existential model of cross-cultural counseling that speaks to the importance of knowing the client as an individual, the minority group from which the client has come, and the universal experiences that are common for all clients.

The chapter concluded with a discussion of the clinician's responsibility to continually be up-to-date on the most current ethical, professional, and multicultural issues. We noted that this is accomplished by being an active member in one's professional associations, attending workshops and continuing education opportunities, and being open to consultation and supervision.

PART TWO

Clinical Skills: Attitudes and Techniques for Effective Counseling

In Chapter 1, we introduced the eight core areas of knowledge and skills for professional counselors and psychotherapists. Of these, the two areas of "attitudes" and "techniques" are critical in developing, maintaining, and deepening the counseling relationship. These clinical attitudes and techniques are the subject of Part II.

Whereas natural helpers may embody some of the attitudes and display some of the techniques addressed in the four chapters of this part, they do not use them in a deliberate and planful manner. And it is likely that the natural helper uses a variety of attitudes and techniques that are deleterious to the helping relationship. Thus, the four chapters of Part II will examine those attitudes and techniques needed by the professional counselor to planfully and intentionally manage the change process.

Chapter 4, "Attitudes and Characteristics of the Effective Clinician," begins by examining attitudes that can have a deleterious effect on the helping relationship. It then goes on to identify and discuss eight attitudes that have been theoretically or empirically shown to be important to positive client outcomes, including being empathic, genuine, accepting, open-minded, cognitively complex, psychologically adjusted, good at relationship building, and competent. The chapter goes on to examine four common concerns of beginning clinicians that sometimes affect their attitudes toward clients, including countertransference, dealing with difficult or resistant clients, the imposter phenomenon, and the white knight syndrome. Finally, this chapter examines how attitudes toward clients from diverse backgrounds can affect our work with them.

Chapter 5, "Foundational Skills," defines the use of nonverbal behavior, silence and pause time, listening, paraphrasing, and empathy. These techniques are considered foundational because they set a tone of acceptance, are core to building rapport and trust, and are key to the client's process of self-examination. Although important throughout the helping relationship, they generally are most crucial near the beginning of the relationship, such as during Stage 1, rapport and trust building, and Stage 2, problem identification.

Chapter 6, "Information Gathering," suggests ways of gathering information that are palatable for the client while simultaneously allowing the clinician to make diagnostic decisions and assist in treatment planning. Particularly important in Stage 2, problem identification, and Stage 3, goal setting and treatment planning, information gathering is critical if clinicians are to understand the depth and breadth of a client's problems. Thus, we discuss the pros and cons of asking questions and distinguish among different kinds of questioning techniques, examine how to gather information quickly and robustly using a structured interview, and look at the use of formal and informal assessment techniques as one method of expediting the gathering of information. We also demonstrate how a case report is a natural outgrowth of the information-gathering process.

Whereas the attitudes and techniques discussed in Chapters 4, 5, and 6 are critical to the helping relationship, the techniques identified in Chapter 7, "Commonly Used Skills," are not necessarily essential. However, their proper use can greatly add to the scope and depth of the helping relationship. Thus, we discuss the proper use of giving, affirmation, encouragement, modeling, self-disclosure, offering alternatives, giving, information, giving, advice, confrontation, and collaboration.

Within all of the chapters of Part II, you will find a myriad of exercises so that you can practice and enhance the attitudes and techniques you are learning. In addition, at the conclusion of each of these chapters, there is a short section that speaks to the importance of continually learning and enhancing your ability to embody the attitudes and techniques necessary for successful client outcomes. We hope that as you read these chapters and do the practice exercises, you will feel that you are well on your way to becoming a professional counselor.

CHAPTER 4

Attitudes and Characteristics of the Effective Clinician

A growing body of evidence indicates that the personal qualitites of helpers are as significant for the positive growth of helpees as are the methods they use.
(Brammer & MacDonald, 2003, p. 26)

As noted in Chapter 1, it is clear that the helping relationship has a positive effect on client change. However, what is it that makes this relationship so special and so effective? Two factors that seem particularly related to such change are the attitudes that the helper embraces and the skills the helper uses. This chapter examines those attitudes that have been shown empirically and theoretically to be related to positive client outcomes. The remainder of Part II will examine critical helping skills needed for an effective helping relationship.

The chapter begins by examining attitudes that can have a deleterious effect on the helping relationship. Then, we examine some attitudes that others have suggested may be important in bringing about a positive helping relationship. Next, we discuss eight attitudes we have identified as theoretically or empirically important to positive client outcomes, including being empathic, genuine, accepting, open-minded, cognitively complex, psychologically adjusted, good at relationship building, and competent. The next section of this chapter reviews four common concerns of beginning clinicians that sometimes affect their attitudes toward their clients. They include countertransference, dealing with difficult or resistant clients, the imposter phenomenon, and the white knight syndrome. Finally, we examine how our attitudes toward clients of color can affect our work with them.

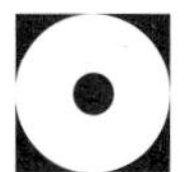

At this point, we recommend that you pause reading the text, turn to the DVD, and view the section entitled:

Clinical Skills, Eight Attitudes and Characteristics

Helper Attitudes

Destructive Attitudes

Although all natural helpers will embrace some helpful attitudes, they generally do not know how to employ helpful attitudes at opportune moments and may at times use destructive attitudes. For instance, natural helpers who cannot show empathy will have difficulty building a trusting relationship, and those who seem judgmental, dogmatic, and nongenuine will bring out defensiveness in the individual they want to help. Natural helpers who do not view situations in a complex manner will understand helpees in a limited way, and those who have significant unfinished emotional business of their own will unconsciously thwart the change process for the individual they are trying to help. Natural helpers who cannot build alliances will have a difficult time forming the kind of relationship necessary to effect change, and those who have not spent time learning effective helping skills can hardly be competent at facilitating change.

In addition, some natural helpers will be critical, disapproving, disbelieving, scolding, threatening, discounting, ridiculing, punishing, sexist, prejudiced, and rejecting toward one's helpee, attitudes that have little place in the helping relationship (Benjamin, 2001). In contrast, professional counselors have learned how to use a wide range of helpful attitudes at critical moments in the helping relationship and have practiced assuming those attitudes in their training programs.

Attitudes That Effect Change

Which attitudes and behaviors should be embraced to effect change in another? Some evidence suggests that certain characteristics historically thought to be important are not. For instance, it seems that the clinician's race, gender, age, cultural background, professional identity, and years of experience appear unrelated to client outcomes (Sexton, Whiston, Bleuer, & Walz, 1997). On the other hand, some have suggested that the clinician's personality has more to do with the effectiveness of psychotherapy than does any specific technique a helper might learn (Oppenheimer, 1998).

A number of studies have examined the qualities that seem important for an effective counseling relationship (Sexton, 1999; Sexton & Whiston, 1991, 1994; Sexton et al., 1997; Wampold, 2001). Based on this research, as well as their clinical and supervisory observations, Hackney and Cormier (2005) present eight characteristics of the effective helper, including: (a) self-awareness and understanding, (b) good psychological health, (c) sensitivity, (d) open-mindedness, (e) objectivity, (f) competence, (g) trustworthiness, and (h) interpersonal attractiveness. Purkey and Schmidt (1996) took a different course and attempted to identify four characteristics of the successful clinician based on what they considered to be ways of living a healthy life. The characteristics they included are:

1. *Being personally inviting with oneself.* This quality has to do with the ability to access one's emotions while at the same time keeping emotional control when assisting clients. It also has to do with keeping oneself intellectually and physically well rounded.

2. *Being personally inviting with others.* This quality has to do with the ability to develop deep, long-lasting relationships and having the ability to celebrate life. It means that in the tradition of Sidney Jourard (1971), we are transparent to others and able to share ourselves with others.
3. *Being professionally inviting with oneself.* This quality means that the counselor is professionally active, views learning as a lifelong process, and is actively seeking new professional development activities.
4. *Being professionally inviting with others.* This characteristic has to do with cooperating with others professionally, contributing to the field, and having a collaborative attitude with both clients and other professionals.

Eight Attitudes to Embrace

Based on the current state of research on counseling effectiveness, we have generated eight helper attitudes and characteristics that we believe are either empirically or theoretically related to counselor effectiveness. Some will sound similar to Hackney and Cormier (2005) or to Purkey and Schmidt (1996), but others will be new. They include:

1. Being empathic
2. Being genuine
3. Being accepting
4. Being open-minded
5. Being cognitively complex
6. Being psychologically adjusted
7. Being good at relationship building
8. Being competent

Being Empathic

Empathy, or the ability to understand the inner world of another, has been discussed for centuries and was spoken of by such philosophers as Plato and Aristotle (Gompertz, 1960). Empathy can be viewed as both a critical attitude that the helper must embrace as well as a critical skill that the helper must learn to master (Orza, 1996). Thus, the importance of being empathic is discussed in this section as a critical attitude, and it is discussed again in Chapter 5 as a foundational skill that can be learned in a systematic fashion.

Empathy is not being sympathetic or identifying with a client's problem. Empathy is, however, feeling a sense of deep understanding toward the client. With respect to the counseling relationship, this understanding is seen as critical for building rapport, eliciting information, and helping the client feel accepted (Egan, 2002; Rogers, 1989a). In addition, empathy has been shown to be related to positive client outcomes (Carkhuff, 2000; Luborsky, Crits-Christoph, Mintz, & Auerbach, 1988; Weaver, 2000).

Carl Rogers felt that being empathic was a core condition to the counseling relationship and should be shown throughout the length of the relationship.

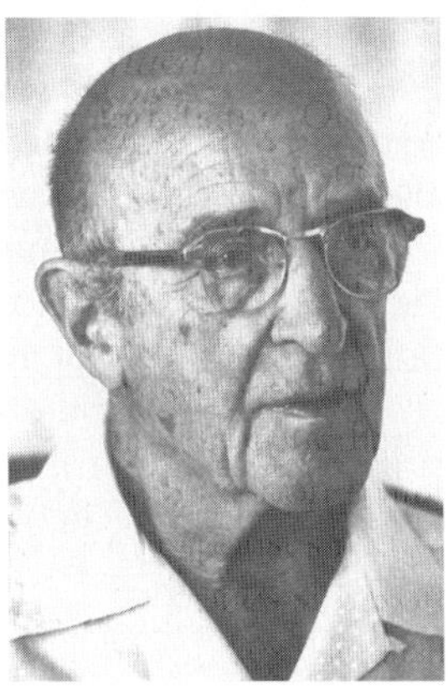

Figure 4.1 Carl Rogers, a leader in the humanistic psychology movement, believed that being empathic was a core condition in the helping relationship.

However, some research (Gladstein, 1983; Kegan, 1982, 1994; Ridgway & Sharpley, 1990) suggests that its importance might be contingent on:

- the stage of the counseling relationship (e.g., more important when building a relationship)
- the kind of client problem (e.g., depression)
- the ability of the clinician to be empathic
- the cognitive complexity of the clinician
- the ability of the client to recognize empathy

EXERCISE 4.1 **Are You Empathic?**

Separate into triads and have one person volunteer to discuss an emotionally charged situation he or she has experienced. This person should be as real as possible in relating the situation while a second person tries to show empathy to that person. The third person should be in charge of audio- or videotaping the discussion. Do this for about 10 minutes. After completing the exercise, all three individuals should listen to or watch the tape together and, using the scale below, rate the individual on each of the eight items listed. Then, determine the person's average score of all eight items. After the first person has finished, have the second and then the third person do the exercise.

1	2	3	4	5
not at all like this (not empathic)		somewhere in the middle		very much like this (empathic)

1. *Talks minimally:* The empathic person will talk considerably less than the individual who is describing the situation.
2. *Asks few questions:* The empathic person will tend to ask few, if any, questions.
3. *Is attentive:* The empathic person "works" on being focused and paying attention.
4. *Does not offer advice:* The empathic person will give little, if any, advice.
5. *Does not judge:* The empathic person will not judge the person he or she is listening to.
6. *Does not interpret:* The empathic person will not analyze and/or interpret the other person's situation.

7. *Does not cut off:* The empathic person will not cut off the other person and will allow himself or herself to be cut off by the person talking.
8. *Shows caring:* The empathic person is able to show, with his or her body language, a sense of caring.

If your average score is higher than 3.5 (i.e., the ratings were mostly 3s, 4s, and 5s), you are doing very well. If however, your average is lower than 2.5 (i.e., the ratings were mostly 1s and 2s), you have more work to do. In Chapter 5, you will have the opportunity to examine in more depth the skill of empathy and be able to fine-tune this important response.

Being Genuine

Genuineness refers to the willingness on the part of the therapist to be authentic, real, open, and periodically self-disclosing within the helping relationship. Genuineness may also be related to emotional intelligence, which is the ability to monitor one's emotions, a quality that counselors and counseling students seem to have more than others (Martin, Easton, Wilson, Takemoto, & Sullivan, 2004). Humanists often speak of the importance of authenticity or genuineness in the establishment of a healthy relationship (Greenberg, 1994; Jourard, 1971; Miars, 2002; Rogers, 1957). On the other hand, they note that those who are nongenuine are closed off to their feelings and live fake, false lives. Rogers (1957) popularized the term *genuineness* (or congruence) and stated that it was a core condition to the counseling relationship, along with empathy and unconditional positive regard. Whereas Rogers and other humanists have sung the praises of genuineness in the relationship, psychoanalysts and some behaviorists have traditionally downplayed the importance of this quality during the helping relationship.

Today's common theoretical approaches stress the importance of sharing parts of oneself to differing degrees. However, Gelso and Carter (1994) suggest that for all theoretical orientations there exists an ongoing "real" relationship in which the client, to some degree, will see the therapist realistically, "even when the therapist tries to hide or make ambiguous his or her self" (p. 298). This real relationship has at its core the ability of the client to recognize the genuine (or nongenuine) self of the counselor. Therefore, Gelso and Carter (1994) suggest that all clinicians realize the importance that genuineness plays in all counseling relationships and in some fashion deal with this critical issue. Although research on the relationship between genuineness and client outcomes has shown mixed results, genuineness is clearly an important quality for all clinicians to acknowledge (Beutler et al., 2004).

Being genuine should not be confused with ongoing self-disclosure on the part of the clinician. Holding back parts of oneself, to some degree, is an important practice for all clinicians at certain times during the relationship. It is critical to remember that the clinician comes to the helping relationship to hear the client and not to reveal his or her own thoughts and feelings to the client.

EXERCISE 4.2 **Genuineness**

In small groups, discuss the following:

1. Have there been times when you believed it was prudent not to be real or authentic with a significant person in your life? Why did you choose to hold back parts of yourself in this situation? Do you believe holding back how you actually felt or thought was harmful or helpful?
2. If you held ongoing negative feelings toward a client, do you believe it would be best to share them? How might you deal with such feelings? Make a list of times that you believe clinicians would be more effective by not being open about such thoughts and feelings. Share your list with the other groups in your class.
3. If you held ongoing positive feelings toward a client, do you believe it would be best to share them? How might you deal with such feelings? Make a list of times that you believe clinicians would be more effective by not being open about such thoughts and feelings. Share your list with the other groups in your class.
4. Are there any times other than ones you have already mentioned that you believe it would be important to withhold your feelings and thoughts from a client?

Being Accepting

Being accepting is the ability to regard clients unconditionally, despite differences in cultural heritage, values, or belief systems. Rogers (1957) called being able to accept clients "without strings attached" unconditional positive regard. Unconditional acceptance of a client does not necessarily mean that one likes or condones everything a person does; however, such acceptance does show a deep understanding for another. For instance, one would assuredly not like the actions of a murderer or rapist; however, being accepting of this client would mean that the counselor has an understanding of the felon's world and how he or she came to be. This acceptance of another person is a likely by-product of the counselor's ability to be nondogmatic, empathic, and open-minded. The manifestation of these attitudes allows the client to feel safe enough to open a window into his or her inner experience, allowing the helper to see the client's hurts and pains. Research on acceptance and positive regard shows a relationship between these characteristics and positive client outcomes (Patterson, 1984; Pope & Kline, 1999).

EXERCISE 4.3 **Being Accepting**

Part I: In class, have a student role-play the following client and watch as a faculty member or another student role-plays the counselor. After the role-play is finished, discuss your reactions to the client and to the counselor. How easy was it for the counselor to respond to the client? How easy was it for you, as an observer, to be accepting of this client?

Client: You are a 33-year-old male who always gets his own way. You are married and have two daughters, aged 15 and 13. You see yourself as the "man of the house" and expect your every wish to be listened to. You sometimes drink heavily, and you're sometimes abusive with your wife. Although not physically abusive to your daughters, you are verbally abusive to them on a regular basis. Your oldest daughter recently discovered she was pregnant, and although she tried to hide the fact from you, you found out and are insistent that she obtain an abortion. You have been referred to counseling by the courts for being abusive to your wife.

Part II: After dividing into dyads, have one student role-play one of the clients that follow while the other role-plays the counselor. After you have completed your role-plays, in small groups discuss any difficulty you had accepting the client. What prevented you from being more accepting? Do you believe acceptance of the client is a prerequisite for successful therapy? Is there anything you can do to be more accepting? If time allows, role-play additional clients.

Client: You are deeply religious, and you believe that anyone who does not believe the same way you do is destined for hell. You are in counseling because your oldest son does not believe the same way you do.

Client: You are gay and have multiple sex partners on an ongoing basis. You would like to discuss the conflict you hold between wanting an ongoing committed relationship and wanting to date many people.

Client: You are heterosexual and have multiple sex partners on an ongoing basis. You would like to discuss the conflict you hold between wanting an ongoing committed relationship and wanting to date many people.

Client: You are a 12-year-old who is diagnosed as having a conduct disorder. You are considered a "bully" at school, rarely listen to others, and are known to provoke fights.

Being Open-Minded

Closely related to the ability to accept others is whether or not an individual is open-minded, or nondogmatic (Rokeach, 1960). Belkin (1988) notes that "open-mindedness in the counseling setting may be defined as freedom from fixed preconceptions and an attitude of open receptivity to that which the client is expressing" (p. 66). The critical difference between acceptance and open-mindedness is that, in addition to having an accepting attitude toward the client, the open-minded counselor is willing to take in the client's perspective and change the way he or she comes to understand the client's situation (see Professional Perspectives 4.1). We believe that it is only through having an open-minded attitude that one can have true empathy for another.

The open-minded clinician is nondogmatic; he or she does not try to convince the client of a certain point of view. Instead, this person is able to hear the client, be with the client, and be open to whatever the client might say. In contrast, dogmatic and closed-minded counselors are poor at showing empathy, are persistent in their way of viewing the world despite evidence to the contrary, and have difficulty forming positive counseling relationships (Allen, 1967; Anderson, Lepper, & Ross, 1980; Kemp, 1962; McAuliffe, Neukrug, & Lovell, 1998; Mezzano, 1969; Russo, Kelz, & Hudon, 1964; Tosi, 1970; Wright, 1975). Probably one of strongest indications that

PROFESSIONAL PERSPECTIVES 4.1
Being Open to a Client's Perspective

I [Ed Neukrug] was working with a client who had some delusional tendencies, when at one point he talked about being able to visualize, while he sat in his home, what people were doing at various parts of the city in which he lived. Although not personally believing in the ability to do "remote viewing," I suspended my disbelief for the session. At the end of the session, the client noted, with a sense of relief, how for the first time he felt a sense of closeness to a therapist. The ability to suspend one's belief in this instance was the beginning of a healing process for this client. By the way, there are those in the scientific field who believe remote viewing is a legitimate phenomenon (see Persinger, Roll, Tiller, Koren, & Cook, 2002).

a person is dogmatic is a belief in absolute truth. Such absolutist, unequivocal thinking is highlighted by Carl Rogers in his review of a book by theologian Reinhold Niebuhr:

> *As I lay the book down, I find that I am impressed most of all by the awesome certainty with which Dr. Niebuhr knows. He knows, with incredible assurance, what is wrong with the thinking of St. Thomas Aquinas, Augustine, Hegel, Freud, Marx, Dewey, and many, many others. He also knows what are the errors of communism, existentialism, psychology, and all the social sciences. His favorite term for the formulations of others is "absurd," but such other terms as "erroneous," "blind," "naive," "inane," and "inadequate" also are useful.* (Rogers, 1989b, p. 208)

EXERCISE 4.4 **Open-Mindedness**

In class, divide into triads. From the list below, find a situation in which one person is "pro" and one person is "con." If everyone in your group is either pro or con the situations listed, try to come up with a situation in which one of you is pro and one is con. Your task is to have one person who is pro and one who is con discuss the situation. The third person is the moderator who should take notes and later give feedback as to how each individual is responding to the role-play. While discussing the situation, try your best to listen to the other person's point of view and reflect back to him or her what you heard. When you have finished, discuss the points listed below. Then, repeat the situation or tackle another situation, but this time the moderator is pro or con and one of the other individuals is the moderator. When you have finished, answer the questions that follow.

Situations: Abortion, Capital Punishment, Torturing of Suspected Terrorists, Euthanasia, Gay Marriages

Questions to Ponder and Discuss

1. Were you able to hear the other person's point of view? If you could, you should have been able to paraphrase what that person had said to you.
2. Did you prevent yourself from getting too emotionally involved so you could hear the person clearly?
3. Were you willing to embrace the other person's opinion, at least for a short while?
4. Did your opinion change at all as a result of your ability to be open-minded to another person's point of view?
5. Do you have a stronger sense of understanding for the other person's point of view?
6. How might being open-minded to another's point of view be beneficial to the client–counselor relationship? Might it be harmful?

Being Cognitively Complex

Cognitive complexity refers to a broad range of cognitive skills related to the manner in which one makes sense of the world. Individuals who are not highly complex see the world as either–or, or right or wrong, generally believe there is a "correct" solution to every problem, are unwilling to question their own beliefs, and may lean toward a dogmatic position with others. In contrast, those who are highly complex are able to understand an individual from both an individualistic and systemic framework, understand the notion that knowledge is not fixed, have the ability to take on multiple perspectives to understanding the world, are willing and open to change based on new knowledge that is presented, and are generally more open and empathic (Benack, 1984, 1988; Bowman & Allen, 1988; Bowman & Reeves, 1987; Kegan, 1982, 1994; King, 1978, 1994; McAuliffe et al., 1998; Neukrug & McAuliffe, 1993; Reeves, Bowman, & Cooley, 1989; Widick, 1977).

In the Piagetian tradition of development (Piaget, 1954), cognitive development theories propose that cognitive complexity is formed in a sequential and hierarchical manner and that all individuals are capable of moving to higher levels of development. For such movement to occur, the individual must learn in an environment that is nurturing and supportive, on the one hand, but also challenging to the individual's view of the world. Counselor training programs hope to offer such an environment—one that supports students, yet challenges them to think about new ways to view the world and new ways of being with one's self and others (McAuliffe, Eriksen, 2001). With cognitive complexity being related to the ability to understand clients from multiple perspectives, you can see why one's ability to think in complex ways is so critical to being an effective helper (Duys & Hedstrom, 2000; Heibert & Johnson, 1994; Sexton, 1999).

EXERCISE 4.5 **Cognitive Complexity**

On your own, read the scenarios that follow and then respond to the Questions for Discussion.

Client 1

Jason Reunter, 13, was brought in for counseling by his father due to feelings of depression and a drop in his grades within the last 6 months. He is the oldest of three children, having two younger sisters, Nicole who is 10 and Stephanie who is 7. Jason has been diagnosed as having attention-deficit/hyperactivity disorder and dyslexia. Until recently, Jason obtained mostly As and Bs in school. Now, he is obtaining mostly Cs. Over the years, Jason has received assistance in a resource room for a math learning disability. He tends to be very well spoken, alert, and is described by teachers as "intellectually sharp." Jason has a fear of doctors and counselors, which his father relates back to Jason's treatment for meningitis when he was 4 years old. The meningitis was successfully treated.

Jason's father, who is divorced, notes that he had always been satisfied in his marriage and was surprised when a couple of years ago his wife noted that she was unhappy. One year ago, he and his wife separated and they recently were divorced. Mr. Reunter believes his wife left him to "discover herself as she moved into a new stage in life" (he references Gail Sheehy's book *Passages*). He notes that a year ago his wife moved in with an "unemployed alcoholic," although she is currently not living with this man. Mr. Reunter has custody of the children, and he states that he is dealing with his own depression related to the loss of his marriage. Mr. Reunter works as a shoe salesman. He wonders if the recent divorce and his own feelings of depression are related to Jason's drop in grades and feelings of depression.

Client 2

Kenny is a 28-year-old male who was referred to this therapist due to feelings of depression as a result of the recent death of a friend from AIDS and the emergence of memories of being molested at a very young child by an adult male relative. In addition, he is currently questioning his sexual identity, which has been homosexual his whole adult life.

Kenny's mood has been depressed. However, despite a suicide attempt by ingestion of pills

(continued)

EXERCISE 4.5 (*continued*)

6 months ago, he currently denies suicidal ideation and states he wants to "move on" with his life. Kenny has had a number of recent experiences, including seeing flashes of white light, black forms, feelings of something crawling on him, and feeling like he was "shocked." He believes that some of this may be related to feelings of guilt that are a result from his strict fundamentalist upbringing. He states that the guilt he has felt from his homosexual lifestyle may have caused him much stress, which manifested in some of the above symptoms. He describes his homosexual relationships as addictive and compulsive in nature. He has never had a long-term relationship.

Kenny is alert, oriented to time, place, and person, and verbal. He is quite open, easily sharing much about his life. His mood is moderately depressed, and he periodically sobs about the death of his friend, the guilt he feels about his homosexuality, and the memories of his sexual molestation. He seems coherent and his thinking seems clear. His conversations are clear and sharp. Although there is no clear indications of verbal or auditory hallucinations, seeing "white lights, black forms, and feelings things crawling on me" should be explored in more depth as possible hallucinatory material. It is unclear whether these are manifestations of a stressful period in his life, medical in nature, or possible hallucinations of a psychotic nature. He currently denies suicidal or homicidal ideation.

On your own, write down responses to the following questions:

1. In Scenario I, who have you identified as the client?
2. What are the major issues that you have identified in each scenario?
3. How might you address each issue that you have identified in each scenario?
4. How do your values affect the kinds of issues you identified in each scenario and the manner in which you decided to address the issues?

In small groups, discuss the following:

1. See if each individual in your group identified the same client in Scenario I.
2. In Scenario I, how might your values have affected the client you identified? How do the values of the different students in your group affect their understanding of the situation?
3. For both scenarios, are there right and wrong ways to make sense of the situation? Why or why not?
4. How does one's understanding of the scenarios affect the manner in which the issues are addressed?
5. In the text we argue that the greater one's cognitive complexity, the broader one's understanding of clients. Using the scenarios given, discuss how this might be the case.

Being Psychologically Adjusted

> *My involvement in this [my own] therapeutic process brought about a turning point in my illness and a radical shift in my personal life. As a therapist myself, I now know how frightening it is for clients to take this step from the known into the unknown, to honestly experience and lovingly evaluate what they feel and who they are.* (Remen, May, Young, & Berland, 1985, p. 89)

With research showing that a well-adjusted counselor may have better client outcomes than counselors who are not well-adjusted (Bellows-Blakely, 2000; Weaver, 2000; Williams, 1999), it is disturbing to find that therapists seem to have more than their share of psychological dysfunction (Gilroy, Carroll, & Murra, 2002; White & Franzoni, 1990). However, with 66% to 84% of various types of therapists having participated in their own therapy (Deutsch, 1984; Gilroy, Carroll, &

Murra, 2001; Neukrug, Millikcn, & Shoemaker, 2001; Neukrug & Williams, 1993; Norcross, Strausser, & Faltus, 1988; Pope & Tabachnick, 1994; Prochaska & Norcross, 1983), it is heartening to see that therapists seem to want to work on their own issues. In fact, some research shows that positive client outcomes may be more likely if a therapist has been in his or her own personal therapy (Bellows-Blakely, 2000; Greenberg & Staller, 1981). It is also interesting that although only a small percentage of professional training programs in the mental health field require participation in therapy (Sherman, 2000), an overwhelming percentage of therapists believe that therapy should be required by training programs, and a majority of therapists think it should be required by state licensing boards (Pope & Tabachnick, 1994).

Participation in one's own therapy has a number of benefits for the budding counselor, including the following:

1. It can assist the counselor in dealing with his or her own personal difficulties. "For a counselor to set themselves up as a helper to others, without having resolved major difficulties of their own, would appear to be farcical" (Wheeler, 1991, p. 199).
2. It enables the therapist to identify and empathize with the experience of sitting in the client's seat by giving the clinician a firsthand understanding of what it's like to be a client.
3. It helps the clinician gain insight and helps to prevent countertransference, which is "the process of [counselors] seeing themselves in their clients, of overidentifying with their clients, or of meeting their needs through their clients," all of which can deleteriously affect the helping relationship (Corey, 2005, p. 21). Preventing or minimizing counter-transference plays an important role in the health and development of the relationship with the client (Gelso & Carter, 1994).
4. It addresses the important professional and ethical responsibility of assuring that one is providing unimpaired services, as noted in the following American Counseling Association [ACA] (1995) ethical code and stressed in all ethical codes: "Counselors refrain from offering or accepting professional services when their physical, mental or emotional problems are likely to lead to harm to a client or others. They are alert to the signs of impairment, seek assistance for problems, and if necessary, limit, suspend, or terminate their professional responsibilities." (Standard C.2.g).

Is therapy the only road to psychological adjustment? Probably not; however, it is a very special relationship not achievable through friendships or other significant relationships. Other activities, such as support groups, meditation, exercise, and journaling, have all been shown to have positive effects on our psychological adjustment. Therapy is not the only way, but it is one of a few activities that together can lead to good mental health, which can result in the helper being more effective (see Exercise 4.6).

EXERCISE 4.6 **Psychological Adjustment**

Here are two examples of methods that can be used to increase one's psychological adjustment. Each example has a cost and impacts on the helper in a specific manner. This can have a specific effect on the counselor–client relationship. Examine the examples and, in the space provided, come up with other examples of your own.

METHOD	COST	IMPACT	EFFECT ON COUNSELOR–CLIENT RELATIONSHIP
1. Personal Therapy	Relatively Costly	Gain clarity about self	Reduce countertransference
		Deal with unfinished business	Reduce countertransference
		Change understanding of self and others	View client in expanded manner
		Learn new skills via modeling	Apply new skills learned
		Increase self-esteem	Helper seen as a strong role model
2. Aerobics	Relatively Inexpensive	Decrease anxiety and depression	Increase clarity of one's understanding of client through reduction in anxiety and depression
		Increase self-esteem	Helper seen as a strong role model
3.			
4.			
5.			

Being Good at Relationship Building

The relationship between the counselor and client may be the most significant factor in creating client change (Safran & Muran, 2000; Sexton & Whiston, 1991; Wampold, 2001; Whiston & Coker, 2000). Gelso and Carter (1994) state that the "working alliance" is related to how the client brings his or her inner experience into the counseling relationship and how the counselor subsequently joins with the client. Such a relationship is closely related to the ability of the client and counselor to build an emotional bond and to work on setting attainable goals. The working alliance exists throughout the stages of the counseling relationship, regardless of whether it is explicitly acknowledged by the counselor and the client.

Most well-known theorists talk about the importance of this alliance. For instance, as early as 1957, Carl Rogers highlighted the notion that the therapeutic relationship was critical to positive client outcomes. William Glasser, the founder of reality therapy, also talks about the importance of the therapist having personal qualities that allow for a good working relationship (Glasser, 2000). Family therapist Salvadore Minuchin (1974) uses the term "joining" to describe the therapeutic relationship: "Unless the therapist can join the family and establish a therapeutic system, restructuring cannot occur, and any attempt to achieve the therapeutic goals will fail" (p. 123). And today, even the behaviorist stresses the importance of the relationship: "The skilled behavior therapist conceptualizes problems behaviorally and makes use of the client/therapist relationship in facilitating change" (Corey, 2005, p. 236).

Although the manner in which a therapeutic relationship is formed is often an outgrowth of one's theoretical orientation, it is likely mediated by the clinician's personality. For example, although psychoanalytic therapy stresses anonymity and distance on the part of the analyst early in the relationship, many analysts are still able to quickly build a strong emotional bond with their clients. Similarly, although humanists stress the importance of the relationship, there are many humanistically oriented therapists who have difficulty maintaining emotional bonds with clients because of their own personality style. The challenge for all clinicians is to have the emotional fortitude to build strong relationships with their clients, to know how to build such bonds within the context of their theoretical framework, and to understand how these bonds dramatically affect work with clients.

EXERCISE 4.7 **The Therapeutic Alliance**

In the space provided, make a list of those qualities you have that would be conducive to building a strong relationship with your clients. How might you use those qualities with clients? Are these qualities unique to your personality style, or can they be adapted by other clinicians? Discuss your list with three to five other students.

1. ______________________________
2. ______________________________
3. ______________________________
4. ______________________________
5. ______________________________
6. ______________________________

Being Competent

Counselor expertise has been shown to be a crucial element for client success in counseling (Whiston & Coker, 2000), and perceived competence has been consistently chosen by therapists as the most important factor in picking a therapist (Grunebaum, 1983; Neukrug et al., 2001; Neukrug & Williams, 1993; Norcross et al., 1988). Thus, it should not be surprising that being competent is the final characteristic we have chosen as crucial for counselors to embrace.

Competent clinicians have a thirst for knowledge. They desire to examine the newest trends, understand the latest approaches, and judiciously be on the cutting edge of the field. Such clinicians exhibit this thirst through their study habits, their desire to join professional associations, their reading of professional journals, their belief that education is a lifelong process, and their ability to view their own approach to working with clients as something that is always broadening and deepening.

Clinicians have both an ethical and legal responsibility to be competent (Corey, Corey, & Callanan, 2003; Welfel, 2002). For instance, the ACA ethical guidelines elaborate on seven areas of competence, including: (a) practicing within one's boundary of competence, (b) practicing only in one's specialty areas, (c) accepting employment only for positions for which one is qualified, (d) monitoring one's effectiveness, (e) knowing when to consult with others, (f) keeping current by attending continuing education activities, and (g) refraining from offering services when physically or emotionally impaired (ACA, 1995a, Standard C.2). Similarly, both the American Psychological Association (2002) and the National Association of Social Workers (1996) highlight competence as a core part of their ethical guidelines. The legal system reinforces these ethical guidelines: "Psychotherapists commit professional malpractice if they are visibly less competent than the average of their peers, . . . One function of lawsuits is to encourage competent therapy" (Swenson, 1997, p. 166). Thus, being competent is our professional responsibility and necessitates that we continue the learning process throughout our lifetime.

EXERCISE 4.8 **Competence**

Using professional ethical guidelines (see Toolbox A), develop a response to each of the following scenarios. In your responses, answer the questions that follow and then discuss your responses with others in class:

1. Is the individual practicing ethically?
2. What action, if any, would you take if you knew of a situation like any of the ones listed?
3. Are there any legal implications to the clinician's actions?

Scenario 1: Jill is doing her internship at a mental health center. There, she develops a close relationship with one of her clients, and she believes that she could help him if he was able to work through some of his deep-seated feelings about his abusive parents. She thus decides to practice a new form of counseling that involves regressing the client back to his first few years of life. Although she has no formal training in this approach, she practices this with her client while under supervision.

Scenario 2: Rich has been in private practice for 25 years and recently has dealt with his own major depression, which included feeling suicidal and having short lapses of memory. He decides to continue working with his clients while undergoing his own treatment, which includes taking antidepressant medication. If he decides to stop seeing clients, he will not be able to support his family.

Scenario 3: A colleague of yours has continued to practice in the same manner as when he first started 30 years ago. He does not belong to any professional association, does not read the professional literature, and never attends any continuing education workshops.

The eight attitudes of being empathic, genuine, accepting, open-minded, cognitively complex, psychologically adjusted, good at relationship building, and competent are qualities to which the effective clinician should strive. Few if any of us are already fully there. More than likely, each of these qualities can be nurtured and developed as we walk down our unique paths in life.

Common Concerns for Beginning Clinicians

Although there certainly are a wide range of issues and concerns for the beginning clinician, four of the more common concerns that can deleteriously affect the clinician's attitude toward the client include countertransference, dealing with difficult or resistant clients, the imposter syndrome, and the white knight syndrome. Although the natural helper has generally not examined how these issues may negatively affect the counseling relationship, the professional counselor has examined each in some detail. Let's review these areas and see how they might impact on the helping relationship.

Countertransference

> *The important point to remember is that self-awareness about how your past injuries become expressed in your interpersonal behavior is critically important to both your personal relationships with fellow students and teachers and to your future work with clients.* (Echterling et al., 2002, p. 174)

The origins of the term *countertransference* can be found in psychoanalytic theory, where it was defined as "the positive or negative wishes, fantasies, and feelings that the counselor unconsciously directs or transfers to the client, stemming from his or her own unresolved conflicts" (Gladding, 2001, p. 33). Today, however, countertransference has taken on a broader definition and has been applied to just about all counseling approaches. The modern-day definition of countertransference suggests that when a client's behavior touches a clinician's "sore spot," the clinician may respond in ways that can have a deleterious effect on the client. What are sore spots? Generally, they are areas in our lives that we have not fully examined or dealt with (i.e., our unfinished business). As noted earlier, this unfinished business can negatively impact the helping relationship when clinicians see themselves in their clients, overidentify with their clients, or meet their needs through their clients (Corey, 2005). Thus, it becomes particularly critical that as clinicians we are clear as to who we are and have worked through our own issues as fully as possible.

The relationship between countertransference and many of the attitudes we have already discussed is clear. Unfinished business causes us psychological maladjustment, which prevents us from being real, clouds our ability to think in a complex way, causes us to be closed and dogmatic, frustrates our ability to be empathic, and prevents us from building a strong alliance with our clients. It is critical that we attend to our issues if we are to be fully effective clinicians.

Dealing with Difficult or Resistant Clients

Once, when I [Ed Neukrug] was attending a workshop on how to work with resistant adolescents, the workshop leader began by saying, "There are no resistant adolescents; there are only resistant therapists." His point was that for every adolescent who was difficult to treat, there would be some clinician who could be successful with him or her, and therefore, one must conclude that all those other clinicians who would have been unsuccessful had not learned how to work effectively with that kind of problem. He suggested that the unsuccessful clinicians' own issues (e.g., countertransference, lack of experience, lack of expertise) probably were getting in the way of working successfully with this difficult client.

Resistance has been defined as "any behavior that moves a client away from areas of discomfort or conflict and prevents the client from developing" (Gladding, 2001, p. 104). Using this definition, there is probably much the clinician can do to increase the chances of a positive counseling relationship. For instance, it can surely be argued that a clinician whose own issues are not impeding client progress, and who has excellent relationship building skills as well as a wide range of clinical skills, can assist the client in moving toward development. Therefore, one must conclude that competence, psychological adjustment, and the ability to build alliances—three critical attitudes discussed earlier—are crucial factors when working with resistant and difficult clients.

Imposter Syndrome

Did you ever dream that you forgot to take one last class to obtain your bachelor's or graduate degree? This somewhat common dream is related to what many of us feel even after we have made a significant accomplishment. The feeling is so common that it has been given a name—the imposter syndrome, or the feeling that although we have gained expertise in a particular area, we still feel as if we are "faking it" or not worthy of what we have accomplished (Harvey & Katz, 1985). Why do so many of us feel this way? Probably because we realize that after going through rigorous training, there is still so much more to learn and we have only touched the surface of what we need to know to be effective with clients. Also, some of us are brought up feeling a sense of lacking—a sense that we are not good enough. Probably, we have gotten this from significant others in our personal lives, and now it spills over into our work life. Thus, we again see that issues of psychological adjustment and competence can affect our feelings about ourselves and how we work with our clients.

White Knight Syndrome

Are you a rescuer? Many of us who have entered this profession started out as rescuers, and many of us still are. But what happens when we are not able to rescue our clients? Do we feel like failures? The white knight syndrome can motivate us to be superb clinicians, but we can also go too far. In some cases, trying too hard can lead our clients to become overly dependent on us and we on them, can cause us to cross boundaries in our effort to reach out to our clients, and can lead to increased stress to the point where we are not working effectively. Are you a rescuer? Consider the importance of this special call we have to our profession but also consider how it might affect your work with your clients (see Professional Perspectives 4.2).

PROFESSIONAL PERSPECTIVES 4.2
A Failed Rescue

Feeling bad for the plight of a client who was depressed and jobless, and knowing that the client installed car radios, I [Ed Neukrug] decided to pay this client to install a needed car radio. Meeting him at the clinic on a Saturday morning, the client showed up at the scheduled time and immediately said, "I got a speeding ticket on my way here—and it's your fault." Well, clearly this attempt to "help" the client erred, and probably a boundary had been crossed.

Each of the four common concerns noted can have a deleterious effect on our work with clients. Consider how each of them might affect the eight attitudes we discussed earlier in the chapter by completing Exercise 4.9.

EXERCISE 4.9 **Possible Effects of Common Beginning Concerns on Critical Attitudes**

In the space provided, write down possible effects that each of the common concerns might have on the attitudes listed. See the example provided under Empathy. Share your thoughts with others in class.

	COUNTER TRANSFERENCE	DEALING WITH DIFFICULT AND RESISTANT CLIENTS	IMPOSTER SYNDROME	WHITE KNIGHT SYNDROME
Empathy	Unfinished issues can prevent one from "hearing" the other in an empathic manner. Other?	Frustration with client issues, especially if they relate to one's own issues, can lead to lack of empathy. Other?	Thoughts about one's ability, or lack thereof, can prevent one from hearing another person. Other?	Trying too hard to understand a client can prevent listening with the "inner ear." Other?
Genuineness				
Acceptance				
Open-mindedness				
Cognitive complexity				
Psychological adjustment				
Relationship building				
Competence				

Attitudes Toward Clients of Color

Awareness that our cultural blinders will inevitably impact what we do and what we say is critical. (Nwachuku & Ivey, 1992, p. 160)

If you were distrustful of therapists, confused about the counseling process, or felt worlds apart from a counselor you were seeing, would you want to go to or continue in counseling? Assuredly not. Unfortunately, this is the state of affairs for many minority clients. Research has consistently shown that clients from nonwhite backgrounds are frequently misdiagnosed, attend counseling at lower rates, terminate counseling more quickly, and find counseling less helpful (Good, 1997; McKenzie, 1999; Phelps, Taylor, & Gerard, 2001; Poston, Craine, & Atkinson, 1991; Solomon, 1992; Yeh & Hwang, 2002). One reason that minority clients fare so poorly is the stereotypic and biased attitudes, usually based on misinformation, held by many clinicians (Arredondo, 1999). For instance, some have suggested the following counselor attitudes play a role in this situation (Midgette & Meggert, 1991; Sodowsky & Taffe, 1991; Solomon, 1992; Yutrzenka, 1995):

1. Holding onto the melting pot myth. Some believe this country is a melting pot of cultural diversity. However, this is not the experience of many minority clients who want to maintain their uniqueness and are reluctant to giving up their special traditions. Thus, the clinician who assumes the client should conform to the values of the majority culture may turn off some clients. Probably, viewing American society as a cultural mosaic, a society with a myriad of diverse values and customs, more accurately represents the essence of diversity that we find today.

2. Having different expectations about counseling than your client. The Western approach to counseling emphasizes autonomy of the individual; stresses the expression of feelings; encourages self-disclosure, open-mindedness, and insight; attempts to show cause and effect; and tends to be neutral regarding religion. However, many minorities do not place the same values on these qualities as do their therapists and are therefore often found entering the helping relationship with trepidation or confusion. Such clients may be disappointed or even emotionally harmed when a counseling relationship does not meet their expectations (Sodowsky & Taffe, 1991; Yutrzenka, 1995). For example, the Asian client who is proud of her ability to restrict her emotions may leave counseling feeling as if she disappointed her counselor who has been pushing her to express feelings.

3. Not understanding the impact of social forces. Although therapists may be effective at attending to clients' feelings concerning how a client was discriminated against, abused, or affected by other "external" factors, many of these same therapists will deemphasize the actual influence these social forces have on clients. By deemphasizing social forces, clinicians are likely to have a difficult time building a relationship with a client who has been considerably harmed by external factors. For instance, the client who has been illegally denied jobs due to his dis- ability may be discouraged when a counselor says, "What have you done to prevent yourself from obtaining the job?"

4. Maintaining an ethnocentric worldview. Clinicians who are not cross-culturally aware falsely assume that their clients view the world in a similar manner as do they or believe that when a client presents a differing view of the world, he or she is emotionally disturbed, culturally brainwashed, or wrong. Although the importance of understanding a client's unique worldview is crucial to every helping relationship, it is particularly significant when working with minority clients whose experience of the world may be particularly foreign to our own. For instance, a counselor may inadvertently turn off a Muslim when she says to her client, "Have a wonderful Christmas."

5. Being ignorant of one's own racist attitudes and prejudices. Of course, the therapist who is not in touch with his or her prejudices and racist attitudes cannot work effectively with minority clients and is like to be harmful to those clients. Understanding our own stereotypes and prejudices takes a particularly vigilant effort because our biases are often unconscious. For instance, the heterosexual counselor who unconsciously believes that being gay is a disease but consciously states he is accepting of all sexual orientations may subtly treat a gay client as if there is something wrong with him.

6. Not understanding cultural differences in the expression of symptomatology. The counselor's lack of knowledge about cultural differences as it relates to the expression of symptoms can seriously damage a counseling relationship and result in misdiagnosis, mistreatment, and early termination of culturally different clients from counseling. For instance, what may be seen as "abnormal" in the United States may be considered quite usual and customary in another culture. Contrast, for example, individuals from European cultures who show grief through depression, agitation, and feelings of helplessness with individuals from Latin cultures who might present mainly with somatic complaints.

7. Not realizing that assessment and research instruments may be culturally insensitive. Although advances have been made, one can still readily find tests that have cultural bias and research that does not control adequately for cultural differences. Consider an item on a test that asks if a person "hears voices." A religious Hispanic client might answer "yes," thinking that she "talks to God"—a normal response in her culture. Although most acculturated Americans might also talk to God, they have learned to deny that they hear voices because that implies psychopathology in this culture.

8. Being unaware of institutional racism. Because institutional racism is embedded in society, and even within the mental health professional organizations (D'Andrea & Daniels, 1991, 1999), it is likely that materials used by clinicians will contain bias, thus giving clinicians a skewed understanding of culturally different clients. Examples are plentiful. For instance, some diagnoses that have been listed in the *DSM-IV-TR* have been shown to be culturally biased; some counseling approaches prominent in American professional journals have been shown to be relatively ineffective when used with clients from some cultures; and, until recently, many clinical training programs have not stressed multicultural issues.

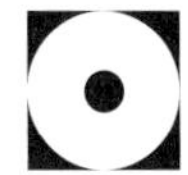

At this point, we recommend that you pause reading the text, turn to the DVD, and view the section entitled:

Cross-Cultural Issues and Attitudes

Clearly, effective cross-cultural therapists must be willing to examine their attitudes in an honest and self-reflective manner and make adjustments to their style of counseling based on what they may find. Examine Exercise 4.10 to review your possible biases and prejudices.

EXERCISE 4.10 **Attitudes Toward Multicultural Counseling**

Reflect on the following eight attitudes that could negatively affect your relationship with a client. Next, complete the columns asking you to show evidence that you do or do not hold each belief. If you do hold the belief, show how you might be able to combat it. Keep in mind that many of us may hold a belief some but not all of the time (see the example under "holding onto the melting pot myth").

Attitudes You Hold Toward Others

COMMON ATTITUDES THAT MAY NEGATIVELY AFFECT THE HELPING RELATIONSHIP	EVIDENCE THAT YOU DO NOT HOLD THIS BELIEF	EVIDENCE THAT YOU DO HOLD THIS BELIEF	WHAT CAN YOU DO TO COMBAT THIS BELIEF?
1. Holding onto the melting pot myth	I attend and embrace celebrations of different ethnic groups (e.g., Ramadan, Chanukah, Christmas, Kwanza).	I sometimes find myself irritated when I see a person wear traditional clothing from their culture and not "American" clothing.	Talk to people who wear traditional clothing to understand the meaning it has for them.
2. Having different expectations about counseling than your client			
3. Not understanding the impact of social forces			
4. Maintaining an ethnocentric worldview			
5. Being ignorant of one's own racist attitudes and prejudices			

6. Not understanding cultural differences in the expression of symptomatology			
7. Not realizing that assessment and research instruments may be culturally insensitive			
8. Being unaware of institutional racism			

LEARNING TO BE A COUNSELOR: An Ongoing Process

In this chapter, we examined a number of attitudes that have been shown to be important to positive client outcomes in the helping relationship. In addition, we reviewed some common issues that might affect our attitudes toward clients in general as well as our attitudes toward clients from diverse backgrounds. Attitudes do not change overnight, and we do not have the expectation that you will read this chapter and suddenly embody the "correct" attitudes that will make you the perfect clinician. However, we do hope that you have reflected on your attitudes and that you have begun a journey to continually review how your attitudes might affect the clients with whom you work. This self-reflection process should start early in your training and ideally stay with you during your whole career.

Chapter Summary

This chapter began by highlighting a number of attitudes that can have a deleterious effect on the helping relationship. We noted the importance of not being judgmental, dogmatic, nongenuine, critical, disapproving, disbelieving, scolding, threatening, discounting, ridiculing, punishing, sexist, prejudiced, and rejecting toward a client. We then delineated a number of attitudes we believed, through empiricial or theoretical evidence, to be related to positive client outcomes in therapy. These included being empathic, genuine, accepting, open-minded, cognitively complex, psychologically adjusted, good at relationship building, and competent. Each of these qualities was defined as it relates to the helping relationship, and you were given the opportunity to reflect on the extent to which you have taken on these qualities.

The chapter then identified four common concerns of beginning clinicians that sometimes affect their attitudes toward their clients and ultimately their success with clients. The first common concern we noted was countertransference, or the process in which the clinician's unfinished business negatively impacts the helping relationship. This includes when clinicians see themselves in their clients, overidentify with their clients, or meet their own needs through their clients. Next, we noted how the clinician's psychological adjustment, ability to build alliances, and attitudes about being competent can affect his or her ability to deal with difficult or resistant clients. The imposter phenomenon was the next common concern we examined. This phenomenon has been defined as the feeling that although we have gained expertise in a particular area, we still feel as if we are "faking it" or not worthy of what we have accomplished. We noted that when these feelings plague beginning clinicians, they can negatively impact the helping relationship. Finally, we noted that the desire to rescue a client, sometimes called the white knight syndrome, can have negative effects on the helping relationship, such as when clinicians overextend themselves and end up fostering a dependent relationship.

As the chapter continued, we discussed eight potentially destructive attitudes that beginning clinicians sometimes hold toward minority clients. These included (a) holding onto the melting pot myth, (b) having different expectations about counseling than your client, (c) not understanding the impact of social forces, (d) maintaining an ethnocentric worldview, (e) being ignorant of one's own racist attitudes and prejudices, (f) not understanding cultural differences in the expression of symptomatology, (g) not realizing that assessment and research instruments may be culturally insensitive, and (h) being unaware of institutional racism. We stressed the importance of taking a self-inventory to examine which of these attitudes, if any, you may hold.

Finally, we highlighted the importance of continually reviewing all of the attitudes we stressed in the chapter. We noted that although this process starts at the beginning of our career, it is a process that should continue throughout one's career in the helping professions.

CHAPTER 5

Foundational Skills: Nonverbal Behavior, Silence and Pause Time, Listening, Paraphrasing, and Empathy

Although good listening skills are considered by almost all natural helpers as critical to effective helping, in actuality, most natural helpers have not developed the ability to apply listening skills, as well as the related foundational skills of paraphrasing and empathy, in helpful ways. As with all of the skills we will examine in Part II, there are specific ways of applying these skills, and the professional counselor has learned how to do this.

This chapter explains the importance of, and how to use, the foundational skills of nonverbal behavior, silence and pause time, listening, paraphrasing, and empathy. The skills in this chapter are considered foundational because they set a tone of acceptance, are core to building rapport and trust, and are key to the client's process of self-examination. Although important throughout the helping relationship, these skills are generally most crucial near the beginning of the relationship and should be continually revisited especially when an impasse is reached (see Chapter 2 Appendix).

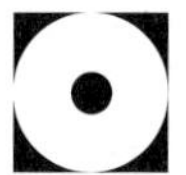

At this point, we recommend that you pause reading the text, turn to the DVD, and view the section entitled:

Nonverbals, Silence and Pause Time

Nonverbal Behavior

> *Yet when humans communicate, as much as eighty percent of the meaning of their messages is derived from nonverbal language. The implication is disturbing. As far as communication is concerned, human beings spend most of their time studying the wrong thing.* (Thompson, 1973, p. 1)

Although nonverbal behaviors are important across all stages of the helping relationship, they are particularly important at the initial stages because they affect how the client initially experiences the counselor and are thus critical for building the therapeutic alliance. Nonverbal behavior is often out of a person's conscious control (Argyle, 1975; Wolfgang, 1985), is difficult to censor, and compared to verbal behavior, is often a more accurate representation of how the client and the helper feel (Mehrabian, 1972). Also, nonverbal behaviors can vary dramatically as a function of culture (Locke, 1999). Helpers communicate nonverbally to their clients in a number of ways, including attire, eye contact, body positioning and facial expressions, personal space, touch, and voice intonations and tone.

Attire

What the clinician wears is an important aspect of a client's initial perception of the helper. Similarly, how a client dresses can be an important message to the clinician. A clinician will often make a determination concerning what to wear based on how important he or she thinks certain kinds of attire are to maintaining a comfortable relationship with clients. Also, a helper's dress will be a function of covert or overt rules of the agency. Ultimately, each helper must determine the importance of these factors and how they will be addressed.

Eye Contact

Eye contact reveals much about the clinician's willingness and desire to work with the individual. Similarly, eye contact gives the clinician information about the willingness of the client to work with the helper. Although intense eye contact will certainly turn off almost any client, the clinician who has trouble with eye contact will have a difficult time building a trusting relationship. Finding the "correct" amount of eye contact that tells a client that the clinician is ready to listen is critical to the helping relationship. As you might expect, the amount of eye contact that is comfortable to a client is sometimes a function of the cultural background of the client as well as whether a counselor and client are of a different ethnic background or gender (Guthmann, 1999).

Body Positioning and Facial Expressions

Body positioning can telegraph whether or not the helper wants to work with the client and has been shown to be related to rapport in the counseling relationship (Sharpley & Sagris, 1995). Often, it has been suggested that the clinician should have both feet touching the ground, be leaning forward slightly, and have his or her arms postured in a manner that suggests a readiness to listen (Brammer & MacDonald, 2003). In addition to body positions, head motions and facial expressions are important to the client's experience of the helping relationship. Is the clinician's head movement saying to the client, "yes, I hear you" and "keep on talking," or is it indicating to the client that the clinician is bored, restless, and/or simply not interested?

Personal Space

The level of comfort with personal space between a clinician and his or her clients can vary dramatically and is mediated to some degree by culture, age, and gender (Evans & Howard, 1973). Clinicians must allow for enough personal space so that the client feels comfortable, yet not so much that the client feels distant from the helper. Although this will generally happen in very subtle ways, the helper should take the lead in creating an appropriate amount of distance.

Touch

Although for some clinicians it may be quite natural to hold a client's hand when he or she is expressing deep pain or to hug a client at appropriate moments, in today's litigious society clinicians must be sensitive to their clients' boundaries, their own boundaries, and the limits of touch according to one's professional ethics (Gabbard, 1995). Brammer and MacDonald (2003) suggest that physical contact be based on (a) an assessment of the client's level of comfort, (b) the clinician's awareness of his or her own needs, (c) what is likely to be helpful within the helping relationship, and (d) risks involved as a function of agency policy, customs, personal ethics, and the law.

Voice Intonation and Tone

Human communication takes place in complex ways, and clinicians need to be aware of the varying levels at which one can communicate, including through voice intonation and voice tone. For instance, all helpers will make a number of guttural responses to clients (e.g., uh huh), often unconsciously, which can go a long way in telling clients whether or not they are being heard. Voice intonation and tone can mean more than what they seem to mean on the surface, and clinicians must be aware that what they say (word meaning) may not always match how they're saying it

EXERCISE 5.1 **Playing with Nonverbal Cues**

In class, find a partner and have one person role-play a client discussing a situation of his or her choice. The other person should attempt to listen to the client while offering very little eye contact. Then, repeat the same role-play and offer too much eye contact. Now switch roles, having the other person in the dyad role-play a client. You may want to continue this exercise trying to exaggerate or minimize other nonverbal cues such as head nodding, saying "uh huh," touching your client, and so forth. After you have finished the role-play, in class discuss the level of comfort you felt with the various types of nonverbal behaviors you expressed and received.

(tone of voice, body language) (Watzlawick, 1967). For instance, an angry person may still mouth the words "I love you," and a clinician, when asked by a client, "Are you attracted to me," may say, "No," but his or her body language may say something else.

A Cross-Cultural Perspective on Nonverbal Behavior

Traditionally, helpers have been taught to lean forward, have good eye contact, speak in a voice that meets the client's affect, and rarely touch the client. However, research suggests that there are cross-cultural differences in the ways that clients perceive and respond to such nonverbal helper behaviors (Morse & Ivey, 1996; Sue & Sue, 2002). Therefore, it is now suggested that helpers be acutely sensitive to client nonverbal differences while being knowledgeable and skilled in culturally appropriate responses.

Culturally skilled helpers are able to engage in a variety of verbal and nonverbal helping responses. They are able to send and receive both verbal and nonverbal messages accurately and appropriately. They are not tied down to only one method or approach to helping but recognize that helping styles and approaches may be culture bound. When they sense that their helping style is limited and potentially inappropriate, they can anticipate and ameliorate its negative impact (Sue, Arredondo, & McDavis, 1992).

Effective cross-cultural clinicians must understand that some clients will expect to be looked at, while others will be offended by eye contact; that some clients will expect the helper to lean forward, while others will experience this as an intrusion; and that some clients will expect the helper to touch them, while others will see this as offensive. In respect to nonverbal behavior, effective helpers keep in mind what works for the many yet are sensitive to what works for the few.

EXERCISE 5.2 **Assessing Nonverbal Behavior**

In class, break up into groups of five students. Have each student, one at a time, role-play a helper while another student role-plays a client. Do this for about 3 or 4 minutes. The other three students are to watch the role-play, and, using the chart below, make comments about the nonverbal behaviors of the student role-playing the helper. After you finish each role-play, give the helper the feedback sheets and discuss what was written.

	POSITIVE NONVERBALS	NEGATIVE NONVERBALS
Attire		
Eye Contact		
Body Language		
Personal Space		
Touch		
Voice Intonation and Tone		

Silence and Pause Time

> *The subconscious is ceaselessly murmuring, and it is by listening to these murmurs that one hears the truth.* (Bachelard, 1960)

Shhhh! Silence is golden to the helping relationship, and you need to know how to use silence effectively. Thus, the professional counselor needs to know

when empty space is facilitative and when it
becomes a bit much.

Silence is a powerful tool in the helping relationship that can be used advantageously for the growth of the client (Hutchins & Cole, 1992; Kleinke, 1994). It allows the client to reflect on what he or she has been saying. It allows the clinician to process the session and to formulate his or her next response. It says to the client that communication does not always have to be filled with words, and it gives the client an opportunity to look at how words can sometimes be used to divert one from his or her feelings. Silence is powerful. It will sometimes raise anxiety within the client—anxiety that, on the one hand, could push the client to talk further about a particular topic but, on the other hand, could cause a client to drop out of treatment. In short, to be an effective listener, you must maintain a certain amount of silence in the helping relationship, for if you are always filling silent spaces, you are not listening.

EXERCISE 5.3 **Silence**

Pair up with another student in class. Have one person role-play a helper while the other role-plays a client. The client should begin discussing a situation and continue talking for a short time, at which point the instructor should say "stop." The counselor should then formulate a response to the client but not say it until the instructor says "go," which will be 30 seconds after the instructor has said "stop." After the counselor gives his or her response, discuss how it felt to wait this amount of time. You may want to continue to do this on your own but, this time, with a few different amounts of "pause times." Make sure each student gets to be the helper.

We're sure that after you complete Exercise 5.3, you will agree that 30 seconds is a very long time to wait before making a response. Although waiting that long is fairly unusual, you probably found that waiting before responding not only allowed you to formulate your response but gave the client an opportunity to think about what he or she said as well as consider what he or she would say next. You might want to continue the role-play after you have finished Exercise 5.3 to find what amount of silence would feel comfortable to you when making a response and, at the same time, be facilitative to the helping relationship.

Silence on the part of the helper or client may be somewhat culturally determined. For instance, some research has found that the pause time for different cultures varies. In fact, Tafoya (1996) notes that Native Americans have at times been labeled reticent to talk and resistant to treatment when in fact the pause time for some Native Americans is longer than other cultural groups. If they had been treated by

Native American helpers, they most likely would not have been labeled in this fashion. As a helper, you may want to consider your pause time to discover your comfort level with silence while at the same time recognize that your client's pause time might vary as a function of cultural heritage.

EXERCISE 5.4 **Pause Time**

In dyads, have one student role-play a client and a second student role-play a counselor. While the client role-plays, the counselor should wait a minimum of 15 seconds before responding. When you have finished your role-play, discuss the following:

1. How comfortable did the counselor feel with pausing a minimum of 15 seconds?
2. How comfortable did the client feel with the counselor's pauses?
3. Could you identify any cross-cultural issues that may have affected the counselor's or client's comfort with pausing (e.g., as a New Yorker, I [Ed Neukrug] have a more difficult time with pause time because the cultural style of many New Yorkers is to quickly fill silent moments).
4. Make a list of advantages and disadvantages you might find to the use of silence and pause time. Share the list in class while the instructor makes a master list.
5. After completing items 1 through 4, discuss how silence and pause time should be used in a deliberate and planful manner within the counseling relationship.

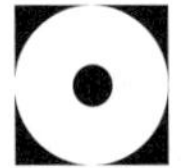

At this point, we recommend that you pause reading the text, turn to the DVD, and view the section entitled:

Listening, Paraphrasing, and Empathy

Listening

Listening looks easy, but it's not simple. Every head is a world. (Cuban proverb)

Listening is much more complex than you might assume. Start by taking the quiz in Exercise 5.5 and begin to examine the many components to listening.

EXERCISE 5.5 **Listening Quiz**

Think back to helping relationships you have been in and answer each item below by placing an X in the appropriate space to indicate how you generally respond to someone.

U = Usually S = Sometimes R = Rarely

U	S	R	
_____	_____	_____	1. When in a helping relationship, I decide what should be talked about.
_____	_____	_____	2. I prepare myself physically by sitting in a way I can make sure I hear what is being said.

____ ____ ____ 3. I try to be "in charge" and lead the conversation.

____ ____ ____ 4. I usually clear my mind and take a nonjudgmental attitude when helping another.

____ ____ ____ 5. I try to tell the other my opinion of what he or she is doing.

____ ____ ____ 6. I try to decide from the other's appearance whether or not what he or she says is worthwhile.

____ ____ ____ 7. I often ask questions about the other's behavior when facilitating a helping relationship.

____ ____ ____ 8. I try to judge from the opening statement whether or not I know what is going to be said.

____ ____ ____ 9. I try to listen intently to feelings.

____ ____ ____ 10. I try to listen intently to content.

____ ____ ____ 11. I try to tell the other person what is "right" about what he or she is saying.

____ ____ ____ 12. I try to "analyze" the situation and give interpretations.

____ ____ ____ 13. I try to use my experiences to best understand the other person's feelings.

____ ____ ____ 14. I try to convince the other person of the "correct" way to view the situation.

____ ____ ____ 15. I try to have the last word.

For items 2, 4, 9, and 10, give yourself 3 points if you listed usually, 2 points if you listed sometimes, and 1 point if you listed rarely. For items 1, 3, 5, 6, 7, 8, 11, 12, 13, 14, and 15, give yourself 3 points if you listed rarely, 2 points if you listed sometimes, and 1 point if you listed usually. An individual who does not have a natural listening style will likely score between 15 and 25. One who has a moderate listening style will likely score between 25 and 35, and one whose natural style is listening will likely score between 35 and 45. If you scored less than 35, you might have to expend a little more effort than others to learn how to listen.

Summarizing some of the reasons it is important to be an effective listener, Scissons (1993) stresses that listening helps to build trust, convinces the client that he or she is being understood, encourages the client to reflect on what he or she has just said, ensures that the clinician is on the right track, and is an effective way of collecting information from a client without the potentially negative side effects of using questions (the use of questions will be discussed in Chapter 6).

Although easy to define, listening is one of the most difficult skills to implement because Americans are rarely taught how to hear another person. In fact, ask an untrained adult to listen to another, and usually he or she ends up interrupting and giving advice. But what exactly are the components of good listening? Complete Exercise 5.6 and come up with your list.

EXERCISE 5.6 **Components of Listening**

In small groups or as a class, list the components of good listening in the space provided. Start by using the definition below and add your thoughts about what makes a good listener.

The dictionary asserts that "to listen" means:

1. To pay attention to.
2. To hear something through thoughtful attention: To give consideration.
3. To be alert, to catch an expected sound.
4. To give close attention in order to hear.

Components of good listening:

1. ______
2. ______
3. ______
4. ______
5. ______
6. ______
7. ______
8. ______
9. ______
10. ______

After coming up with your components of good listening, take a look at those that we have composed and see if they are similar. A good listener:

1. minimally talks
2. concentrates on what is being said
3. does not interrupt
4. does not give advice
5. gives and does not expect to get
6. accurately hears the content of what the helpee is saying
7. accurately hears the feelings of what the helpee is saying
8. is able to nonverbally communicate to the helpee that he or she has been heard (e.g., head nods, uh huhs, body language, etc.)
9. asks clarifying questions such as, "I didn't hear all of that. Can you explain that in another way so I'm sure I understand you?"
10. does not ask other kinds of questions

Hindrances to Effective Listening

Even when we "know" how to listen, a number of factors can prevent our ability to listen effectively. Take part in Exercise 5.7 and see what hindrances to listening you come up with. Then examine those we've identified.

EXERCISE 5.7 **Hindrances to Listening**

In class, break into triads. Within your group, have each person take the number 1, 2, or 3. From the topics listed below (or other topics of the instructor's choice) the instructor will assign one of the topics to persons 1 and 2. Number 1 should be "pro" the situation, and number 2 should be "con." One of you start debating the situation while the other listens. When the first person is finished, the second person should repeat back verbatim what he or she heard. Do not reflect or paraphrase—repeat back verbatim. Then, debate back and forth, taking turns listening and repeating verbatim until the instructor tells you to stop. Number 3 is an objective "helper," to give feedback if needed. As the objective observer, also give feedback concerning each person's body language. When you have finished this first situation, numbers 2 and 3 should do the second situation (2 is pro, 3 is con), and then numbers 3 and 1 do the third situation (3 is pro, 1 is con) with the person who is not in the role-play acting as the objective helper.

When you have finished, the instructor will ask for feedback concerning what obstacles prevented you from hearing the other person. List these "hindrances to listening" on the board. Make sure you discuss some of the following items: preoccupation, defensiveness, emotional blocks, and distractions.

Some Possible Situations: Abortion, Capital Punishment, Gays in the Military, Affirmative Action, Torture of Terrorist Suspects, Gay and Lesbian Marriages, Tax Cuts for the Wealthy, Euthanasia

From Exercise 5.7, you likely discovered that some potential hindrances to listening include the following:

1. *preconceived notions:* having preconceived notions about the client that interfere with the helper's ability to hear the client
2. *anticipatory reaction:* anticipating what the client is about to say and not actually hearing the client
3. *cognitive distractions:* thinking about what you are going to say and therefore blocking what the client is saying
4. *personal issues:* having personal issues that interfere with your ability to listen (you are too depressed to hear the client)
5. *emotional response:* having a strong emotional reaction to your client's content and therefore not being able to hear the client accurately
6. *distractions:* being distracted by such things as noises, temperature of the office, hunger pains, and so forth

What other hindrances did you discover besides those that are listed?

Preparing Yourself for Listening

When you are ready to listen, the following practical suggestions should assist you in your ability to effectively hear a client (Egan, 2002; Ivey & Ivey, 2003):

1. *Calm yourself.* Prior to meeting with your client, calm yourself down—meditate, pray, jog, or blow out air, but calm your inner self.
2. *Stop talking and don't interrupt.* You cannot listen while you are talking.
3. *Show interest.* With your body language and tone of voice, show the person you're interested in what he or she is saying.

4. *Don't jump to conclusions.* Take in all of what the person says, and don't assume you understand the person more than he or she understands himself or herself.
5. *Actively listen.* Many people do not realize that listening is an active process that takes deep concentration. If your mind is wandering, you are not listening.
6. *Concentrate on feelings.* Listen, identify, and acknowledge the person's feelings.
7. *Concentrate on content.* Listen, identify, and acknowledge what the person is saying.
8. *Maintain appropriate eye contact.* Show the person with your eyes that you are listening, but be sensitive to cultural differences in the amount of eye contact given.
9. *Have an open body posture.* Face the person and show the person you are ready to listen through your body language but be sensitive to cultural differences.
10. *Be sensitive to the amount of personal space.* Be close enough to the client to show that you are ready to listen but have a sense of the amount of personal space that is comfortable to your client.
11. *Don't ask questions.* Questions are often an indication that you are not listening. Try to avoid questions unless they are clarifying ones (e.g., Can you tell me more about that?).

Paraphrasing

Paraphrasing what a client has said is one way of showing that you have listened well. Paraphrasing is repeating back to the client the same meaning just communicated to you—usually in condensed form. Generally, a student should paraphrase in one or two sentences. Questions should not be asked and interpretations should not be made. This is simply reflecting back what the client has said to you. The following is an example of a client statement followed by a paraphrase.

Client: *Recently, Jason has been particularly mean to me. He seems to be on edge all of the time, and sometimes he yells at me uncontrollably. We've been together for 13 years, and I've seen him this way before; however, it hasn't been this bad for a while. It makes me feel scared to be around him—although he has never physically hurt me, and I do love him.*

Student: *So you're saying that Jason has been on edge recently and has been yelling at you quite a bit. Although you're not scared for your physical safety, it is scary being around him.*

The student's paraphrase gets to the gist of what the client has said and does not add any extraneous information. It simply acknowledges to the client that you were listening. Some stems that you might use when paraphrasing back to a client include:

1. So you're saying that . . .
2. You just said that . . .
3. I heard you saying that . . .
4. If I heard you right, you are saying that . . .
5. What you're saying is . . .

Paraphrasing is an important basic tool to begin with as you move to the even more important skill of empathic responding. Practice paraphrasing in Exercise 5.8 and, after you have mastered this skill, move onto the next section on empathy.

EXERCISE 5.8 **Practicing Paraphrasing**

Pair up with two other students in your class to practice your paraphrasing skills. Have one person role-play a client while the other paraphrases what the client says. The third person will be an observer who can give feedback as to how well the listener heard what the client said. The paraphraser should first prepare for listening, as noted earlier. Then, he or she should make sure that there are as few hindrances to listening as possible. Next, this person should try to paraphrase what his or her partner has said. After the first role-play, have different students play the client, paraphraser, and observer. Then, do a third role-play giving the last student an opportunity to be the person who paraphrases. Of course, while paraphrasing, try to be cognizant of the nonverbal behaviors between the counselor and the client.

Empathic Understanding

Listed as one of the important critical attitudes in Chapter 4, empathy is also an important skill in the helping relationship. As such, it can be systematically learned, although some of us have more "natural empathy" than others.

Empathy has been alluded to for centuries as an important helping skill (Gompertz, 1960), but it wasn't until the 20th century that empathy was formally incorporated into the helping relationship. Probably, the person who has had the greatest impact on our modern-day understanding and use of empathy is Carl Rogers.

> *The state of empathy, or being empathic, is to perceive the internal frame of reference of another with accuracy and with the emotional components and meanings which pertain thereto as if one were the person, but without ever losing the "as if" condition.* (Rogers, 1959, pp. 210–211)

Empathy is the act of showing clients that they have been heard. This can be done in many ways, including the use of what has become known as reflective or active listening as well as through paraphrasing. However, good empathic responses are much more than being an active listener or paraphrasing what the client said. In fact, many master therapists become very creative and mix reflective listening responses with metaphors, analogies, and self-disclosure in an attempt to let clients know that they have been heard accurately and their feelings have been understood (Neukrug, 1997).

The popularity of Rogers' use of empathy during the 20th century eventually led to the development of a popular five-point scale to measure empathy. Known as

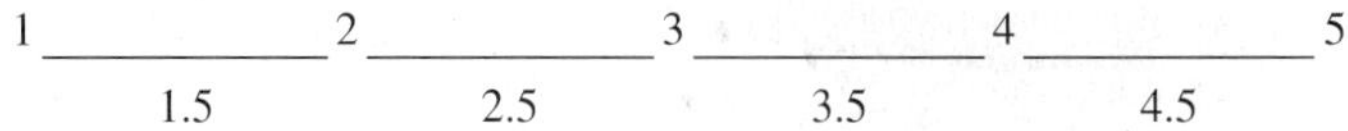

Carkhuff's Accurate Empathy Scale

Level 1
The verbal and behavioral expressions of the first person either *do not attend to* or *detract significantly from* the verbal and behavioral expressions of the second person(s) in that they communicate significantly less of the second person's feelings than the second person has communicated himself [or herself]. . . .

Level 2
While the first person responds to the expressed feelings of the second person(s), he [or she] does so in such a way that he [or she] *subtracts noticeable affect from the communications* of the second person. . . .

Level 3
The expressions of the first person in response to the expressed feelings of the second person(s) are essentially *interchangeable* with those of the second person in that they express essentially the same affect and meaning. . . .

Level 4
The responses of the first person *add noticeably* to the expressions of the second person(s) in such a way as to express feelings a level deeper than the second person was able to express himself [or herself]. . . .

Level 5
The first person's responses *add significantly* to the feeling and meaning of the expressions of the second person(s) in such a way as to (1) accurately express feelings levels below what the person himself [or herself] was able to express or (2) in the event of ongoing, deep self-exploration on the second person's part, to be fully with him [or her] in his deepest moments. . . . (Carkhuff, 1969, pp. 174–175)

Figure 5.1 The Carkhuff Scale

the Carkhuff Scale, after its developer, this instrument has been widely used in the training of helpers (Baumgarten & Roffers, 2003; Egan, 2002; Gazda et al., 1999; Ivey & Ivey, 2003). Numerous research studies have indicated that good empathic ability is related to progress in the helping relationship (Carkhuff & Berenson, 1977; Elliott, Greenberg, & Lietaer, 2004; Neukrug, 1980; Truax & Mitchell, 1971).

The Carkhuff Scale ranges from a low of 1.0 to a high of 5.0 with 0.5 increments (Figure 5.1). Any responses below 3.0 are considered subtractive or nonempathic, whereas responses of 3.0 or higher are considered additive or empathic.

As is obvious in Figure 5.1, the Carkhuff Scale defines level 1 and level 2 responses as detracting from what the person is saying (e.g., giving advice, not accurately reflecting feeling, not including client's content in the response), with a level 1 response being way off the mark and a level 2 only slightly off (Carkhuff & Berenson, 1977; Neukrug, 1980). For instance, suppose a client said, "I can't seem to get along with anybody. People at work seem to avoid me, and my family, well, they just are judgmental and yell at me. Life really sucks." A level 1 response might be, "Well, why don't you do something to make your life better—try harder to get along with people" (giving advice and being judgmental). A level 2 response might be, "You are having a kind of bad time right now" (does not reflect the intensity of the feeling and is not specific enough about the content). On the other hand, a level 3 response accurately reflects the affect and meaning of what the helpee has said.

Using the same example, a level 3 response might be, "Well it sounds like the criticism and yelling at home, as well as people avoiding you at work, are making for a really bad time right now."

Level 4 and level 5 responses reflect feelings and meaning beyond what the person is saying and add to the meaning of the person's outward expression. For instance, in the same example, a level 4 response might be, "It sounds like you're feeling pretty estranged from everybody at home and at work" (expresses a new feeling, estrangement, which the client didn't outwardly state). Level 5 responses are usually made in long-term therapeutic relationships by expert helpers. They express to the helpee a deep understanding of the feelings (e.g., intense pain, or joy) he or she feels as well as a recognition of the complexity of the situation. In the example, a level 5 response might be, "I hear how estranged you feel from those around you—family, coworkers, friends—and am aware of how isolated, alone, and fragile you feel day to day" (expresses deeper understanding of client's aloneness and insecurity).

Usually, in the training of helpers, it is recommended that they attempt to make level 3 responses. A large body of evidence suggests that such responses can be learned in a relatively short amount of time and are beneficial to clients (Carkhuff, 2000; Neukrug, 1980, 1987). However, for effective empathic responding, it is not only crucial to "be on target" with the client's feelings and the content but also to reflect these feelings at a moment when the client can absorb the helper's reflections. For instance, you might accurately sense a deep sadness or anger in a client and reflect this back. However, if the client is not ready to accept these feelings at the time you reflect them back, then the response is considered subtractive.

Making Empathic Responses: A Step-by-Step Approach

Whereas some natural helpers might make good empathic responses, they do not do so on a consistent basis and do not have a reliable method by which to make such responses. Because empathy is such a critical factor in the helping relationship, the professional counselor must be able to make an empathic response whenever he or she deems it necessary and important to do so. To learn how to make these responses, we have devised a step-by-step method of developing your skills. The steps include: Step I: Learning the Components, Step II: Making Formula Responses, Step III: Making Conversational Responses, Step IV: Making Advanced Empathic Responses.

Step I: Learning the Components

A number of guidelines can help you in learning to make effective and purposeful empathic responses. These include the following:

1. *Listen:* Attend to the basic listening skills noted earlier.
2. *Pause:* Wait for a natural pause on the part of the client before responding, and allow some pause time after your client pauses.

3. *Condense:* If the client has spoken for a rather lengthy amount of time, try to focus on what you believe to be the most important aspect of the client's content.
4. *Question Not:* Do not put your response in question form.
5. *Be Short:* Generally, do not make your response more than one sentence or two short sentences.
6. *Reflect Content:* Accurately reflect back the content of what the client said.
7. *Reflect Feelings:* Accurately reflect back the feelings expressed by the client.
8. *Be Specific:* Don't add any extraneous material (e.g., interpretations), and do not reflect back feelings the client has not presented to you (although sometimes client feelings are communicated in various ways: voice inflection, body language, etc.).
9. *Make a Level 3 Response:* Try to shoot for Carkhuff level 3 responses, not higher. Generally, higher level responses will come naturally if you're shooting for a level 3 response.
10. *Obtain Client Feedback:* The client is the best person to let you know if your response was "on target." If it wasn't, then the client will likely tell you directly or indirectly (e.g., he or she may not respond to your response).

So, Step I involves memorizing the components just listed. Here's a quick summary of all of the components:

> *Listen, pause, and condense what the client said. Don't ask questions and keep responses short. Reflect content and feelings and be specific. Make level 3 responses and get client feedback.*

Step II: Making Formula Responses

When first practicing empathic responding, it is suggested that clinicians make a response that attends to each of the components just listed and use paraphrasing while doing so. Called a "formula response," these empathic responses sometimes seem stilted or artificial but tend to be a good way to start. By beginning in this manner, it is assured that each response encapsulates all of the components listed. Sometimes, it is suggested that the clinician use the following model in making a response:

> You feel *place feeling word here* because (or "and") *place content here.*

For instance, in the example given earlier, look at how one might make a formula response to the client.

> Client: *Recently, Jason has been particularly mean to me. He seems to be on edge all of the time, and sometimes he yells at me uncontrollably. We've been together for 13 years, and I've seen him this way before; however, it hasn't been this bad for a while. It makes me feel scared to be around him–although he has never physically hurt me, and I do love him.*

Clinician: You feel *scared* because *Jason is yelling at you and seems out of control.*

Notice how some other feeling words could have been used (e.g., nervous, upset), but we chose to go with the same word the client was giving. Also, more of the content could have been reflected; however, it's often good to keep things as short as possible just as long as the meaning is more or less the same. Lengthy responses tend to make clients wander. Try Exercise 5.9 to practice these kinds of responses. By the way, did you make any assumptions about the gender of the client in our example?

EXERCISE 5.9 **Making Basic Empathic Formula Responses**

Using a formula response, respond to the scenarios that follow. In the first few scenarios, use the feeling words given to you by the client. As the scenarios continue, they become more complex and you may have to imply feelings or make a response to a client who is presenting more than one feeling. Try to stay within the format even as the scenarios get more complicated.

1. **Client:** I am considering leaving my wife. I'm constantly belittled by her. I think I need some time on my own.

   Clinician: You feel ______________________
   because (and) ______________________
   ____
   ____

2. **Client:** My boyfriend just asked me to marry him. I'm ecstatic and can't wait for the wedding.

   Clinician: You feel ______________________
   because (and) ______________________
   ____
   ____

3. **Client:** I'm suspicious about all that the government is doing to maintain our status in the world. I think it's all about oil. What do you think?

   Clinician: You feel ______________________
   because (and) ______________________
   ____
   ____

4. **Client:** I hate my teacher, and I hate all of the kids in the class. I just want to go home.

   Clinician: You feel ______________________
   because (and) ______________________
   ____
   ____

5. **Client:** John is cheating, and I don't care about him anymore. I just want him to get out of my life. We've been together for 6 years and finding a gay man in this town is so hard.

   Clinician: You feel ______________________
   because (and) ______________________
   ____
   ____

6. **Client:** On the one hand, I'm happy I'm pregnant. On the other hand, it's scary being a single parent. I'm not sure I can handle all of the responsibility.

   Clinician: You feel ______________________
   because (and) ______________________
   ____
   ____

In Exercise 5.9, were you able to identify the feeling correctly and then reflect back the content accurately? Before you move on to the next exercise, you might want to pair up with another student in class and further practice your formula responses as you role-play a counselor and a client.

You probably noticed in Client 6 that the client presented more than one feeling. How did you deal with this? In point of fact, people are pretty complex and it is extremely common that a client will present two or more feelings about a situation. Sometimes they'll present opposing feelings, and it is the clinician's responsibility to reflect back to the client in ways that capture the client's meaning. There are a few ways of doing this, and as you look at the following examples, consider the complexity required to show a client that you really hear him or her.

Client: *My best friend is leaving town, and I'm going to miss her so much. We do everything together. I even stay at her place a few nights a week. On the other hand, I am excited about the possibility of making new friends and forming new relationships.*

Example 1
Using the "you . . . feel" formula twice, in succession.

Clinician: You feel *sad* because *your best friend is leaving*, yet you also feel *excited* because *you might make new friends after she leaves.*

Example 2
Stating both feelings up front and following with content related to both feelings.

Clinician: You feel *both sad and excited—sad* because *your friend is leaving* and *excited about the potential of meeting new people.*

Example 3
Acknowledging two or more feelings and following up with each feeling and its associated content.

Clinician: You feel *a couple of feelings—sad* because *your friend is leaving* and *excited about the potential of meeting new people.*

Now is your chance. In the next eight examples, you will find a client expressing multiple feelings (see Exercise 5.10). Applying one or more of the examples just presented, make your responses to the clients. Or if you can find other ways of responding while maintaining the basic "you . . . feel" formula, feel free to do so.

EXERCISE 5.10 **Making Basic Empathic Formula Responses: Multiple Feelings**

Using one or more of the formula responses just discussed, or coming up with your own formula response, reflect the multiple feelings presented to the following scenarios.

1. **Client:** My best friend is leaving town, and I'm going to miss her so much. We do everything together. I even stay at her place a few nights a week. On the other hand, I am excited about the possibility of making new friends and forming new relationships.

   Clinician: ______________________________

   ____

2. **Client:** Although I'm HIV positive, I'm maintaining a positive attitude toward life. Once in a while, I get the doldrums, but generally, I expect to live a relatively long and satisfying life.

   Clinician: ______________________________

   ____

3. **Client:** My dad has Alzheimer's. Sometimes I wake up in the middle of the night screaming—scared that he's going to die. And the thought of him not being here seems to always stay with me. I hate to admit it, but once in a while, I wish this would all be over with. It's taking such a toll on me and my family.

   Clinician: ______________________________

4. **Client:** I'm not using any more and I feel much better about myself. Since rehab, my life has changed dramatically. My family likes me. I'm more productive at work. But sometimes I still get that urge.

   Clinician: ______________________________

5. **Client:** I'm torn between my wife and my girlfriend. I love my wife because she represents stability for me, and she is good to me. But all my passion is with my girlfriend. I want to leave my wife, but what will others think?

   Clinician: ______________________________

6. **Client:** I often sit around and wonder what my life is all about. What meaning does it have for me, and where am I going? Then reality hits, and I'm suddenly realizing that I need to get back to my work. Do you think I'm nuts?

   Clinician: ______________________________

7. **Client:** I love mommy but not daddy. I want my mommy to snuggle with me.

   Clinician: ______________________________

8. **Client:** I'm trying to figure out what to major in. On the one hand, I love psychology, but I think it's more realistic to go into business, even though I don't have strong feelings for that field. What do you think?

   Clinician: ______________________________

Step III: Making Conversational Responses

As helpers become more comfortable with formula responses, they can begin to make empathic responses using their unique conversational style. Such responses infuse your natural personality style into the response. However, they do so *while maintaining the critical components of an empathic response:* reflection of feelings and content. There are a multitude of ways to respond to a client using your unique conversational style. For instance, in the example given earlier, you could make the following empathic responses:

> Client: *Recently, Jason has been particularly mean to me. He seems to be on edge all of the time, and sometimes he yells at me uncontrollably. We've been together for 13 years, and I've seen him this way before; however, it hasn't been this bad for a while. It makes me feel scared to be around him—although he has never physically hurt me, and I do love him.*
>
> Clinician: *It sounds really scary to be around Jason right now, even though you're not particularly nervous for your physical safety.*

or

> Clinician: *Frightened and fearful—those are the feelings I hear when you talk about how out of control Jason is right now.*

or

> Clinician: *I think that situation sounds particularly scary. I would imagine that you feel on edge all of the time with Jason's acting out the way he is.*

As we repeat the scenarios from Exercises 5.9 and 5.10, this time practice making empathic responses using your unique conversational style in Exercise 5.11. Remember, you need to reflect back to the client the fact that you have heard his or her feelings and meaning while at the same time having your unique conversational style come through. This is often not an easy task.

EXERCISE 5.11 **Making Conversational Responses**

Make a conversational response to each of the following:

1. **Client:** I am considering leaving my wife. I'm constantly belittled by her. I think I need some time on my own.

   Clinician: ______________________________
   ____

2. **Client:** My boyfriend just asked me to marry him. I'm ecstatic and can't wait for the wedding.

   Clinician: ______________________________
   ____

3. **Client:** I'm suspicious about all the government is doing to maintain our status in the world. I think it's all about oil. What do you think?

   Clinician: ______________________________
   ____

4. **Client:** I hate my teacher, and I hate all of the kids in the class. I just want to go home.

   Clinician: ______________________________
   ____

5. **Client:** John is cheating, and I don't care about him any more. I just want him to get out of my life. We've been together for 6 years and finding a gay man in this town is so hard.

   Clinician: ______________________________
   ____

6. **Client:** On the one hand, I'm happy I'm pregnant. On the other hand, it's scary being a single parent. I'm not sure I can handle all of the responsibility.

   Clinician: ______________________________
   ____

7. **Client:** My best friend is leaving town, and I'm going to miss her so much. We do everything together. I even stay at her place a few nights a week. On the other hand, I wonder what new people I might connect with after she's gone.

   Clinician: ______________________________
   ____

8. **Client:** Although I am HIV positive, I am maintaining a positive attitude toward life. Once in a while, I get the doldrums, but generally, I expect to live a relatively long and satisfying life.

   Clinician: ______________________________
   ____

9. **Client:** My dad has Alzheimer's. Sometimes I wake up in the middle of the night screaming—scared that he's going to die. And the thought of him not being here seems to always stay with me. I hate to admit it, but once in a while, I wish this would all be over with. It's taking such a toll on me and my family.

   Clinician: ______________________________
   ____

10. **Client:** I'm not using any more and I feel much better about myself. Since rehab, my life has changed dramatically. My family likes me. I'm more productive at work. But sometimes I still get that urge.

    Clinician: ______________________________
    ____

11. **Client:** I'm torn between my wife and my girlfriend. I love my wife because she represents stability for me, and she is good to me. But all my passion is with my girlfriend. I want to leave my wife, but what will others think?

    Clinician: ______________________________
    ____

12. Client: I often sit around and wonder what my life is all about. What meaning does it have for me, and where am I going? Then reality hits, and I'm suddenly realizing that I need to get back to my work. Do you think I'm nuts?

Clinician: ______________________________

13. Client: I love mommy but not daddy. I want my mommy to snuggle with me.

Clinician: ______________________________

14. Client: I'm trying to figure out what to major in. On the one hand, I love psychology, but I think it's more realistic to go into business, even though I don't have strong feelings for that field. What do you think?

Clinician: ______________________________

Step IV: Making Advanced Empathic Responses

There are actually many ways to respond empathically to a client, and some responses can bring about deeper levels of understanding than either a formula response or an empathic response that uses your unique conversational style (Neukrug, 1997). Three kinds of responses that are often used by seasoned clinicians are (a) reflecting feelings at deeper levels than the client has outwardly expressed because you are able to sense deeper feelings; (b) using a metaphor, analogy, or visual image to show the client you have heard him or her; and (c) reflecting back contrasting feelings. Because advanced empathic responses bring deeper understanding to the client, they are generally rated 3.5 or 4.0 on the Carkhuff scale.

REFLECTIONS OF DEEPER FEELINGS Sometimes when listening to a client, the clinician will sense the presence of deeper feelings than the client is expressing. Such a response is based on both a general understanding of human interaction and on one's intuitive sense about the specific client. To do this effectively, however, the clinician must be careful to not reflect back an interpretation of the client's situation or a feeling based on overly identifying with the client's situation. The clinician must actually be "sensing" these deeper feelings. Using our example, let's see how a clinician might respond to our client.

> Client: *Recently, Jason has been particularly mean to me. He seems to be on edge all of the time, and sometimes he yells at me uncontrollably. We've been together for 13 years, and I've seen him this way before; however, it hasn't been this bad for a while. It makes me feel scared to be around him—although he has never physically hurt me, and I do love him.*
>
> Clinician: *It sounds really scary to be around Jason right now, and I think I'm also hearing how hurt you feel—hurt that he's broken your trust in the relationship.*

In this example, look at how the helper reflected back the new feeling, "hurt," which was not explicitly expressed by the client. Ideally, the helper picked up on underlying feelings and did not reflect "hurt" because he or she assumed that's what the client was feeling.

REFLECTIONS USING ANALOGIES, METAPHORS, AND VISUAL IMAGES Other times, a helper might use an analogy, metaphor, or visual image to bring forth deeper meanings to the client. It is our belief that metaphors, analogies, and visual images are assimilated by a person in different and deeper ways than formula responses or even conversational responses; thus, they can make a greater impact on the person. For instance, in the same situation, the clinician might say:

> Clinician: *The feelings you have about your relationship with Jason make me think of a house with a shaky foundation.*

or

> Clinician: *When you just told me what you're going through, I felt my stomach twist and turn—I imagine this is how you must be feeling.*

REFLECTIONS THAT POINT OUT CONTRASTING FEELINGS Sometimes when a client expresses opposing feelings, the helper can point out these contradictory emotions. Such a response acknowledges these mixed feelings and, in a subtle manner, says to the client that life is filled with complex feelings. Then, look at the helper response:

> Client: *Recently, Jason has been particularly mean to me. He seems to be on edge all of the time, and sometimes he yells at me uncontrollably. We've been together for 13 years, and I've seen him this way before; however, it hasn't been this bad for a while. It makes me feel scared to be around him—although he has never physically hurt me, and I do love him.*
>
> Clinician: *Right now, I hear that you have a couple of feelings—you feel scared because Jason is out of control with his anger, and yet you still feel like you love him. It must be difficult having these somewhat opposing feelings.*

It is generally recommended that beginning clinicians stick to making formula or conversational responses because making an advanced response is an art that comes with being a seasoned professional. However, making advanced responses adds depth to the kinds of responses available to the clinician, and as you feel more comfortable, you might want to begin to try making these kinds of responses.

For Exercise 5.12, in small groups, you will have the opportunity to formulate some advanced responses; however, if you are having trouble coming up with an advanced response, keep in mind that a good formula response will be helpful to a client.

EXERCISE 5.12 **Making Advanced Empathic Responses**

Divide into groups of four or five in your class, and using the same scenarios as earlier, try to make one of the three types of advanced empathic responses just noted. After you have finished, discuss in class how effective such responses might be.

1. **Client:** I am considering leaving my wife. I'm constantly belittled by her. I think I need some time on my own.

   Clinician: ______________________________

   ____

2. **Client:** My boyfriend just asked me to marry him. I'm ecstatic and can't wait for the wedding.

   Clinician: ______________________________

3. **Client:** I'm suspicious about all the government is doing to maintain our status in the world. I think it's all about oil. What do you think?

   Clinician: ______________________________

4. **Client:** I hate my teacher, and I hate all of the kids in the class. I just want to go home.

   Clinician: ______________________________

5. **Client:** John is cheating, and I don't care about him any more. I just want him to get out of my life. We've been together for 6 years and finding a gay man in this town is so hard.

   Clinician: ______________________________

6. **Client:** On the one hand, I'm happy I'm pregnant. On the other hand, it's scary being a single parent. I'm not sure I can handle all of the responsibility.

   Clinician: ______________________________

7. **Client:** My best friend is leaving town, and I'm going to miss her so much. We do everything together. I even stay at her place a few nights a week. On the other hand, I wonder what new people I might connect with after she's gone.

   Clinician: ______________________________

8. **Client:** Although I am HIV positive, I am maintaining a positive attitude toward life. Once in a while, I get the doldrums, but generally, I expect to live a relatively long and satisfying life.

   Clinician: ______________________________

9. **Client:** My dad has Alzheimer's. Sometimes I wake up in the middle of the night screaming—scared that he's going to die. And the thought of him not being here seems to always stay with me. I hate to admit it, but once in a while, I wish this would all be over with. It's taking such a toll on me and my family.

   Clinician: ______________________________

10. **Client:** I'm not using any more and I feel much better about myself. Since rehab, my life has changed dramatically. My family likes me. I'm more productive at work. But sometimes I still get that urge.

    Clinician: ______________________________

11. **Client:** I'm torn between my wife and my girlfriend. I love my wife because she represents stability for me, and she is good to me. But all my passion is with my girlfriend. I want to leave my wife, but what will others think?

    Clinician: ______________________________

12. **Client:** I often sit around and wonder what my life is all about. What meaning does it have for me, and where am I going? Then reality hits, and I'm suddenly realizing that I need to get back to my work. Do you think I'm nuts?

    Clinician: ______________________________

13. **Client:** I love mommy but not daddy. I want my mommy to snuggle with me.

    Clinician: ______________________________

14. **Client:** I'm trying to figure out what to major in. On the one hand, I love psychology, but I think it's more realistic to go into business, even though I don't have strong feelings for that field. What do you think?

    Clinician: ______________________________

Practicing Empathic Responses

In this chapter, you have learned how to make formula responses, empathic responses using your unique conversational style, and advanced empathic responses. All of these responses are critical to the helping relationship. Clinicians often rely on the tried-and-true formula response when an empathic response using your conversational tone or an advanced response does not come to mind. On the other hand, empathic responses using your conversational style are the mainstay of the skills repertoire of many seasoned clinicians, and they show clients that the clinician hears them very deeply. Advanced responses help clients see themselves in even deeper and more complex ways. Now complete Exercises 5.13, 5.14, 5.15, and 5.16, and try to make several of these three different types of response. Process the exercises when you are done.

EXERCISE 5.13 **Empathic Bombardment**

Your instructor will sit in the middle of the classroom. Form two circles around him or her. The instructor will role-play the client while the first circle will be helpers. The second circle will be observers who will rate the responses of the helpers. All observers should have a pencil and a piece of paper. The instructor will role-play a situation, and any person in the first circle can respond, but only with one of the three kinds of empathic responses (formula, conversational, or advanced). The instructor will turn to the helper who is responding and, meanwhile, the observers will write down the response and rate it on the Carkhuff scale. After you have done this exercise for a few minutes, observers can share their ratings of the various responses. Then, do another role-play with the observers and helpers switching roles.

EXERCISE 5.14 **Practicing Empathic Responding**

The following scenario involves a client named Alicia. For each of the client statements, make a formula, conversational, and/or advanced response. When you have finished, share you responses in small groups and/or in class.

1. **Alicia:** I'm not sure why I came to see you, except that I know that I'm feeling depressed.

   Formula Response: You feel ________ because (and) ________ Conversational or Advanced Response:

   ____

2. **Alicia:** I've felt this way for a while but can't figure out what's going on. Everything seems to be okay in my life. I guess I must just have one of those depressive personalities.

   Formula Response: You feel ________ because (and) ________ Conversational or Advanced Response:

   ____

3. **Alicia:** Well, I have two great kids, a husband, a good job, and a good life. I have nothing to complain about. Things really should be great.

   Formula Response: You feel ________ because (and) ________ Conversational or Advanced Response:

   ____

4. **Alicia:** To be honest, maybe my marriage isn't the best. It's not like my husband is mean or anything. And I don't think he would ever cheat on me. But he doesn't *really* seem to love me. I mean, I think we just go through the motions much of the time. What kind of marriage is that?

   Formula Response: You feel ________ because (and) ________ Conversational or Advanced Response:

   ____

5. **Alicia:** Maybe I've just been hiding my head in the sand. I have been under this delusion that everything is fine, when in fact it's not. Maybe we need marriage counseling to sort some of this stuff out. But I'm scared of what he'll say to me — or maybe what I might say to him.

   Formula Response: You feel ________ because (and) ________ Conversational or Advanced Response:

   ____

6. **Alicia:** I appreciate you listening to me today. I really feel that I at least have a little bit of a sense of where I'm going. Should I come back next week?

   Formula Response: You feel ________ because (and) ________ Conversational or Advanced Response:

   ____

EXERCISE 5.15 **More Practice with Empathy**

The following scenario involves a client named William. For each of the responses, make a formula, conversational, and/or advanced response. When you have finished, share you responses in small groups and/or in class.

1. **William:** My doctor referred me to you because of my high blood pressure and because I told him I was feeling stressed out.

   Formula Response: You feel ________ because (and) ________ Conversational or Advanced Response:

   ____

2. **William:** So, what can you do for me? I need to take care of this stress in my life, and I want a plan to fix it. What do you think? What ideas do you have?

   Formula Response: You feel ________ because (and) ________ Conversational or Advanced Response:

   ____

3. **William:** I've been stressed for a number of years. Well, I guess now that my kids are grown, I'm realizing it. I used to not worry about it — you know, I was driven. Driven to do well at work, provide for my family—the usual stuff. But now I look back on my life and I'm wondering why. But let's get back to the basics. How can you help me?

   Formula Response: You feel ________ because (and) ________ Conversational or Advanced Response:

   ____

4. **William:** I had an affair a few years back. And to be honest, it was the best thing in my life. It made me feel alive. I stopped seeing her—well, at least sexually, but she's still on my mind. My wife knew about the affair and was, of course, pretty upset. But she wasn't about to leave me. She loved me, and in a way, I loved her. But even after all these years, I still think about the other woman. I don't think that will ever change.

   Formula Response: You feel ________ because (and) ________ Conversational or Advanced Response:

   ____

(*continued*)

EXERCISE 5.15 *(continued)*

5. **William:** Sometimes I think that maybe I should leave my wife, but my kids would go crazy. They didn't know about the other woman, and they see me as the Rock of Gibraltar. If I would ever leave her, they would never talk to me again. And people at work would have a fit. They wouldn't believe it. Everyone thinks I'm the pillar of the community. They even named the street where I live after me.

   Formula Response: You feel ________ because (and) ________ Conversational or Advanced Response: ________

6. **William:** Well, I've just told you a whole lot of things today, and I come back to my original question. What are you going to do for me? Are you just going to sit there and listen? I need some real help.

   Formula Response: You feel ________ because (and) ________ Conversational or Advanced Response: ________

7. **William:** Well, maybe there isn't just one answer to this dilemma. Maybe just talking about it would be helpful. I'll try this for a little while, but I make no promises.

   Formula Response: You feel ________ because (and) ________ Conversational or Advanced Response: ________

EXERCISE 5.16 **Practicing Advanced Empathic Responses**

Either at home or in class, practice role-playing a clinician for 30–60 minutes. During that time, attempt to use formula responses, conversational responses, and advanced responses. In small groups or as a class, compare and contrast these three types of responses.

Final Thoughts

Empathy is probably the most important helping skill for any mental health professional. It is the skill that works best in building the relationship, is crucial for maintaining a bond with the client, and can help the client understand deeper parts of himself or herself. It is a skill that we are always getting better at as we continue in our careers.

LEARNING TO BE A COUNSELOR: An Ongoing Process

Making the shift from being a natural helper to a professional counselor entails letting go of one's haphazard method of responding to individuals and taking on a deliberate and systematic counseling approach. In learning how to listen, paraphrase, and make an empathic response, you are on your way to doing this. Often, we have found students struggling with this first step as they fall back on their natural style and begin to ask questions, give advice, and offer judgments. We encourage you to fight this urge and continually practice these important foundational skills. You will find that, over time, the urge to be your natural self will give way to an urge to be a professional counselor. In fact, over time, you will find that your natural self has changed and has merged with your professional self; that is, making foundational responses will become natural.

Chapter Summary

This chapter examined the important foundational skills of nonverbal language, silence and pause time, listening, paraphrasing, and empathy. Relative to nonverbal behavior, we found that a number of nonverbal behaviors can influence the trust and rapport found in the helping relationship. Some of these include attire, eye contact, body positioning and facial expression, personal space, touch, and voice intonation and tone. We defined each of these behaviors and noted that they are often mediated by the cultural background of the client and the clinician.

We next defined silence and pause time. We highlighted the fact that silence can be very powerful because it gives time for the client and the helper to review what has been said in an interview. We noted that sometimes clients will want to fill the silent void and may feel an urgency to talk more fully about a topic. Pause time, which is related to silence, is the amount of time a helper allows between responses. We stressed that pause time is a cross-cultural issue in that individuals from different cultures may have varying pause times.

Listening was highlighted as one of the most important helping skills and as a skill that does not come easily to many individuals. We delineated a number of components to listening, including minimally talking, concentrating, not interrupting, not giving advice, giving–not getting from the client, accurately hearing content and feelings, nonverbally letting your client know you heard him or her, asking clarifying questions to make sure you heard accurately, and not asking other types of questions. We went on to note that there are a number of hindrances to listening, which may include preconceived notions, anticipatory reactions, cognitive distractions, personal issues, emotional responses, and other distractions. We also noted the importance of preparing adequately prior to listening.

Paraphrasing, the next foundational skill, was defined as repeating back to the client the same meaning he or she has just communicated to you—usually in condensed form. We noted that this skill is important to learn prior to learning the critical skill of empathy.

We stressed that empathy is probably the most important skill for the helper. We first defined empathy as the ability to perceive the internal world of the client—as if one were the person, "without losing the 'as if' feeling." We noted that empathy became increasingly important as a helping skill during the 20th century. Popularized by Carl Rogers, empathy was operationalized by Carkhuff when he developed a five-point scale that delineated different kinds of empathic responses. We noted that those who make a level 3 or above empathic response have been shown to be helpful to clients, whereas those who make less than a level 3 response may be harmful to clients. We showed that level 1 or 2 responses are judgmental or off the mark in reflecting affect and meaning. On the other hand, a level 3 response was defined as accurately reflecting the affect and content of what the client is saying. Level 4 was defined as reflecting feelings and meanings beyond those of which the client is aware, and level 5 was shown to occur when clients, in their deepest moments of pain, recognize that the helper hears them.

As we continued our discussion of empathic responding, we offered four steps to the learning of empathy that included Step I: Learning the Components, Step II:

Making Formula Responses, Step III: Making Conversational Responses, and Step IV: Making Advanced Empathic Responses. We discussed how formula responses have a preconceived structure (e.g., you feel . . . because . . .) and require the helper to paraphrase content and meaning. Conversational responses, on the other hand, reflect content and meaning but do so in a more natural conversational tone and can be quite creative. We defined advanced empathic responses as reflections that bring even deeper levels of understanding than either formula or conversational responses. Three kinds of advanced responses highlighted were (a) reflecting feelings at deeper levels than those expressed outwardly by the client because you sense the presence of deeper feelings; (b) using a metaphor, analogy, or visual image to show the client you have heard him or her; and (c) reflecting back contrasting feelings. Although advanced empathic response are usually rated at level 3.5 or 4.0 on the Carkhuff scale, we stressed that making a good level 3.0 conversational response has been shown to be related to positive counseling outcomes.

Throughout this chapter, we offered numerous exercises to practice the skills presented, and we concluded the chapter by noting that the more you practice empathic responding, the easier it becomes to make these kinds of critical responses. Eventually, our hope is that empathic responding will become part of your natural style.

CHAPTER 6

Information Gathering: Questions, Structured Interviews, Assessment Procedures, and Writing a Case Report

Until recently, mental health professionals had the luxury to slowly develop a relationship and gather information. However, today, clinicians must quickly gather information in an effort to show funding agencies and insurance companies that they are rapidly on their way to the development of treatment strategies. Such accountability, these overseers believe, will help clients reach their goals more quickly, reduce caseloads, and graduate clients from counseling in a relatively short amount of time. Although the efficacy of such briefer treatment can be debated, it is clear that gathering information in an effort to expedite client progress has become a critical part of what the clinician does.

Although natural helpers often apply information-gathering techniques, they do so in a chaotic fashion. In this chapter, we suggest systematic ways of gathering information that will be palatable to the client. Thus, we discuss the pros and cons of asking questions and distinguish among different kinds of questioning techniques, paying particular attention to direct questions, closed questions, open questions, tentative questions, and "why" questions. Then, we examine how to gather information quickly and robustly using a structured interview. In this process, we highlight the importance of using a professional disclosure statement and obtaining informed consent prior to conducting the interview and how to conduct a mental status exam during the structured interview. Next, we examine how the use of formal assessment techniques, such as personality tests, and the use of informal assessment techniques, such as a genogram, can expedite the gathering of information. The chapter concludes with a brief discussion about the importance of finding the balance between the information gathering process and the use of our foundational skills.

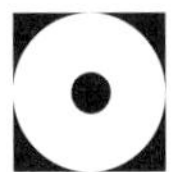

At this point, we recommend that you pause reading the text, turn to the DVD, and view the section entitled:

Information Gathering

Questions

There is no dispute that the use of questions is critical if one is to gather meaningful information in a relatively short amount of time. In addition, questions can serve a multitude of purposes, including uncovering historical patterns, revealing underlying issues, challenging the client to change, and encouraging the client to deepen his or her self-exploration (Kleinke, 1994). However, despite the ability of questions to help the clinician quickly delve into the world of the client, the use of questions is often challenged and viewed negatively by training programs (Benjamin, 1987). This is because the use of questions can be detrimental to building a trusting counseling relationship and ultimately to ensuring positive client outcomes (Kleinke,1994; Orlinsky & Howard, 1986).

Although some clients, under some circumstances, will flourish through the clinician's use of questions, many clients will feel defensive, challenged, put off, and misunderstood when barraged with questions (Byrne, 1995; Cormier & Nurius, 2003). Too often, beginning clinicians will prematurely ask a question when there is a lengthy pause, ask a question when at a loss for another, better type of response, ask a question that is irrelevant to the topic, or use a question that leads to client defensiveness. In a more positive light, the appropriate use of questions can assist clients in identifying issues, help clinicians quickly move toward the establishment of goals, and be important in the eventual development of treatment plans. When using questions, it is important that the clinician monitor the type of question being asked to maximize the potential for benefit. Let's examine different kinds of questions and when some would be more effective than others, including direct questions, closed questions, open questions, tentative questions, and why questions.

Direct Questions

A direct question is one in which the clinician attempts to get specific information about a topic. Thus, questions such as, "How many years have you been in the relationship?" or "Can you tell me when you started to feel depressed?" are direct questions because they focus on obtaining targeted information about specific subjects. Often, direct questions will be used near the beginning of the helping relationship, such as during an intake interview. The key for the clinician is to balance the use of foundational skills, in an effort to build a supportive relationship, with the use of questions and other techniques that are critical in the assessment process.

EXERCISE 6.1 **Asking Direct Questions**

Part I: Which of the following are direct questions?

1. How do you feel about that?
2. Why do you think that was so important?
3. How do the children respond when you get drunk?
4. Can you tell me more about that?
5. What specifically about the marriage makes you feel so discontent?

Questions 3 and 5 are direct questions because they focus on content, or subject matter—the drinking and the marital situation.

Part II: Find a partner in class and have one person role-play a client with a specific problem while the other person role-plays a clinician who uses direct questions to delve deeper into the problem. Feel free to also intersperse foundational skills. When finished, switch roles. Then, in small groups, discuss the level of ease you had in the use of direct questions and the positive and negative aspects of their use.

Closed Questions: Delimiting Content and Affect

If a question is asked in a manner that delimits the kinds of responses available to the client, it is said to be a closed question. Closed questions can delimit content or affect. For instance, the closed content question, "Did the children get money or toys from their relatives?" limits the kinds of response options available to the client (although clients can, of course, transcend the questions—e.g., "Well, actually, they didn't get either."). Similarly, the closed affect question, "Did you feel sad or relieved when you separated from you partner?" limits possible client responses, as there may be many other client feelings that the clinician is not highlighting (e.g., angry, upset, annoyed, joyful, etc.) because he or she is using a closed question.

Closed questions are helpful if you want to gather information very quickly and you are pretty confident that the response will likely be one of the options you offer. However, closed questions run the risk of corraling the client into talking about a particular point and/or pushing the client to choose one of the options given in the question. What if the first client above did not wish to discuss what the children received from their relatives or if the second client has more prevalent feelings about the separation that were not highlighted because a closed question was used?

EXERCISE 6.2 **Contrasting Closed Questions with Empathic Responses**

Have the class divide into groups of six to eight students. In these small groups, have one student volunteer to talk about some kind of life dilemma or difficulty while the others form a circle around him or her (of course, the student should feel comfortable sharing this information). Then, the students in the circles should ask closed questions about the presenting issue of the student volunteer. Do this for about 5 or 10 minutes, at which point the instructor should say "switch." At this point, the students in the circles should stop asking questions and make only empathic responses. When you are finished, discuss the following questions as a group:

1. How did the client experience the first half of the exercise?
2. How did the client experience the second half of the exercise?

(continued)

EXERCISE 6.2 *(continued)*

3. Was it easier to ask questions or to make empathic responses?
4. Were there better types of questions that could have been used?
5. Did questions need to be asked at all?
6. Could better empathic responses have been made?
7. Do you think it would be better to ask a closed question or to make an empathic response?

Open Questions

In contrast to direct or closed questions, open questions enable the client to have a wide range of responses. For instance, a client could be asked questions like, "Can you tell me more about that?" "What do you think that was all about?" "How do you make sense of that?" or "What are you feeling now?" Open questions can be very powerful in that they allow clients the freedom to respond in a multitude of ways. This creates an environment in which the client can direct his or her own session, and thus, this type of question is seen as more "client-centered" than a closed question (Tamase & Arake, 1993; Tamase, Baker, & Ivey as cited in Daniels, 2003). However, in contrast to direct or closed questions, because they allow the client to discuss any of a number of issues, this response can be burdensome if one is in the position of needing to gather information quickly.

EXERCISE 6.3 **Practicing Open Questioning**

Your instructor should break the class into triads. Within your triad, identify a clinician, client, and observer. The client is to choose a topic of his or her choice, and the clinician should respond by asking only open questions. The observer is there to assist the clinician should she or he have difficulty with the task. Also, if the observer believes the clinician did not respond with an open question, he or she should stop the interview and the three students should discuss what possible open questions could be asked. Then, resume the exercise. After doing this for 5–10 minutes, change roles and have the client be the clinician, the observer be the client, and the clinician be the observer. Then, after another 5–10 minutes, do the exercise one last time, changing roles again. In class, discuss the relative ease or difficulty of asking open questions.

Tentative Questions

Tentative questions are asked in a manner that invites the client to tell the clinician if he or she is on target with the response made. Tentative questions are not as effective when the clinician wants to gather information quickly, but they can be quite powerful when the clinician is helping the client examine himself or herself. Tentative questions can take many different forms. The following section examines one type of tentative question, which we call "empathy with a twist of doubt," and this is followed by some other forms of tentative questions.

Empathy with a Twist of Doubt

We have found that when counselors and therapists attempt empathic responses, sometimes they will respond using an empathic format with an inflection in their voice that turns the response into a question. Generally, this is done when the clinician has doubt about whether or not he or she heard the client correctly. For instance, suppose you are with a client who is expressing feelings about a relationship. You think you hear sadness but are not sure. Thus, you add inflection at the end of what would have been an empathic response and say, "It sounds like you feel sad about where your relationship is going?" Although purists would say that this response is not an empathic response, it certainly has many of the same components.

Sometimes beginning counselors convert a perfectly good empathic response into a question because they are apprehensive and tentative about their ability in general, as opposed to being unsure about what they have heard in any one particular instance. This practice should be monitored and avoided if possible. However, if a clinician is unsure of the feelings expressed by the client and wants to test the waters, a tentative "empathic response" could be quite effective because it allows the client to ponder what the clinician has said without making the client feel defensive.

Other Types of Tentative Questions

In addition to making a tentative response that uses empathy as its base, you can make direct, closed, and open questions more palatable by asking them in tentative ways. For instance, rather than asking the direct question, "Can you tell me the names of the people in your family and their ages?" you could ask, "Would you mind telling me about your family members, like their names and ages?" Or rather than asking the closed question, "How sad and depressed do you feel about your divorce?" a clinician could respond with the following tentative question: "I'm wondering if you might be feeling sad and depressed right now about your divorce?" These tentative questions reduce the impact of the inquiry and give the client the opportunity to back out of responding to the question if feeling uncomfortable. Even open questions can be asked tentatively. For instance, rather than saying, "What are you feeling about the divorce?" you could ask, "I would guess that you might have some feelings about the divorce?" In this case, you probably notice that the original question was actually turned into one of those "empathic responses with a twist of doubt." Finally, when making responses to clients, sometimes clinicians will add a short question at the end such as, "Is that true?" This is another method of making a response more palatable to the client.

EXERCISE 6.4 **Developing Tentative Questions**

Part I: As a class, come up with different beginning phrases that might start a tentative question. For instance, in the examples above, we began the responses by stating, "I wonder if you . . . ," and with "I would guess that you. . . ." Write the phrases in the spaces provided.

1. ______________________________

2. ______________________________

3. ______________________________

(continued)

EXERCISE 6.4 *(continued)*

4. ______________________________

5. ______________________________

6. ______________________________

Part II: Pair up with two other students and take turns role-playing and practicing using tentative questions. Have the student who is not involved in the role-play make a list of the questions made by the counselor; then, at the end of the role-play, discuss the kind of questions made and assess their effectiveness. Also, monitor how easy or difficult it was making responses using tentative questions while avoiding other types of questions.

Why Questions

Have you ever been asked the question, "Why do you feel that way?" Did it make you feel defensive? Because "why" questions do tend to make a person feel defensive, it is generally recommended that clinicians use other kinds of questions or empathic responses (Benjamin, 1987). In actuality, if clients could honestly answer why, the why question would be the most powerful question used in the helping relationship. However, clients use the helping relationship to find the answer why. If they knew why, they wouldn't be in the clinician's office. Although we have found that after forming an alliance with a client, we might periodically be able to slip in a "soft" why question and say something like, "Why do you think that is?" we try to use this type of question sparingly so as not to make a client feel on guard.

Professional Perspectives 6.1 offers a quick comparison of the different kinds of questions thus far examined in this chapter.

PROFESSIONAL PERSPECTIVES 6.1

Summarizing Direct, Closed, Open, Tentative, and Why Questions

TYPE OF QUESTION	DEFINITION	EXAMPLES
Direct Question	A question that focuses on specific content in an effort to obtain information quickly.	"If you decide to keep the child, how will you care for it?"
Closed Question: Delimiting Content	A question that focuses on a particular topic or point of view and forces the client to pick between choices given.	"Do you think you will live with your parents or on your own after the child is born?"
Closed Question: Delimiting Affect	A question that forces the client to pick between feeling choices assumed by the clinician.	"Did you feel happy or sad when you found out that you were pregnant?"

TYPE OF QUESTION	DEFINITION	EXAMPLES
Open Question	A question that allows the client to respond in a myriad of ways.	"So how do you feel about the fact that you may be pregnant?" "Can you tell me more about that?"
Tentative Question	A question that is asked in a manner that invites the client to tell the clinician if he or she is on target with the response made. Empathic responses can be made into tentative questions, or other kinds of questions can be asked in a tentative fashion.	"Sounds like you are feeling happy about how you are succeeding at work?" "Is it that you have a lot of mixed feelings about being pregnant?"
Why Question	A question in which the intent is to have the client delve deeply into self. However, clients often feel defensive with why questions, and they should generally be avoided.	"Why do you think your partner reacts in the manner that she does?" "Why do you feel that way?"

When to Use Questions

Direct and closed questions are good to use when gathering specific information quickly, thus expediting a session. In this age of accountability and brief therapy, such questions come in quite handy at the beginning of therapy, when gathering information during an intake interview, or when conducting a structured interview (see p. 127 of this chapter). In contrast to direct and closed questions, open and tentative questions are seen as more effective in facilitating a deeper helping relationship and should generally be used when there are fewer time constraints or intermittently during the information-gathering phase of the helping relationship to help build the counselor–client alliance.

Although questions can be helpful in uncovering patterns, inducing self-exploration, and in challenging the client to change, their careless use can be detrimental. For instance, the overuse of questions can set up an atmosphere some consider derogatory, in which "the interviewee submits to this humiliating treatment only because he expects you [the clinician] to come up with a solution to his problem or because he feels that this is the only way you have of helping him" (Benjamin, 1987, p. 72). Some suggest that questions can lead to an authoritarian atmosphere that fosters dependence on the clinician (Byrne, 1995; Cormier & Nurius, 2003). Still others believe that asking a question is not as helpful as making an empathic response (Neukrug, 2003a, 2003b, 2004; Rogers, 1942). This is because a good empathic response is seen as empowering—it allows clients to feel as if they are discovering answers on their own. In fact, an empathic response can often be made in place of a question.

Although much more can be said about the different uses of questions in the interviewing process, suffice it to say that one should be careful whenever questions are asked. Keeping this in mind, Benjamin (1987) suggests the following when asking questions:

- Are you aware of the fact that you are asking a question?
- Have you weighed carefully the desirability of asking specific questions and challenged their usage?
- Have you examined the types of questions available to you and the types of questions you personally tend to use?
- Have you considered alternatives to the asking of questions?
- Are you sensitive to the questions the interviewee is asking, whether he or she is asking them outright or not? And, most significantly,
- Will the question you are about to ask inhibit the flow of the interview?

EXERCISE 6.5 **Identifying Types of Questions**

Decide if the following are direct, closed, open, or tentative questions. Also, discuss whether some questions could be a combination of questions. Finally, offer alternative responses to the one given in the question.

TYPE OF QUESTION OR RESPONSE

Example 1

Question: Did you feel sad or angry about your daughter running away? — Closed Question

Alternative Response: It sounds like you had some strong feelings about your daughter's behavior. — Empathy

or

Example 2

Question: What did you do about the pregnancy? — Direct Question

Alternative Response: You must have had some difficult decisions to make about the pregnancy. Is that true? — Tentative Question

Question 1: Did you feel apprehensive or calm about the licensing exam? ____________

Alternative Response: ______________________________ ____________

____

Question 2: How did you feel about your friend's diagnosis? ____________

Alternative Response: ______________________________ ____________

____

Question 3: How angry were you when your friend did that to you? ____________

Alternative Response: ______________________________ ____________

____

Question 4: How often do you get into it with your wife? ____________

Alternative Response: ______________________________ ____________

____

Question 5: Is it that you were feeling pretty upset about being betrayed? ____________
Alternative Response: ____________________________ ____________

____

Question 6: How many times a week do you have a panic attack? ____________
Alternative Response: ____________________________ ____________

____

Question 7: Would you like to tell me more about that? ____________
Alternative Response: ____________________________ ____________

____

Question 8: Might you have some strong feelings about the accident? ____________
Alternative Response: ____________________________ ____________

____

Question 9: Do you think it will take days or months to get over this? ____________
Alternative Response: ____________________________ ____________

____

Question 10: How many times have you been in counseling and who did you see for counseling? ____________ ____________
Alternative Response: ____________________________

____

Question 11: Why did you believe that talking with your wife would alleviate the problem? ____________ ____________
Alternative Response: ____________________________

____

Question 12: It seems like you tried particularly hard to mend the pain between you and your mom. Did I get that right? ____________ ____________
Alternative Response: ____________________________

____

Conducting a Structured Interview

The use of questions is particularly helpful when conducting a structured interview, which by its very nature is an information-gathering process. Often, the structured interview is conducted when clients first contact an agency, during their initial intake interview. The structured interview has as its basis a preset format that gives the clinician a mechanism to gather information in a consistent, concise, and expeditious manner, and it has become an important precursor to developing treatment goals and treatment plans. Prior to conducting the structured interview, the clinician should offer the client a professional disclosure statement and obtain informed consent for treatment.

Professional Disclosure Statements and Informed Consent

As noted in Chapter 2, generally, when initially meeting a client, the clinician first introduces himself or herself and then discusses the nature of the interview. Often, this is done by offering clients a *professional disclosure statement,* which is a statement, often in writing, describing the nature of the helping relationship (see American Mental Health Counselors Association, 1987; Corey, Corey, & Callanan, 2003). The professional disclosure statement usually includes information about the helping process, the clinician's theoretical orientation and credentials held, the purpose of the interview, relevant agency rules, limits to confidentiality, legal issues, fees for service, and other important information relative to the helping relationship (Corey et al., 2003). The agency itself can develop a professional disclosure statement, but if your place of employment does not have such a statement, develop your own and/or encourage your agency to adopt one (see Exercise 6.6).

EXERCISE 6.6 **Developing a Professional Disclosure Statement**

Using the outline below, develop your own professional disclosure statement. Keep the statement under one page and have a place for your client to sign. After you are finished, meet in small groups and receive feedback about your statement. Your instructor may ask for students to volunteer to read their professional disclosure statements to the class.

Explanation of the helping process:

Clinician's theoretical orientation:

Credentials held:

Relevant agency rules:

Limits to confidentiality:

Relevant legal issues:

Fees for service:

Other:

PROFESSIONAL PERSPECTIVES 6.2
Informed Consent

Informed Consent

I have read the professional disclosure statement provided by ______________, and I understand all aspects of it or have asked my therapist to explain those aspects that were not clear to me. This includes an understanding of the helping process, knowledge of the credentials and relevant background of the clinician with whom I am working, agency rules and legal issues, fees for services, and the limits of confidentiality. I willingly agree to participate in counseling and realize that I can stop counseling at any point in its process.

____
Clinician's Signature and Date

____
Client's or Parent's Signature and Date

After the client has reviewed the professional disclosure statement, the clinician should have him or her give *informed consent* to partake in the interview. Such consent requires the client to give verbal or written permission to participate in the helping interview. Professional Perspectives 6.2 offers an example of an informed consent statement that can be used with a client. However, you would probably want to develop your own based on the unique needs you may have in your clinical setting. After you have reviewed the informed consent statement, go on to Exercise 6.7.

EXERCISE 6.7 **Informed Consent Form**

Using the professional disclosure statement presented in Exercise 6.6, sit down with a student in class and role-play a beginning helping relationship. As you begin, offer the professional disclosure statement to your client, and after he or she has read it and following any discussion that has taken place about it, obtain informed consent from your client.

After giving the client a professional disclosure statement and obtaining informed consent, the clinician is ready to gather information. Some information can be gathered by having the client fill out forms; other information requires that the clinician ask questions.

The Use of Questions in Conducting the Interview

To make the information-gathering process as smooth as possible, it is important to ask questions in a manner that is comfortable for the client and at the same time accomplishes the task of gathering information. Although any type of question already discussed in this chapter can be used, attention should be paid to how the client is responding. For instance, clients will often respond in a more pleasant fashion to open and tentative questions as opposed to direct and closed questions. However, because direct and closed questions are generally more efficient at gathering information quickly, they are sometimes preferred. We urge you to find a balance between the use of these different types of questioning techniques because it is as important to build and maintain a strong relationship with your client as it is to gather information.

As noted earlier, in addition to asking questions during the interview, it is imperative that one regularly use foundational skills. Asking questions of a sensitive nature often touches on a client's emotionally raw areas. Thus, it is crucial that the clinician listen attentively and be empathic when painful issues arise. In fact, it is sometimes important to delay the gathering of information because it is more humane to be empathic to a particular issue than it is to gather the information. In addition, empathy at this stage will help build the relationship and can help gather information that might not be gained through the rather sterile question-and-answer process. Again, the bottom line is for each clinician to find a balance among using questions, being empathic, and gathering information in a manner helpful to the client.

How to Gather Information

You have handed out your professional disclosure statement, obtained informed consent, and now you're ready to gather the information. A good method is to have a preset process that allows you to go down a list and obtain specific information. These days, there are a number of computer programs that can assist you in doing this. For instance, one such program (Schinka, 2003) has the clinician or the client complete 120 items that asks clients to divulge information about a wide range of personal items and provides a computer-generated report that covers such areas as the client's presenting problems, legal issues, current living situation, tentative diagnoses, emotional state, treatment recommendations, mental status, health and habits, disposition, and behavioral/physical descriptions. These case reports have become so sophisticated that they are often a great help to clinicians when they prepare their own reports.

Although these computer-generated case reports can be helpful, there is still value to the tried-and-true method of conducting a clinical interview. The benefits of such an interview are many and include:

1. setting a tone for the types of information that will be covered during the sessions to come
2. allowing the client to become desensitized to information that can be very intimate and personal
3. allowing the clinician to assess the nonverbals of the client while he or she is talking about sensitive information, thus giving the clinician a sense of those items that might be important to focus on
4. allowing the clinician to learn firsthand the problem areas of the client; this can help the clinician remember the client in a more detailed and personal manner, which is not accomplished through a computer-generated report
5. giving the client and clinician the opportunity to study each other's personality style to assure that they can work together

When you are ready to gather information, Drummond (2004) suggests the following guidelines before and during the interview:

1. Have a clear idea of why the individual is being interviewed. The kinds of questions asked depend on the types of inferences, decisions, or descriptions to be made after the interview. Better information results from specific goals.
2. Be concerned about the physical setting or environment for the interview. Interviews will go better if the environment is quiet and comfortable. If the room is noisy or has poor lighting, it may detract from the quality of the information gained. Comfortable and private facilities permit the client to relax without the confidentiality and privacy of the interview being threatened.
3. Establish rapport with the interviewee. Good rapport helps the interviewee to be cooperative and motivated.
4. Be alert to the nonverbal as well as verbal behavior of the client. How a person says something may be as important as what is said.
5. Be in charge and keep the goals of the interview in mind. Have the interview schedule readily available but do not suggest answers. Give the client time to answer and do not become impatient during periods of silence. (p. 276)

What to Assess

Whether you are using a computer-generated report or are conducting a clinical interview, there are a number of areas that most clinicians will assess when conducting a structured interview, including demographic information, reason for referral or contact, family of origin background, current family background, cross-cultural issues, educational and vocational background, medical/psychiatric history, substance abuse history, legal issues and history, and mental status. Information gathered from these categories as well as the diagnosis and the summary, conclusions, and recommendations for treatment are usually included in a case report (see Professional Perspectives 6.3). This report is often assessed by funding agencies and supervisors, can be helpful in remembering important client issues, and is helpful in treatment planning.

Although all aspects of the structured interview are critical to fully understanding your client and coming up with treatment options, the mental status exam has become an increasingly important aspect of the clinical interview and deserves special attention.

The Mental Status Exam

In this age of diagnosis, brief treatment, and the necessity of developing treatment plans for which one is accountable, the mental status exam has become one aspect of information gathering that has gained increasing importance (Aiken, 2003). A mental status exam is an assessment of the client's appearance and behavior, emotional state, thought components, and cognitive functioning. This assessment is used to assist the clinician in making a diagnosis and in treatment planning (Polanski & Hinkle, 2000). A short synopsis of each of the four areas of the mental status exam follows.

APPEARANCE AND BEHAVIOR This part of the mental status exam reports the client's observable appearance and behaviors during the clinical interview. Thus, such items as manner of dress, hygiene, body posture, tics, significant nonverbals (eye contact, wringing of hands, swaying), and manner of speech (e.g., stuttering, tone) are often reported.

EMOTIONAL STATE When assessing emotional state, the client's affect and mood are examined. The affect is the client's current, prevailing feeling state (e.g., happy, sad, joyful, angry, depressed, etc.) and may also be reported as constricted or full, appropriate or inappropriate to content, labile, flat, blunted, exaggerated, and so forth. The client's mood, on the other hand, represents long-term, underlying emotional well-being and is usually assessed through client self-report. Thus, a client may seem anxious and sad during the session (affect) and report that his or her mood has been depressed.

THOUGHT COMPONENTS The manner in which a client thinks reveals much about how he or she comes to understand and make meaning of the world. Thought components are generally broken down into the content, and the process, of thinking. Clinicians will often make statements about thought content by addressing whether the client has delusions, distortions of body image, hallucinations, obsessions, suicidal or homicidal ideation, and so forth. The kinds of thought processes often identified include circumstantiality, coherence, flight of ideas, logical thinking, intact as opposed to loose associations, organization, and tangentiality.

COGNITION Cognition includes a statement as to whether the client is oriented to time, place, and person (knows what time it is, where he or she is, and who he or she is); an assessment of the client's short- and long-term memory; an evaluation of the client's knowledge base and intellectual functioning; and a statement about the client's level of insight and ability to make judgments.

Although much more can be said about each of the four areas, when incorporating a mental status exam into a case report, all four areas are usually collapsed into a one- or two-paragraph statement about the client's presentation. Generally, a statement about the client's demeanor, orientation, affect, intellectual functioning, judgment, insight, and suicidal or homicidal ideation is included. However, many times, other areas are only reported if significant. Thus, referring back to Sienna, our case illustration from Chapter 2, let's look at an example of a mental status exam:

Sienna was appropriate in dress and appearance and her eye contact seemed appropriate. She was oriented by time, place, and person. She presented with a low mood and her affect was depressed. She seemed somewhat fatigued and was a bit slow in her verbal responses. There was no apparent delusions or hallucinations. Sienna appeared to be above average intellectually and her memory was intact. Her judgment seemed good, her insight was high, and she appeared motivated for treatment. She reported occasional, passing thoughts of "wanting to die" but denies any immediate plan to act on these thoughts and does not appear to be an immediate risk for self-harm.

EXERCISE 6.8 **Writing a Mental Status Report**

Keeping the elements of the mental status exam in mind, one student in class should volunteer to role-play a client being interviewed by a counselor for an intake interview. (It might also help if the student chose to reflect a diagnosis in *DSM-IV-TR*.) After the role-play is complete, all other students in class should write a mental status report. Share your reports with the instructor and come up with one mental status report for the class. Compare your report to the final version produced in class. This type of role-play can be repeated in small groups if you would like to gain further practice writing mental status reports.

PROFESSIONAL PERSPECTIVES 6.3
Outline for Structured Interview and Subsequent Case Report

DEMOGRAPHIC INFORMATION

Name of Client: ______________________

Date of Birth: ______________________

Address: ______________________

Phone (home and work): ______________________

E-mail Address: ______________________

Current Place of Employment: ______________________

Financial Status: ______________________

Disability: ______________________

Language Spoken: ______________________

Race/Ethnicity/Cultural Background*: ____________

REASON FOR REFERRAL OR CONTACT

1. Who referred the client to the agency?
2. What is the main reason the client contacted the agency?

FAMILY OF ORIGIN BACKGROUND

1. Relationship with parents or guardians with whom client grew up
2. Relationship with siblings when growing up
3. Relationship with significant others when growing up

CURRENT FAMILY BACKGROUND

1. Relationship with significant individuals in client's family or extended family (e.g., spouse, significant other, children and stepchildren, others living in current home)
2. Significant events related to family or extended family

CROSS-CULTURAL ISSUES (e.g., client believes he or she is being discriminated against)

EDUCATIONAL AND VOCATIONAL BACKGROUND

1. Describe current employment of client
2. Describe educational background of client
3. Describe vocational background of client
4. Describe educational and vocational background of parents, siblings, and spouse if significant

MEDICAL/PSYCHIATRIC HISTORY

1. Health of client
2. Health-related issues of significant others
3. History of prior counseling if any
4. History of psychiatric admissions if any

(*continued*)

PROFESSIONAL PERSPECTIVES 6.3 (*continued*)

SUBSTANCE ABUSE HISTORY
1. Alcohol
2. Drug Use
3. Eating Disorders
4. Smoking

LEGAL ISSUES AND HISTORY
1. Contact with police
2. Current legal problems if any
3. History of any acting out or violent behavior

MENTAL STATUS
1. Appearance and behavior
2. Emotional state
3. Thought components
4. Cognitive functioning

TENTATIVE *DSM-IV-TR* DIAGNOSIS (see Chapter 8)
Axis I: Clinical Disorders and Other Conditions That May Be a Focus of Clinical Attention:
Axis II: Personality Disorders and Mental Retardation
Axis III: General Medical Conditions
Axis IV: Psychosocial/Environmental Stressors
Axis V: GAF Score (at intake)

SUMMARY, CONCLUSIONS, AND RECOMMENDATIONS
This section offers a brief summary of information gathered in the report, offers tentative hypotheses about the client's state of well-being, and often results in a series of possible treatment options.

* Some clinicians only use this category if they believe it is relevant to the client's situation. Others regularly use this category.

EXERCISE 6.9 **Practicing Structured Interviews**

Each student in the class should find a partner. Have one student role-play a clinician while the other role-plays a client. Each clinician should first present his or her professional disclosure statement to the client and follow that by giving the client a copy of an informed consent form. Have the client sign the form. Then, using your foundational skills (listening and empathy) and your questioning skills, go through the structured interview format listed in Insert 6.3. After you have completed gathering information from your client, ask for feedback about his or her experience of the process. The following questions might facilitate the feedback process.

1. Did your client understand your professional disclosure statement?
2. Did your client understand the informed consent form?
3. Did your client feel comfortable during the session?
4. Would your client recommend a greater or lesser use of questions?
5. Did your client feel "heard" during the session?
6. Did your client experience the clinician as caring, open, nondogmatic, accepting, and real?
7. Were you able to "build an alliance" with your client through this process?
8. Other feedback?

Administering Assessment Procedures

The process of gathering information can often be maximized and expedited through the use of assessment techniques (Mehr, 2004; Neukrug & Fawcett, 2005). Because gathering information quickly was not stressed in the past, assessment techniques did not have the same urgency that they have today. Assessment techniques are generally classified as "formal" or "informal," and there are advantages to each type. Formal assessment techniques, such as standardized, norm-referenced tests, are often used when one wants to gather very focused information and when it is important to compare clients to their peer group within the general population. Informal assessment techniques are generally more open to interpretation and allow for a wide range of client responses.

Formal Assessment Techniques

Generally, when we talk about formal assessment instruments, we mean the administration of tests that are valid, reliable, practical, cross-culturally fair, and specific to the issue at hand. Today, there are literally hundreds of potential assessment instruments that can be administered. Generally, clinicians will administer specific tests based on the information they would like to obtain. Some of the more popular test categories that might be administered include:

1. a test to assess psychopathology and assist in diagnostic formulations (e.g., MMPI-II)
2. a test to measure depression and suicidal ideation (e.g., the Beck Depression Inventory—BDI)
3. a test to assist in helping individuals understand personality styles and relationship issues (e.g., the Myers–Briggs)
4. a test to assess substance abuse (e.g., Michigan Alcoholism Screening Test—MAST)
5. a test that can be used to assess personality style and to assist the client in the self-discovery process (e.g., the California Psychological Inventory—CPI)
6. an intelligence test to assess general intellectual functioning, brain damage, and learning disabilities (e.g., WISC-III, the Stanford-Binet)
7. a projective test to assess underlying personality components (e.g., the Rorschach, the Thematic Apperception Test—TAT)
8. an interest inventory to assist in career exploration (e.g., the Strong)

Although this text will not focus on the use of formal assessment instruments, in your training you will likely be exposed to many tests that can be used in this process. As you continue to learn about testing in other courses, consider which ones might be useful to you when working with clients.

Informal Assessment Techniques

A large number of informal assessment techniques can also be used, especially when you are looking to gather a wide range of information and want the client to have greater freedom of response during the assessment process. A few examples of such instruments include clinician-made ratings scales, sentence completions, client diaries, client autobiographies, observation of clients, interviewing others about clients (parents, significant others), drawings (e.g., asking clients to draw a picture of their family), and genograms. The genogram, we believe, needs special attention because it is a method of quickly uncovering a number of inherited and learned traits that might be critical toward your work with your clients.

Genogram

Genograms are an excellent tool to examine, in detail, a family's functioning over a number of generations. Although the basic genogram includes such items as dates of birth and death, names, and major relationships including breakups or divorces, usually the therapist will also ask the family to include such things as where various members are from, who might be scapegoated and/or an identified patient, mental illness, disabilities, cultural or ethnic issues, physical diseases, affairs, abortions, and stillbirths (Figure 6.1).

EXERCISE 6.10 **Completing a Genogram**

Using the items identified and the genogram in Figure 6.1 as a model, complete a genogram of your family, or, if you're working with a client or, a fellow student, complete a genogram of that person.

Timing of Assessment Techniques

Assessment techniques can be administered at varying times during the interview, and their administration should be based on one's counseling philosophy and the needs of the counseling setting. For instance, administering some assessment measures prior to starting the helping relationship has the following advantages:

- They do not interfere with the building of the helping relationship or a natural flow that has begun to develop.
- They can help to identify problem areas quickly and thus focus the clinical interview.
- They can quickly identify problem areas that may be missed during the clinical interview because clients might reveal something on a written measure that they would not reveal face to face (e.g., suicide ideation, alcoholism, abuse).
- They can help set a tone that anything is fair game to discuss.

On the other hand, offering assessment measures during or after the clinical interview has begun, has the following advantages:

- Assessment techniques can be tailored to the specific issues at hand—issues that were raised during the clinical interview.
- In some cases, the building of rapport early in the relationship can raise the likelihood that clients will be more honest when taking the assessment instruments.
- Assessment instruments can give the client and the clinician a needed break in the sometimes arduous interviewing process.

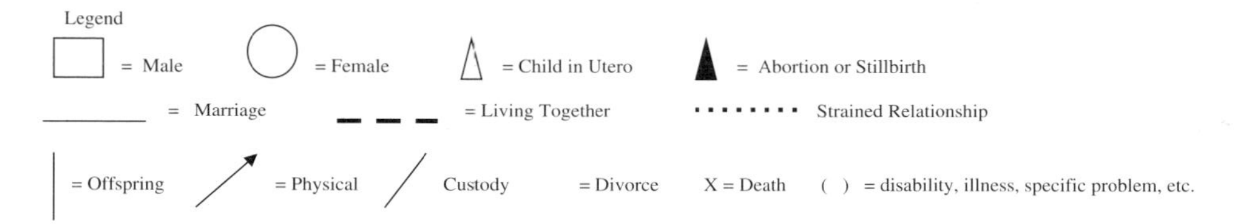

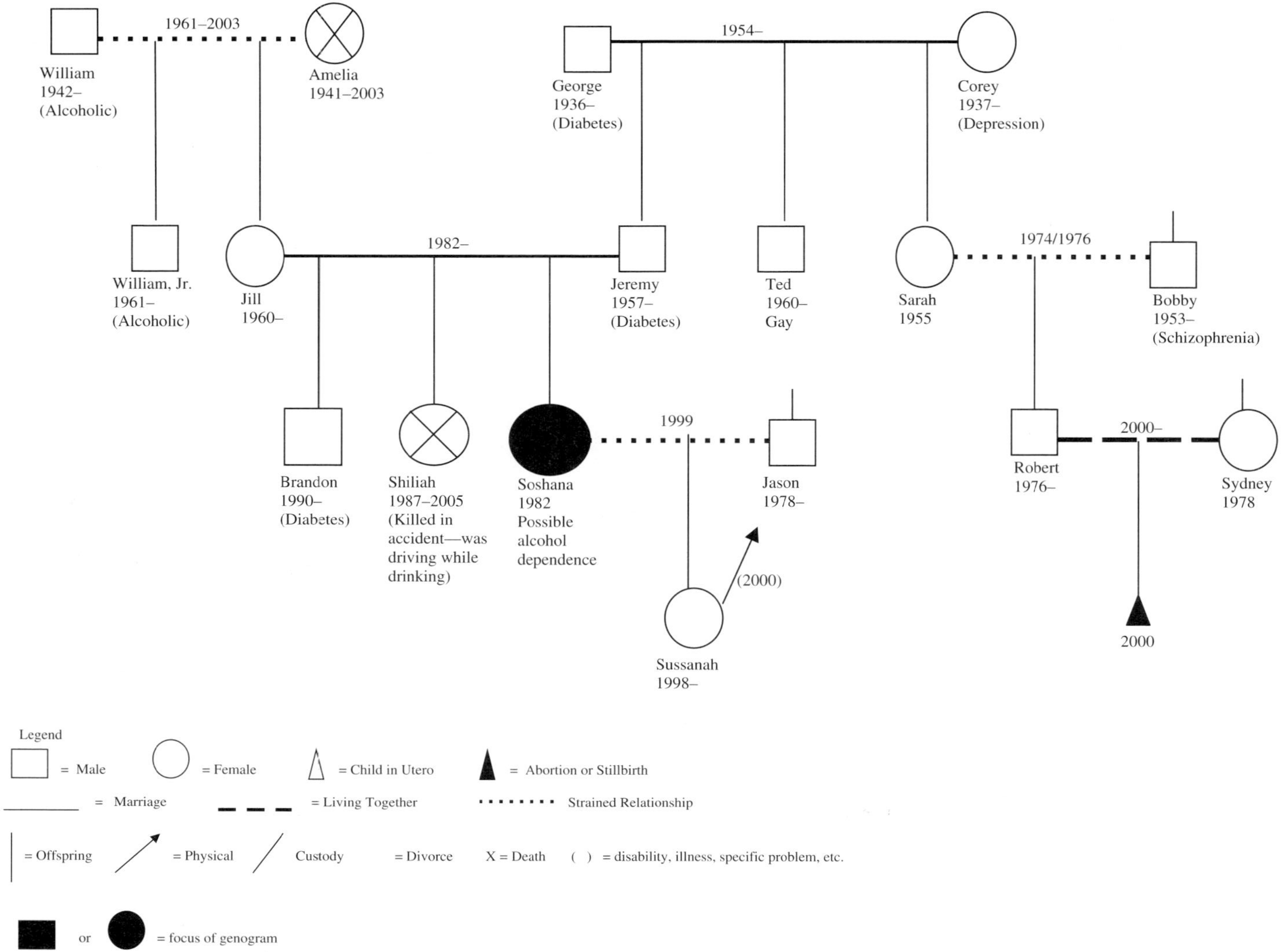

Figure 6.1 Soshana's Genogram

Writing a Case Report

One natural outgrowth of the information-gathering process is the integration of all the information gathered into a case report. Today, reports are often carefully scrutinized because they are the mechanism used by the interviewer to communicate his or her assessment to others and are often used by funding agencies and supervisors when evaluating a clinician's work. Thus, when writing a report, the interviewer needs to make the report clear, concise, and easy to understand (Harvey, 1997; Neukrug & Fawcett, 2005).

Due to laws, such as the Family Educational Rights and Privacy Act of 1974, the Freedom of Information Act, and the Health Insurance Portability and Accountability Act (HIPAA), clients will often have access to their records. Therefore, it is suggested that a report be written so that a non–mental health professional could understand it and with the expectation that the client or the client's parents might have access to it. Thus, the following is often recommended for writing reports (Drummond, 2004; Harvey, 1997; Neukrug & Fawcett, 2005):

1. Keep sentence lengths relatively short.
2. Minimize the number of difficult words.
3. Reduce the use of jargon and acronyms.
4. Omit passive verbs.
5. Increase the use of subheadings.
6. Don't be judgmental.
7. Only label when necessary and beneficial to the client's well-being.
8. Describe behaviors that are representative of client issues.
9. Dont be afraid to take a stand if you feel strongly that the information warrants it (e.g., the information leads you to believe a client is in danger of harming self).
10. Point out both strengths and weaknesses of your client.

Lengths of case reports will vary depending on the purpose of the report, the agency, and your writing style. Typically, an initial intake summary may be between one and four pages long. Toolbox C shows an example of an initial intake summary using the categories suggested in this chapter. Chapter 11 on case management presents some additional examples of case reports and case notes. Exercise 6.11 gives you an opportunity to practice writing a report. Use the sample case report in Toolbox C as a model when completing this exercise.

Pulling It All Together

In this chapter, we discussed the use of a number of information-gathering techniques that are critical to the work of the counselor. The use of questions, the structured interview, and assessment procedures are all critical to successfully understanding the client and making plans for change. Exercise 6.11 gives you the opportunity to practice all of these skills.

EXERCISE 6.11 **Pulling It All Together**

Part I: Practicing the Structured Interview

In class, the instructor should ask students to break into dyads. In your dyads, have one student be the counselor and the other the client. The role-play should be audio- or videotaped. Then, spend a minimum of 45 minutes conducting a structured interview with the client, starting with giving your professional disclosure statement and obtaining informed consent. In conducting the interview, balance your use of questions with your foundational skills and use assessment instruments if appropriate and available. If time allows, switch roles. Then, prior to the next class, have each student critique the tape. At the next class, students can discuss how they did.

Part II: Writing an Intake Report

Now that you have gathered all of the information from the structured interview, you may want to practice writing an intake report using the same headings from the structured interview and then adding the five axes diagnosis, the summary, conclusions, and recommendations. Toolbox C offers an example of such a report using Sienna as our client.

LEARNING TO BE A COUNSELOR: An Ongoing Process

The natural helper knows how to ask questions—perhaps too well. Thus, we learned in Chapter 5 the importance of learning how not to ask questions. Now, here we are again learning how to ask questions. But this time there's a twist. Professional counselors have a specific method to their madness! This clinician knows when to ask questions, knows how to use them appropriately, and knows which questions to ask. It is not a haphazard use of questions as with the natural helper, and it is always with an eye toward balancing the use of questions with foundational skills, such as empathy. This process of knowing how, when, and what questions to use and how to balance their use with other skills occurs over one's professional life. We are always trying to find the best and most efficient ways to simultaneously gather information and to build the relationship—the best ways to obtain an in-depth understanding of our clients while maintaining a strong alliance that can help lead the client toward change. This is a never-ending process.

Chapter Summary

In this chapter, we discussed some important ways to gather information from a client. Examining the use of questions, we explored when questions should be used, if used at all, and then we examined different kinds of questions. First, we looked at direct questions, such as when the clinician is attempting to obtain specific information from a client. Next, we looked at closed questions that delimit content and closed questions that delimit affect. Such questions limit the kinds of responses the client can make. Open questions, or questions that enable a wide range of client responses, were the next kind of question we examined. We noted that empathic responses could be converted to a tentative question by adding an inflection at the end of the response. We suggested this might be done when a clinician is not sure he or she has heard the client accurately. We also noted that regardless of the type of question being asked, it can be asked in a tentative manner that tends to "sit" better with the client. Finally, we examined the use of why questions, suggesting that they probably should be used very sparingly if at all.

We suggested when to use different types of questions. We noted that direct and closed question are best when you need to gather specific information rather quickly, thus expediting a session. In contrast, we suggested that open and tentative questions are seen as more effective at facilitating a deeper helping relationship and should generally be used when there are fewer time constraints. We noted that sometimes the use of questions may lead to a helping relationship that is authoritarian in nature and/or may foster a dependence on the clinician as the client is more likely to rely on the clinician for lending direction to the helping relationship. We ended this section by offering some pointers a clinician can use when deciding whether or not to use a question.

The next part of this chapter examined how to conduct a structured interview as one method of obtaining information from your client. Prior to conducting a structured interview, however, we noted the importance of distributing to the client a professional disclosure statement. Such a statement should explain the clinician's theoretical orientation, credentials held, relevant agency rules, limits to confidentiality, relevant legal issues, and fees for service. After giving a professional disclosure statement, we noted the importance of obtaining informed consent from the client for counseling.

In conducting a structured interview, we suggested that to make the information-gathering process as smooth as possible, it is important to use questions but to ask them in a manner that is comfortable to the client. Because direct and closed questions tend to be quicker in obtaining information, we suggested they are often more efficient than open or tentative questions at gathering needed information. However, we urged clinicians to find a balance between the use of these different types of questioning techniques and the use of one's foundational skills because it is as important to maintain a strong relationship with your client as it is to gather information.

When gathering information, we suggested that clinicians could use a computer-generated report but noted that there may be some advantages to conducting a clinical interview instead of, or along with, a computerized evaluation. These included the fact that a clinical interview helps to set a tone, allows the client to become desensitized to the sharing of very intimate information, allows the clinician to assess the nonverbals of the client, allows the clinician to hear and ultimately remember the problem areas presented firsthand and in a detailed and personal way, and helps the clinician and client decide whether or not they can work with one another.

The chapter next examined the mental status exam, an increasingly important aspect of the structured interview. We highlighted and discussed four areas of the mental status exam, including appearance and behavior, emotional state, thought components, and cognitive functioning.

We noted that the mental status exam is one of a number of areas addressed in the structured interview, which generally should include all of the following: demographic information, reason for referral or contact, family of origin background, current family background, cross-cultural issues, educational and vocational background, medical/psychiatric history, substance abuse history, legal issues and history, and mental status. We also suggested that a case report can be generated from the information gained and that this report often includes all of the above areas as well as a tentative diagnosis, summary, recommendations, and treatment plans.

We next discussed the importance of the administration of assessment procedures in the information-gathering process. We noted that assessment has become increasingly important because it can expedite this process. We discussed the advantages of offering assessment prior to and at the beginning of the helping interview. We then distinguished between formal and informal assessment techniques, noting that formal assessment techniques usually include standardized, norm-referenced tests and that informal techniques involve clinician-made assessments that allow the client a wide range of responses. We listed some of the more popular formal assessment techniques, as well as some common informal assessment techniques, with particular emphasis on the genogram.

The case report, we noted, is a natural outgrowth of the information-gathering process and, in these days of accountability, increasingly important to the overall case management process. We thus offered a number of important points to consider when writing the report, including keeping sentences short, minimizing difficult words, reducing the use of jargon and acronyms, omitting passive verbs, using subheadings, not being judgmental, being careful about labeling, describing representative client behaviors, taking a stand when necessary, and pointing out both strengths and weaknesses.

As the chapter ended, we suggested that the professional counselor should know when to ask questions, how to use them appropriately, and which questions to ask. We highlighted the fact that asking questions is not haphazard, as it is with the natural helper, and that it always is with an eye toward balancing the use of questions with foundational skills, such as empathy. We suggested that the professional counselor is always improving his or her ability at finding this important balance.

CHAPTER 7

Commonly Used Skills: Affirmation Giving, Encouragement, Modeling, Self-Disclosure, Confrontation, Offering Alternatives, Information Giving, Advice Giving, and Collaboration

In contrast to the critical skills and attitudes identified in Chapters 4, 5, and 6, not all clinicians consider the commonly used skills in this chapter essential to the helping relationship. However, most of them are used by clinicians, and they often enhance the helping relationship by adding to its scope and depth.

Whereas the natural helper might use many, if not all, of the skills discussed in this chapter in a haphazard manner, the professional counselor understands the positive and negative aspects of their use and thus employs them in a deliberate manner and only when it appears as if they will be helpful. The important, but not necessarily essential, skills we look at in this chapter include affirmation giving; encouragement; modeling; self-disclosure; confrontation; the problem-focused skills of offering alternatives, information giving, and advice giving; and collaboration.

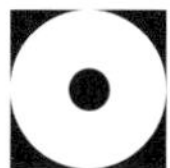

At this point, we recommend that you pause reading the text, turn to the DVD, and view the section entitled:

Affirmation Giving and Encouragement

Affirmation Giving

"Good job making it this far in the book!" You have just been affirmed, and hopefully, it felt good. Affirmations are a natural part of being human. Unfortunately, many of us, and particularly many of our clients, have not been affirmed enough by significant persons in our lives. This often results in low self-esteem and difficulty, or even the inability, to affirm others. Clients need to learn how to affirm themselves, and self-affirmation often has its beginnings in affirmation by others. The clinician can be a significant person to bring such affirmations to clients. Fleeting statements such as "good job" and "I'm happy for you," or strong handshakes, warm hugs, and approving smiles, are just a few of the ways clinicians affirm their clients. Whether called reinforcement, or a genuine positive response to a client's work in therapy, such responses can greatly affect the client.

For years, the affirmation of clients was viewed negatively by many of the traditional psychotherapeutic approaches because it was seen as potentially fostering an external locus of control (Benjamin, 1987). More recently, however, the role of the clinician has changed and broadened, and from most theoretical perspectives, affirmations are now regularly seen as a genuine and caring response to a client that can encourage work in therapy. As you practice this skill, reflect on how comfortable you are giving and receiving such positive feedback (see Exercise 7.1).

EXERCISE 7.1 **Giving Affirmations**

Part I: The instructor should have the class mingle in an open space. Go up to other students in class and tell them something that you like about them. It could be the way they interact in class, how they dress, how they present themselves, and so forth. See how it feels to offer other persons in class an affirmation.

Part II: Write down your name in large letters on an envelope handed out by the instructor. The instructor will find some place to post the envelopes, and during the days or weeks that follow, any student can place an affirmation in your envelope. The affirmation giver can either state his or her name or not, but whatever is written must be an affirmation—nothing negative. Periodically, the instructor can process the kinds of affirmations, if any, students are receiving and how they feel about receiving or not receiving affirmations.

Part III: Break into dyads and role-play a client–counselor situation in which a client is working on specific goals. During the role-play, attempt to affirm the client's goal-seeking behaviors. In small groups, discuss how productive such affirmations were.

Encouragement

Although similar to affirmations, encouragement is focused more on helping a client achieve a specific goal. For instance, a clinician might encourage a client whose goal is to attend Alcoholics Anonymous meetings by saying something like, "I know you're nervous about going, but I also know that you can do it." Like affirmations, encouragement was not stressed in counseling for many years. Today, encouragement is seen as an intervention that can be periodically rather potent (Orlinsky, Ronnestad, & Willutzki, 2004), and most theoretical perspectives view it as an important and genuine way to help a client reach goals in therapy (see Exercise 7.2).

EXERCISE 7.2 **Encouraging One Another**

Break down into dyads and have one person discuss a real situation in which he or she is struggling (e.g., losing weight, finding a job, communicating more with a loved one, etc.). The "counselor" should encourage the client by saying things like, "I know you can do it," "I have confidence that you have the personal fortitude to do this," and so forth. After a few minutes, switch roles. After you have completed the exercise, form groups of eight to ten students and discuss how it felt to be encouraged by another person.

Remaining in your groups, have one student agree to share a personal life problem with everyone else in class. Have that person sit in the middle of the room, and when appropriate, any class member can encourage him or her. Class members should only say something if it feels genuine. If time allows, other members of the group can sit in the middle and share their life issue. After the exercise is completed, the "client" should discuss how it felt to receive such encouragement.

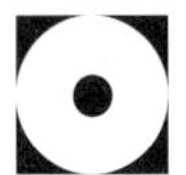

At this point, we recommend that you pause reading the text, turn to the DVD, and view the section entitled:

Modeling and Self-Disclosure

Modeling

Irrespective of one's theoretical orientation, clinicians will act as models for their clients regardless of whether or not they want to be (Brammer & MacDonald, 2003). Clinicians are constantly modeling for their clients. If they are empathic, then clients may learn how to listen to loved ones more effectively. If they are assertive, then clients may learn how to positively confront someone in their lives. And if they can show a client how to resolve conflict, then clients may learn new ways of dealing with conflict in their lives. By using modeling, clinicians can be change agents in two ways: inadvertently or intentionally.

PROFESSIONAL PERSPECTIVES 7.1

Too Much of a Good Thing?

When I [Ed Neukrug] was working with a 16-year-old who had low self-esteem, poor social skills, and few friends, I would affirm the client and encourage him to try out new behaviors. For instance, I would encourage him to go to the movies, just so he would be getting out of his house, and to call a fellow student, in an effort to make friends. In addition, I would encourage him to make positive self-affirmations that he would practice at home. Thus, he would often be saying to himself things like, "I'm worthy and I'm capable." In fact, it began to be a little bit of a joke, when he began to address me as "Stuart Smalley," the guy from *Saturday Night Live* who used an overdose of self-affirmations. Finally, when ending counseling, he gave me a Stuart Smalley audiotape to remind him how much he had been encouraged to make those self-affirmations.

Inadvertent Modeling

Inadvertent modeling is the unplanned adoption of behaviors exhibited by the clinician on the part of the client. The majority of modeling that occurs in the therapeutic relationship is inadvertent. The inadvertent model does not purposefully set out to change specific client behaviors. Instead, this clinician acts as a model through his or her "way of being" in the counseling relationship. In this instance, clients pick up behaviors through passive observation of the therapist. For instance, the humanistically oriented therapist models through the manner in which he or she builds a relationship (e.g., empathy, genuineness, etc.). The behaviorally oriented therapist models through the use of behavioral strategies with the client (e.g., use of operant or classical conditioning techniques or social learning), and the psychodynamic therapist models through the use of such techniques as empathy, analysis, and interpretation. For instance, imagine a clinician who is showing good attending behavior, such as eye contact and silence with a client. The client might learn how to do similar attending to loved ones by having experienced it with the clinician.

Modeling seems most effective when the model has perceived power, status, competence, and knowledge (Baum & Gray, 1992). Because it is common for clients to look up to clinicians, even idealize them, the behavior of clinicians may be perceived powerfully by clients (Brammer & MacDonald, 2003). Therefore, clinicians should not underestimate inadvertent modeling because it will occur in all helping relationships. Exercise 7.3 helps you look at how you have inadvertently modeled from others.

EXERCISE 7.3 **Inadvertent Modeling**

On the top row of the grid are individuals who have been a model for one of the authors. In the space provided in the second row, qualities modeled from these significant people by the author have been listed. In the third row, qualities observed in others that the author would like to integrate into his personality are listed. Examine the completed grid, and in the spaces provided in the second grid, fill in the appropriate spaces yourself, listing individuals you have modeled or would like to model. If you have additional names you would like to add to your grid, create a new grid on a blank piece of paper.

(continued)

EXERCISE 7.3 *(continued)*

PERSON YOU MODELED

	My Father	Roger: My First Therapist	My Wife	????
Qualities Modeled from the Person Listed	Integrity: My father always appeared honest and thoughtful.	Empathy: He was great at exhibiting empathy and I learned how to be empathic with othersby being in counseling with him.		
Qualities Viewed That You Would Like to Model	Patience: He was always soft-spoken and didn't jump into making rash decisions.		Slow Eating: My wife eats slowly and savors every bite. I eat too fast and too much.	

PERSON YOU MODELED

Qualities Modeled from the Person Listed				
Qualities Viewed That You Would Like to Model				

Intentional Modeling

Intentional modeling is the planned viewing and subsequent adoption of desired behaviors by clients. Many clinicians use intentional modeling as an important tool in their arsenal of behavioral change methods. Intentional modeling offers clinicians a number of ways to have clients adopt targeted behavior, including: (a) through the deliberate display of specific behaviors on the part of the clinician (e.g., expressing empathy, being nonjudgmental, being assertive), (b) through the use of role-playing during the session (e.g., the clinician might role-play job interviewing techniques for the client), and (c) by teaching the client about modeling and encouraging him or her to find models outside of the session to emulate (e.g., a person who has a fear of speaking to a large group might choose a speaker he or she admires and view the specifics of how this individual makes a speech) (Perry & Furukawa, 1986).

Intentional modeling involves a two-part process that starts with observing a targeted behavior and then moves to practicing that behavior. Thus, clients need to have appropriate models to imitate and need to practice the desired behavior within and/or outside the session. With intentional modeling, any targeted behaviors the client wishes to acquire need to have a high probability of being adopted. As an example, a client who has a fear of making speeches would first need to find a model to emulate. After observing this model, the client would make a list of those speech-making qualities he or she would like to emulate. Then, the client would practice the emulated qualities with a predetermined number of people or groups, moving from low-anxiety situations to more challenging ones. For instance, he or she might first make a speech to his or her clinician, then to some trusting friends, then to a small group of trusted colleagues, and so forth—perhaps asking for feedback along the way to sharpen his or her performance. Using these "baby steps" assures that there will be a high probability that the client will successfully adopt the targeted behavior, in this case, making speeches.

Intentional modeling is a powerful tool that can be used by clinicians to effectively change client behavior. This kind of modeling necessitates a trusting relationship, should be carefully and deliberately planned, and requires a thorough assessment of the client's needs to assure the appropriate choice of targeted behaviors. Therefore, intentional modeling is generally not used at the beginning of the helping relationship, as it takes time to build rapport and establish an accurate assessment of the client and his or her situation (see Exercise 7.4).

EXERCISE 7.4 **Intentional Modeling**

Part I: In the space provided, list some qualities you would like to adopt, as identified in Exercise 7.3. Then, write out specific ways that you could practice exhibiting those identified qualities. In small groups, share the qualities and discuss your specific plan for acquiring them. Some groups might want to meet on an ongoing basis to encourage the acquisition of the qualities and to assure that each student is following through on his or her plan. In your small groups, you might also want to discuss how these qualities might work positively for you as a clinician. If you do meet in small groups, don't forget to affirm and encourage one another.

QUALITIES YOU WOULD LIKE TO OBTAIN	MECHANISM FOR ACQUIRING THE QUALITIES LISTED
1.	1.
	2.
	3.

(*continued*)

EXERCISE 7.4 *(continued)*

2.
1.
2.
3.

3.
1.
2.
3.

4.
1.
2.
3.

Part II: Using the vignettes that follow, develop a way that you can intentionally model a behavior that would be of use with the client.

Vignette 1: Mary has come to counseling because she feels as if she is a "doormat" for others. She describes herself as "Cinderella" in that others always tell her what to do and how to do it. She rarely, if ever, challenges what others say to her. She is married and has two children. She describes her husband as "demanding," the type of man that "wants his dinner when he wants it," and she states that he is totally in charge of the financial situation in the home. She reports having little money to purchase needed items like clothes for the children.

Vignette 2: Juan sees himself as unlovable. He has strong feelings for his partner but states that he cannot express them to him. He states that he does not feel like he can express loving feelings to others because he does not love himself. He describes his low self-esteem as stemming from a distant mother and a verbally abusive father who often would tell Juan he was "useless."

Vignette 3: Jillian believes that she can no longer effectively parent her three children, ages 8, 7, and 4. She describes her children as out of control and states they do not respond to her angry tone. She states that she tries to put them in time out, but that does not work. She now believes that her only resort is to punish them by taking privileges away and through spankings.

Part III: In dyads, discuss a counselor–client situation in which you believe intentional modeling might be effective. Then, break into dyads and role-play the situation. Discuss the effectiveness of this process in small groups.

Self-Disclosure

Self-disclosure on the part of the clinician is the revealing of parts of oneself in an effort to strengthen the counseling relationship, help the client feel comfortable with self-disclosure, and offer a new way of being in relationships. If applied properly, clinician self-disclosure can be important and helpful for clients (Kleinke, 1994; Pennebaker, Colder, & Sharp, 1990; Pennebaker & Susman, 1988). However, clinicians should recognize that research on its efficacy has shown it to be at best a mixed bag (Orlinsky et al., 2004). This may be due to the fact that clients would rather talk about themselves than learn through the experience of others. When practicing self-disclosure, it is critical to assure that self-disclosure is not the result of unfinished business on the part of the clinician who needs to discuss his or her own issues. This kind of

PROFESSIONAL PERSPECTIVES 7.2
Inappropriate Self-Disclosure

A former student of mine [Ed Neukrug] was in therapy with a psychiatrist, who, over time, increasingly began to disclose his problems to her. One day, she heard that he had hanged himself. Following his death, she revealed that she felt intense guilt that she hadn't saved his life. What a legacy to leave this student. Clearly, the psychiatrist's self-disclosure was unhealthy and unethical.

self-disclosure is inappropriate and unethical, as indicated by the American Psychological Association Code of Ethics (2003) as well as related ethical codes (see Professional Perspectives 7.2).

> *When psychologists become aware of personal problems that may interfere with their performing work-related duties adequately, they take appropriate measures, such as obtaining professional consultation or assistance, and determine whether they should limit, suspend, or terminate their work-related duties.* (Section 2.06.b)

Although you should be wary about the use of self-disclosure, when used appropriately and in a well-timed manner, it can add to the repertoire of clinical techniques and lead to positive client outcomes. Kleinke (1994) identifies two types of self-disclosure: *content self-disclosure*, when one reveals information about himself or herself, and *process self-disclosure,* when one reveals information about how the clinician is feeling toward the client at the moment.

Content Self-Disclosure

In contrast to natural helpers, who periodically self-disclose aspects of their lives without considering the reasons or outcomes, content self-disclosure involves a deliberate decision on the part of clinicians to reveal some aspect of their lives in an effort to enhance the helping relationship. Appropriate content self-disclosure can show the client that the clinician is "real" and thus create a stronger alliance with the client. In addition, such disclosure can create deeper intimacy, which ultimately could foster deeper self-disclosing on the part of the client. Finally, content self-disclosure can offer the client new behaviors to model. An example of content self-disclosure might be the following:

> Clinician: *You know, when I was younger, I also had panic attacks. Although very scary, through my own therapy, I found that my panic attacks were messages to myself about aspects of my life that I needed to change. Perhaps this could be the case with your panic attacks?*

Notice in the example how the clinician finishes the self-disclosure with a "tentative" question. This is an important technique as it brings the situation back to the helpee, and its intent is to offer a mechanism for developing new understanding of self, not new understanding about the clinician. Such self-disclosure should be done very carefully because some clients might think less of the clinician, believing that a clinician should have his or her act together, whereas others might feel put off by a clinician's temporary focus on self (see Professional Perspectives 7.3).

PROFESSIONAL PERSPECTIVES 7.3

Content Self-Disclosure with a Client

When I [Ed Neukrug] was working with a client who was sharing some information about her problem with compulsive overeating, I had considered sharing some of my past difficulties with the same issue. I believed the client might feel an increased bond as a result of the sharing. For about 2 months, I considered sharing this issue and finally noted to her during a session that "I had struggled with compulsive overeating also." Her response: She looked at me and, without skipping a beat, continued to talk about herself, as if I had never said anything. She wanted to talk about herself, and my issues were irrelevant to her purposes in the helping relationship.

Process Self-Disclosure

Similar to the concept of "immediacy," process self-disclosure involves the clinician's sharing a moment-to-moment experience of self in relation to the client (George & Cristiani, 1994). Such process comments can have a number of positive effects. For example, they can help clients see the impact they have on the clinician and, ultimately, on others in their lives. They can help a client see how moment-to-moment communication can enhance relationships. Finally, process self-disclosure can act as a model for a new kind of communication that can be generalized to important relationships in the client's life.

Some have warned clinicians to be careful about when to share moment-to-moment feelings with clients. For instance, Rogers (1957) pointed out that clients were rapidly changing as they shared deeper parts of themselves, and as they changed, the clinician's feelings toward them would likely change. Thus, he suggested that most of the time it was probably more helpful to share longer term feelings, as these are more meaningful to the relationship.

When to Use Self-Disclosure

Regardless of the kind of self-disclosure, its effectiveness has been found closely related to the expectations clients have about how appropriate self-disclosure is to the therapeutic process and to what they expect to gain from it (Derlega, Lovell, & Chaikin, 1976; Neimeyer, Banikiotes, & Winum, 1979; Neimeyer & Fong, 1983). Therefore, the degree to which the clinician self-discloses should be directly proportionate to how much the client expects self-disclosure to be a part of the helping process. In general, self-disclosure needs to be done sparingly, at the right time, and only as a means for client growth—not to satisfy the clinician's needs (Evans, Hearn, Uhlemann, & Ivey, 2004). A general rule of thumb is: If it feels good to self-disclose, don't, because you're probably meeting more of your needs than the needs of your client (see Exercise 7.5). Finally, we agree with Kahn (1991),who states that,

> *I try not to make a foolish fetish out of not talking about myself. If a client, on the way out the door, asks in a friendly and casual way, "Where are you going on*

your vacation?" I tell where I'm going. If the client were then to probe, how "Who are you going with? Are you married?", I would likely respond, "Ah . maybe we'd better talk about that next time." (p. 138)

EXERCISE 7.5 **Practicing Self-Disclosure**

Part I: Students should pair up based on whether or not they have had one of the following problem situations in their lives.

1. Divorce
2. Getting fired
3. Being "dumped" by a significant other
4. Problem pregnancy
5. Trust issues with a friend
6. Parenting issues
7. Financial problems
8. Marital problems
9. Disliking parent(s)

Now, in your dyad, have one person act as counselor while the other plays the client. The client should talk about the chosen situation for about 5–10 minutes, during which the clinician should attempt to make at least one self-disclosing response that relates to the situation. If possible, the response should be given in a manner that facilitates the client's exploration of self. After you are finished, if time allows, switch roles. In class, address the following questions:

1. Was the self-disclosure on the part of the clinician helpful?
2. Did the client develop a greater alliance with the clinician as a result of the self-disclosure?
3. Did the self-disclosure change the focus of the session in any manner?
4. Did the self-disclosure result in the relationship feeling too "friendly"?
5. Were there better responses than self-disclosure?

Part II: With another student in class, role-play a client–counselor situation for at least 15 minutes. During that time, when appropriate, attempt to use content and/or process self-disclosure. In class, discuss the same questions noted in Part I.

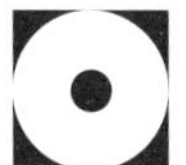

At this point, we recommend that you pause reading the text, turn to the DVD, and view the section entitled:

Offering Alternatives, Information Giving, Advice Giving

Problem-Focused Skills

Problem-focused skills, such as offering alternatives, giving information, and giving advice, can be particularly helpful in guiding a client toward reaching goals or assisting a client in finding some thoughtful short-term solutions (Kleinke,1994). Because students enter the helping professions wanting to help, these responses are often seen as a quick fix and are generously used by students ("I too can be Dr. Laura or Dr. Phil"). In contrast, the experienced professional counselor is wary of overusing problem-focused skills because they tend to encourage an overreliance on the helper, thus fostering dependence (Benjamin, 1987; Kleinke, 1994), and research has shown that the overuse of these types of responses is not particularly helpful to the counseling relationship (Kleinke, 1994; Orlinsky et al., 2004). Thus, the experienced professional counselor knows how to assess whether or not the use of these skills will be helpful and employs them only in a deliberate and purposeful manner.

Offering Alternatives

Offering alternatives is a mechanism for the clinician to extend realistic choices when assisting a client toward achieving his or her goals. This kind of response suggests that there may be a number of ways to tackle the problem and provides a variety of options from which the client can choose. Compared to information giving and advice giving, offering alternatives has the least potential for harm because it does not presume there is one solution to the problem. It also has the least potential of setting up the helper as the final expert and, to some degree, allows the client to pursue various choices while maintaining a sense that he or she is directing the session. Finally, of the three types of problem-focused responses, it is the least judgmental.

Offering alternatives should be used only when the clinician (a) believes the client has not considered the alternatives about to be offered, (b) is confident that the client is ready and willing to work on the alternatives about to be offered, and (c) believes the alternatives about to be offered fit into the treatment plan (see Exercise 7.6).

EXERCISE 7.6 **Practicing Offering Alternatives**

Form triads and in each group have one student be a counselor, one a client, and one an observer who will assist the counselor if needed. The client should talk for a few minutes about a real or made-up problem, and the counselor is to offer possible alternatives to the client. It is probably best if at first you use your basic listening and empathy skills in an effort to fully understand the problem being presented. Then, after you understand the problem, offer alternatives. The observer can suggest alternatives to the counselor if he or she is having difficulty coming up with some. After a few minutes, if time allows, switch roles. If you have additional time, you can switch roles again. After you have finished, discuss in your triad the questions listed. Students in each triad may want to share their responses with the whole class.

1. How easy or difficult was it for the counselor to come up with alternatives?
2. Did the client already know the alternatives being offered?
3. Was offering alternatives helpful?
4. Would other techniques have been more helpful than offering alternatives?
5. How did the client react to being offered alternatives?
6. Did offering alternatives change the tone of the counseling relationship? If so, how?

Information Giving

Information giving is a response that offers the client important "objective" information. The key to making a successful information-giving response is to offer useful information of which the client is truly unaware and which the client is likely to use to his or her benefit. This may not be as easy as it seems, as clients often know more than clinicians might suspect. Because information-giving responses assume that the helper has some valuable information that the client needs, these responses tend to set up the helper as the expert, increasing the potential for the client to become dependent on the relationship.

Information giving should be used only when the clinician (a) believes that the client does not have the information about to be given, (b) is confident that the client is ready and willing to work on the information about to be offered, and (c) believes the information about to be offered fits into the original treatment plan (see Exercise 7.7).

EXERCISE 7.7 **Information Giving**

Part I: Have a student who is an expert in some area of counseling (e.g., problem pregnancy, substance abuse, etc.) role-play a clinician while another student role-plays a client who has a problem in the area in which the clinician is an expert. At some point during the role-play, the clinician should offer information to the client. Then, in small groups or as a class, assess the following:

1. Ask the role-play client if the information given was helpful.
2. Was the information given new to the client?
3. Discuss the timing of the information giving. Was it given too early? Too late? At just the right time?
4. Should information have been given at all?
5. What alternatives were there, if any, to information giving?
6. Do you think that information giving could lead to a dependent counseling relationship?
7. Did offering information change the tone of the counseling relationship? If so, how?

Part II: Break into triads and have one person role-play a clinician, one a client, and a third be an observer. At some point in the role-play, the clinician should offer information to the client. Answer the same questions as in Part I.

Offering Advice

Many receive advice, only the wise profit from it. (Chinese fortune cookie)

The third problem-focused response, offering advice, occurs when the helper offers his or her expert opinion in hopes that the client will follow the suggestions. As with the previous two kinds of problem-focused responses, this kind of response has the potential for developing a dependent relationship, as the client could end up relying on the helper to solve problems. In addition, advice giving may resemble control issues from the client's family of origin (e.g., parents giving advice or telling a child what to do) and is a value-laden response. Some consider advice giving a response that should be avoided (see Benjamin, 1987). However, this response has the potential of assisting a client in finding solutions quickly. And you should keep in mind that there are many ways to give advice. For example, a helper need not act like a tyrant while giving advice (see Exercise 7.8).

Advice giving should be used only when the clinician (a) believes that the advice about to be offered has not been considered by the client, (b) is confident that the client is ready and willing to work on the advice about to be offered,

(c) believes the advice about to be offered fits into the original treatment plan, and (d) thinks the client is not working on deep-seated family of origin issues related to criticism and control.

EXERCISE 7.8 **Advice Giving**

Part I: Have one student sit in the middle of three concentric circles. The student in the middle is to role-play a client problem. The innermost circle is to offer advice in a gruff, authoritarian manner. For instance, students in this circle might start responses with statements like, "You should . . . !" or "It's imperative that you . . . !" The middle circle is to offer advice in a milder form but still with a dogmatic tone. Some examples of how these students might start responses include: "Why don't you . . . ?" or "You might want to . . ." The outermost circle is to offer advice in a mild, tentative way while attempting to avoid being authoritarian. Students in this circle might start their responses with statements like, "I've been wondering if you ever thought about . . . "or "Have you ever given thought to . . . ?"

You may want to have a few students take turns sitting in the middle of the circles. After you have done this exercise for 10 or 15 minutes, the students who sat in the middle should share how they experienced each of the circles. Also, individuals in the circles might want to share how they experienced the exercise.

Part II: Break into triads and have one person role-play a clinician, one a client, and a third be an observer. At some point in the role-play, the clinician should offer advice to the client. After you have finished, respond to the following questions:

1. Was the advice given helpful to the role-play client?
2. Was the advice given not previously considered by the client?
3. Was the advice given in a well-timed fashion (e.g., when the client could take it in)?
4. Should advice have been given at all?
5. What alternatives were there, if any, to advice giving?
6. Do you think that advice giving could lead to a dependent counseling relationship?
7. Did offering advice change the tone of the counseling relationship? If so, how?

Final Thoughts on Problem-Focused Responses

As the helper moves from offering alternatives to giving information to giving advice, the responses become more value laden and helper centered, and thus the responses become potentially more destructive (Doyle, 1998) (Figure 7.1). Therefore, the decision as to whether any of these responses is used within the clinical relationship should be based on a careful understanding of the client's needs and whether an alternative response could be more effective for the client. Meichenbaum (cited in Kleinke, 1994) notes that when the helping relationship is at its optimal, the timing of this kind of response should be such that the client is "one step ahead" of the solution offered (p. 87). Thus, in essence, the client is gaining so much from the helping relationship that he or she is coming up with solutions prior to the helper suggesting them.

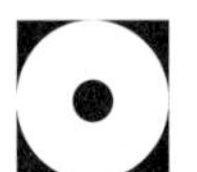

At this point, we recommend that you pause reading the text, turn to the DVD, and view the section entitled:

Confrontation

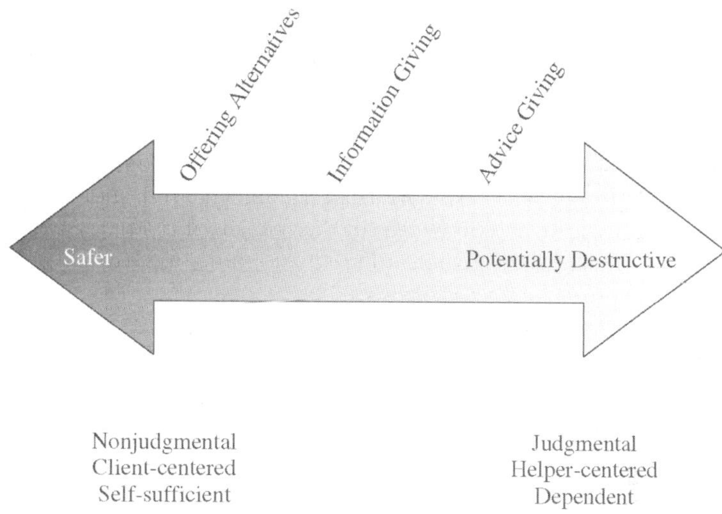

Figure 7.1 Comparison of Damaging Effects of Problem-Focused Strategies

Confrontation

Support, Then Challenge

Although the natural helper generally views confrontation as an aggressive challenge in an effort to change the client's point of view, the professional counselor views it as a gentle push that offers feedback to the client and invites the client to gain an alternative understanding of his or her current situation (Byrne, 1995; Thompson, 2002; Toth & Erwin, 1998). Thus, confrontation is not (a) yelling at a client, (b) telling a client what to do, (c) acting as if you are the authority figure who has "the answer," (d) laying guilt trips on a client for not accomplishing his or her goals, or (e) acting cynically toward a person and treating a client like he or she is not worthwhile.

Confrontation first involves building a trusting and caring relationship, often through the use of your foundational skills. The building of such a relationship is then followed by gentle prodding that carefully pushes the client toward change. This mild confrontation reduces the likelihood that any psychological harm will occur to the client (Egan, 2002; Kleinke, 1994; Young, 1992). Such support, *then* challenge, offers the best potential for clients to hear feedback about themselves and eventually change their perception of reality (Neukrug, 1997, 2002, 2004).

Identifying Client Incongruencies

Confrontation in the helping relationship can assist clients to see incongruencies among their words, feelings, and/or behaviors. Hackney and Cormier (2005) and Neukrug (2003) have highlighted what they describe as discrepancies between a client's (a) *values* and *behavior*, (b) *feelings* and *behavior*, (c) *idealized self* and *real self*, and (d) *expressed feelings* and *underlying feelings,* of which the client is unaware. Let's briefly examine each of these potential client discrepancies followed by ways of confronting them.

Discrepancy between a Client's Values and Behavior: When a client expresses a specific value and his or her actions do not match that expressed value, an incongruency exists. For instance, suppose a client has been an antiabortion advocate and then tells you that her 15-year-old daughter is pregnant and she is "making her" get an abortion.

Discrepancy between a Client's Feelings and Behavior: Sometimes a client might assert certain feelings and then act in a manner that seems to indicate otherwise. For instance, suppose a client says he loves his partner and then goes on to note how often he beats her and cheats on her.

Discrepancy between Idealized Self and Real Self: Some clients might idealize the ways in which they would like to act and then find excuses for why they do not actually act in that manner. For instance, a client might state that he wants to be more real in relationships and then state that he can't be honest with people because if he was really honest, others would not like him. Or a client might state, "I want to communicate effectively with others" but then finds reasons for not acting in that manner: "If only I had more time to work on my communication problems."

Discrepancy between Expressed Feelings and Underlying Feelings: A fourth type of discrepancy is between a client's verbal expression of feelings and the underlying feelings to which a client won't admit or is not currently aware. An example is a client who states she is feeling anxiety related to her marriage and yet seems to be holding back tears.

Challenging Client Incongruencies

Pointing out a discrepancy can help a client see the incongruency in how the client lives in the world. A number of ways exist to point out discrepancies in relatively gentle ways, including you–but statements, gently asking the client to justify the discrepancy, reframing, using satire or irony, and higher level empathy.

1. *You–But Statements*. You–but statements contrast one aspect of the client's feelings, beliefs, or values with another aspect that contradicts the first (Hackney & Cormier, 2005). For instance, to a client who states he believes in honesty but is having an affair, the clinician might state:

Clinician: *You say that you believe in honesty, but you seem to be hiding a serious matter from your wife.*

2. *Gently Asking the Client to Justify the Discrepancy.* A second method of gently confronting a client's discrepancy is by using a tentative question to ask the client to explain the apparent contradiction.

Clinician: *Help me understand how, on the one hand, you say you are honest, and on the other hand, you're hiding an affair from your wife?*

PROFESSIONAL PERSPECTIVES 7.4
Confronting Sally

Sally was in a verbally abusive relationship. Even though she had no major bills, she insisted that she could not leave the relationship and live on her "meager" $70,000 dollar salary. Clearly, her verbal statement that she could not leave the relationship did not match the reality that one could live on this amount (certainly, most of us would be happy to live on this amount). After building a relationship using empathy, Sally had her perception of her situation gently challenged by using many of the techniques above. Using you–but statements, the obvious discrepancy between her salary and her ability to live on her own was highlighted. Asking her to explain her understanding of this situation was a second method used, and it assisted her in seeing that her logic did not hold up. Using higher level empathy helped her see a deeper issue—that she felt as if she was a failure in the relationship and was scared to be alone (she was a recovering alcoholic and was concerned she would start drinking again if alone). Ultimately, Sally was encouraged to work on communication issues with her lover, while at the same time her situation was reframed so she could believe that she could live on her own if she eventually chose to do this. The result for this client was that she became a more assertive woman who improved her communication with her lover and could realistically see her choices about staying in the relationship or finding a place on her own.

3. *Reframing*. A third way of confronting a discrepancy is by reframing, which is offering the client an alternative way of understanding his or her situation. This new understanding can offer alternative issues for the client to work on.

   Clinician: *Even though honesty is important to you, sometimes other values seem to take priority. In this case, your fear of your marriage disintegrating, should your wife find out about the affair, seems more important than being honest.*

4. *Using Satire or Irony*. The use of satire or irony in an effort to highlight the absurdity of a discrepancy is a fourth way to challenge a client, although it is a potentially harsher confrontation than those previously listed and should be carefully considered before using. For instance, continuing with the example, you might say:

   Clinician: *Well, I guess it's okay in this instance to be dishonest. After all, you're saving your wife from those painful feelings. Aren't you???*

5. *Higher Level Empathy*. The final way of challenging a client's discrepancy is through the use of higher level empathic responses. By reflecting back to clients their underlying, out-of-awareness feelings and conflicts, this kind of response challenges clients to expose deeper parts of themselves. For instance, in the same example:

   Clinician: *You must be feeling quite conflicted. On the one hand, you say you believe in honesty, but on the other hand, you are hiding an affair. I guess I sense there is more to this story for you.*

EXERCISE 7.9 **Responding to Discrepancies**

Using the discrepancy categories discussed earlier in the chapter—(a) values and behavior, (b) feelings and behavior, (c) idealized and real self, (d) expressed and underlying feelings—generate a list of client scenarios that accentuate each of these scenarios. The instructor should summarize the scenarios on the board.

Next, have students form small groups, with each group representing one of the five ways to confront discrepancies (see below). In your small groups, come up with responses to the client scenarios using the confrontational technique assigned to your group and write them in the space provided. When you have finished in your groups, pick a spokesperson to share the responses. If time allows, have each group take one or more of the other confrontational techniques and make additional responses to the scenarios. Share them in class.

Group 1: You–But Statements:

Group 2: Asking the Client to Justify the Discrepancy:

Group 3: Reframing:

Group 4: Using Satire or Irony:

Group 5: Higher Level Empathy:

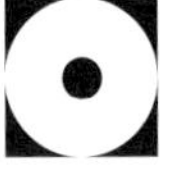

At this point, we recommend that you pause reading the text, turn to the DVD, and view the section entitled:

Collaboration

Collaboration

Collaboration in the counseling relationship involves communicating to your client that you value his or her feedback and that you want to come to a mutually agreed upon decision about the next phase in treatment (Dinnebeil, Hale, & Rule, 1996). Here, the clinician is asking for feedback from the client as to his or her assessment of the counseling relationship thus far and uses techniques that lead to a mutual decision about the future of treatment. Collaboration uses a combination of techniques and follows a format that generally reflects the following:

1. The use of foundational skills to offer a summary of what has been discussed thus far.
2. Asking the client, through the use of questions, how he or she feels about the course of treatment thus far.
3. Asking the client, through the use of questions, about the direction he or she would like to take in treatment.
4. Sharing with the client your own thoughts about which areas might be important to focus on (advice giving).
5. Having an honest discussion concerning any discrepancies between items 3 and 4, which leads to a mutual decision about the course of treatment.

Collaboration can and often does occur throughout the helping relationship and is often most useful at transitional points, such as (a) after rapport and trust building and prior to problem identification, (b) after problem identification and prior to the development of treatment goals, (c) after the development of treatment goals and prior to treatment planning, and (d) during the closure stage prior to ending counseling.

Collaboration after Rapport and Trust Building and Prior to Problem Identification

At this transition point, the clinician may be wise to check in with the client to make sure he or she is satisfied with what has occurred thus far and to assure that the client feels good about moving forward. Clinicians might say something like:

> Clinician: *So far we've talked about ______________, and I was wondering what you thought of the process thus far.*

After the client responds, the clinician might say:

> Clinician: *What thoughts might you have about where we should go at this point?*

Then, after the client responds, the clinician might respond with:

> Clinician: *Well, let me share some of my ideas about where we might go.*

This can be followed by a discussion that leads to a mutual understanding of the next phase of treatment.

Collaboration after Problem Identification and Prior to the Development of Treatment Goals

Clients who don't agree with treatment goals do not make progress. Thus, it is critical that the clinician and the client are in agreement concerning which areas to focus on. In this case, the clinician would first summarize the problems identified, and then the client and clinician would jointly decide on treatment goals. Applying our collaboration guidelines to our case illustration of Sienna from Chapter 2, a clinician might say something like the following:

> Clinician: *Well, Sienna, it seems like you have identified a number of issues in your life. You initially noted that you were feeling depressed and not sure why. Included with this were some periodic thoughts of wanting to kill yourself, although you didn't think you would really do that. Some specific issues you then identified were sadness about moving away from home, confusion about whether you wanted to continue in a relationship with your boyfriend, problems with your roommate, finding school more work than you thought it would be, and difficulty concentrating. Later, you began to believe that you were emotionally dependent on others and also stated that you were somewhat confused about what values you embraced.*
>
> *Maybe we can focus on the areas you would like to discuss, and then I would like to share some of my thoughts on what I think might be*

PROFESSIONAL PERSPECTIVES 7.5
A Woman with a Bridge Phobia

I [Ed Neukrug] once worked with a middle-aged women who initially came to therapy because of a bridge phobia. This phobia was debilitating in that she often would have to drive major distances out of her way to arrive at a destination because she was trying to avoid driving over a bridge. After conducting an initial assessment, a number of other issues arose, including unfinished feelings concerning the suicide of her father, whose body she found after he shot himself; unresolved issues with her grown children; and existentially based issues around meaningfulness in life. After identifying these four issues (bridge phobia, father, children, meaningfulness), in collaboration with the client, it was decided not to work on the bridge phobia initially. What followed, for the next year, were weekly sessions that focused on the other three issues. Most of this counseling was done through an insight oriented approach, which was a mixture of person-centered and psychodynamically oriented counseling. Then, one day in therapy, the client stated, "Okay, I'm ready to work on my bridge phobia." At this point, the focus and type of therapy quickly changed, and a number of behavioral strategies were employed. After a couple of months working on the bridge phobia, the client was able to overcome her phobia and freely drove over any bridge. With some follow-up care, the bridge phobia was successfully cured. About a year later, this client sent a letter saying, "I now go to a 'survivor of suicide' group, and every time I go over a bridge to get there, I think of you." What nice feedback!

important. We can, hopefully, then decide on which goals might be best to focus on. Let's start by you highlighting the areas you think would be most important to focus on.

Sometimes, a problem area identified by a client is not an issue that the client wants to work on. In this case, it is important that the clinician understand the reasons a client might want to put off working on a particular area. It is also important to remember that sometimes clients might not be agreeable to focus on certain areas at first but, at a later date, might be open to examining that area (see Professional Perspectives 7.5).

Collaboration after the Development of Treatment Goals and Prior to Treatment Planning

After treatment goals are jointly identified, a collaborative process occurs to determine a treatment plan. Thus, the clinician might say, something like:

Clinician: *Let me summarize some of the jointly identified goals that you and I decided to focus on, including ____________. Let's talk about how we can tackle some of the goals and work on making some changes in your life. I have some thoughts, but I would like to hear what you think before I share them.*

Then, after the client and clinician share thoughts and ideas, the two should mutually agree on the treatment plan (Young & Long, 1998). It is critical that this is a joint decision, as clients do not always agree with a clinician's thoughts about treatment. For instance, a clinician might think an antidepressant medication would be helpful for Sienna, but she might have strong negative feelings about taking such medication and be adverse to such a referral. Or as in the example noted in Insert 7.5, although the client initially identified a problem driving over bridges, this is not an area that she wished to focus on initially. The clinician therefore has a responsibility to discuss this issue at length with the client and come up with a mutually agreed on plan. This process allows the client to "buy into" the treatment plan and is more likely to lead to success.

Transition Out of the Closure Stage

Collaboration is also very common as you near the end of the helping relationship. At this point, the clinician might say something like:

> Clinician: *Well, we certainly have examined some important issues in your life and, I believe, have made some progress. For instance, we ______________. What are your thoughts about what we have done?*

And after the client responds, the clinician might share some of his or her thoughts about the progress made and then say something like:

> Clinician: *We're going to be ending counseling soon, and I would gather you have some thoughts and feelings about that. I too have some thoughts and feelings. Maybe we can discuss those and make sure that we're in sync with how we are going to say our good-byes, discuss any unfinished business that may be lingering, and address any ideas we both might have about follow-up or future counseling.*

EXERCISE 7.10 **Practicing Collaboration Skills**

Break into dyads and have one student role-play a counselor and the other a client. The counselor should practice applying the collaborative guidelines noted earlier in one or more of the transition points identified: (a) after rapport building and prior to problem identification, (b) after problem identification and prior to the development of treatment goals, (c) after the development of treatment goals and prior to treatment planning, and (d) during the closure stage prior to ending counseling. After the role-play is complete, review the process with the client to make sure he or she felt heard and included in this process.

Pulling It All Together

Now that we have examined attitudes, foundational skills, information gathering, and commonly used skills, you have all that is necessary in your beginning journey to being an effective clinician. Now it's time to practice this array of attitudes and techniques. But before we practice, let's revisit the attitudes and skills needed.

In Chapter 3, we highlighted eight important attitudes that every clinician should embrace prior to imparting on a counseling relationship. These included being empathic, genuine, accepting, open-minded, cognitively complex, psychologically adjusted, good at relationship building, and competent. Chapter 4 examined the foundational skills needed by every clinician, which include the proper use of nonverbal behavior, silence and pause time, listening, paraphrasing, and empathy. As we moved on to Chapter 5, we suggested ways of gathering information and examined how the use of different types of questions could be helpful, such as direct questions, closed questions, open questions, and tentative questions. Also in Chapter 5, we discussed how to conduct a structured interview, mental status exam, and what assessment procedures might come in handy when collecting information. Finally, in this chapter, we explored a number of commonly used skills that can be employed during the counseling relationship, including affirmation giving, encouragement, modeling, self-disclosure, offering alternatives, information giving, advice giving, and collaboration. Now, examine Exercise 7.11 and do some role-playing to practice all of the skills you have learned thus far.

EXERCISE 7.11 **Practicing Attitudes and Skills**

Break into dyads and try an ongoing counselor and client role-play that begins with the rapport and trust building stage and continues to the goal setting and treatment planning stage. It is suggested that you audio- and/or videotape the role-play. This might mean that you and your fellow student would be doing an ongoing role-play over a number of sessions. During class or at home, while listening to or viewing the tape, the two of you should complete the rating scale below. Make sure that time is also given for the client to take on the role of counselor.

Rating Scale

1 = Showed Exemplary Ability (only to be used if counselor has mastered this skill)

2 = Showed Appropriate Use (clearly knows the attitude or skill, but needs some practice)

3 = Needs Improvement (needs to work on this attitude or skill)

4 = Not Exhibited

	RATING	DESCRIPTION OF RESPONSE	COMMENTS
Attitudes			
Empathic			
Genuine			
Accepting			
Open-Minded			
Cognitively Complex			
Psychologically Adjusted			
Relationship Builder			
Competence			
Foundational Skills			
Nonverbal Behaviors			
Silence and Pause Time			
Listening			

	RATING	DESCRIPTION OF RESPONSE	COMMENTS
Paraphrasing			
Empathy			
Gathering Information			
Use of Structured Interview			
Use of Questions			
Direct Questions			
Closed Questions			
Open Questions			
Tentative Questions			
Commonly Used Skills			
Affirmation Giving			
Encouragement			
Modeling			
Self-Disclosure			
Confrontation			
Offering Alternatives			
Information Giving			
Advice Giving			
Collaboration			

LEARNING TO BE A COUNSELOR: An Ongoing Process

The natural helper may use most, if not all, of the skills highlighted in this chapter. Certainly, even prior to being counseling students or working clinicians, we all have affirmed and encouraged others' behaviors, been models for others, self-disclosed in an effort to offer a new perspective to loved ones, confronted others because we thought we could help push them to change, and offered alternatives, information, and advice because we cared and hoped others would listen to what we had to offer. However, generally, the natural helper haphazardly uses these approaches to try to get a person to change.

Professional counselors know when and how to use these skills appropriately. And as professional counselors continue on their professional journey, they fine-tune the use of these skills. Some of us will use some of these skills more frequently than others. However, whether one professional counselor uses advice giving frequently and another does not use it at all, both will decide with consciousness and a deliberateness that the natural helper does not employ.

Chapter Summary

This chapter looked at some commonly used skills that are often employed by clinicians but may not be critical to the helping relationship. We first examined the use of affirmation giving, noting that such a humane response can be motivating to some clients. Encouragement, similar to affirmation giving but with a focus on reaching goals, was examined next. Then, we reviewed two types of modeling: inadvertent and intentional. Inadvertent modeling is the unplanned adoption by the client of some of the clinician's behaviors and is a by-product of the helping relationship because the clinician is seen as an important person in the client's life. Often, clients will inadvertently adopt behaviors that are related to the clinician's style of counseling. In contrast, intentional modeling is the planned viewing and subsequent adoption of desired behaviors by clients. Intentional modeling allows clients to adopt any of a number of targeted behaviors in one of the following ways: through the deliberate display of specific behaviors on the part of the clinician, through the use of role-playing during the session, or by teaching the client about modeling and encouraging him or her to find models outside the session to emulate.

The next part of the chapter examined self-disclosure on the part of the clinician, or the revealing of parts of oneself in an effort to strengthen the counseling relationship, help the client feel comfortable with his or her own self-disclosure, and offer a new way of being in relationships. We noted two types of self-disclosure: content self-disclosure, occurring when clinicians reveal factual information about themselves, and process self-disclosure, occurring when clinicians reveal information about how they are feeling toward the client at the moment. We noted that although self-disclosure can be helpful, it should be done only when the clinician believes the client will benefit and when it is not a result of the clinician's own unfinished business.

The problem-focused skills of offering alternatives, information giving, and advice giving were the next commonly used skills examined. We encouraged clinicians to be careful with these kinds of responses, as they will sometimes lead to defensiveness and dependence on the part of the client. We noted that as clinicians move from offering alternatives to giving information to giving advice, they become more value laden in their response mode and more helper centered; thus, the response becomes potentially more destructive.

Next, we examined the commonly used skill of confrontation. We noted that in contrast to the natural helper, who might view confrontation as an aggressive challenge to the client, the skilled clinician sees confrontation as a gentle push to help clients understand deeper parts of themselves. We noted that clinicians will frequently examine and confront four aspects of the client's presentation, including discrepancies between (a) values and behavior, (b) feelings and behavior, (c) idealized self and real self, and (d) expressed feelings and underlying feelings. We next identified a number of relatively gentle ways to raise consciousness concerning a client's discrepancies, including you–but statements, gently asking the client to justify the discrepancy, reframing, satire or irony, and higher level empathy.

Collaboration in the counseling relationship was one of the last skills examined in this chapter. We noted that collaboration involves communicating to clients that you value their feedback and that you want to come to a mutually agreed on decision about the next phase in treatment. We highlighted the fact that collaboration is often best used during transition points in the helping relationship and generally follows a format in which the clinician (a) uses one's foundational skills to summarize what has been discussed thus far, (b) asks the client, through the use of questions, how he or she feels about the course of treatment thus far, (c) asks the client, through the use of questions, about the direction he or she would like to take in treatment, (d) shares with the client his or her own thoughts about which areas might be important to focus on (advice giving), and (e) has an honest discussion concerning any discrepancies between items (c) and (d), which leads to a mutual decision about the course of treatment.

As we neared the conclusion of the chapter, we listed and suggested that you practice all of the attitudes and skills examined thus far in the text. These consisted of the attitudes emphasized in Chapter 4 of being empathic, genuine, accepting, open-minded, cognitively complex, psychologically adjusted, good at relationship building, and competent; the foundational skills of nonverbal behavior, silence and pause time, listening, paraphrasing, and empathy highlighted in Chapter 5; the usefulness of different types of questions, including direct questions, closed questions, open questions, and tentative questions; and the use of the structured interview, discussed in Chapter 6; and the skills of affirmation giving, encouragement, modeling, self-disclosure, confrontation, offering alternatives, information giving, advice giving, and collaboration discussed in this chapter. Finally, we concluded the chapter by noting that in contrast to the natural helper, the professional counselor has learned how to effectively use skills and is continually analyzing the efficacy with which they are being used within his or her own counseling style.

PART THREE

Clinical Tools: Managing the Change Process

In Chapter 1, we introduced four clinical tools that are part of the core areas of knowledge and skills for professional counselors and psychotherapists: diagnosis, case conceptualization, treatment planning, and case management. These clinical tools are the subject of Part III.

Just as the helper attitudes and helping skills we have been discussing in Part II are needed to make the helping relationship successful, the four types of clinical tools of Part III are needed to manage the change process planfully and intentionally. Professional counselors can apply these four tools to the client's problems in a logical order.

The first clinical tool is discussed in Chapter 8, "Diagnosis: Developing *DSM-IV-TR* Skills." Diagnosis is an important tool that is needed to identify and describe the client's concerns. In addition, diagnosis, as defined through the use of the *Diagnostic and Statistical Manual–Text Revision (DSM-IV-TR)*, offers mental health practitioners from varying disciplines a common language when discussing client concerns. Diagnosis starts early in the helping process during Stage 1, the rapport and trust building stage, and is fully implemented in Stage 2, problem identification. Diagnosis can be useful for conceptualizing client concerns and when devising treatment strategies, so you will see it brought into discussions in Chapters 9 and 10, which cover these areas. Finally, diagnosis is also important for case management, especially when describing changes in client behaviors and progress toward treatment goals. Thus, it will also be mentioned in Chapter 11, which discusses the case management process.

The next clinical tool, discussed in Chapter 9, is case conceptualization. Conceptual skills are needed to understand and explain what has led to the client's difficulties, so the helper and client know what areas will need to be addressed to resolve the difficulties. As with diagnosis, case conceptualization takes place early in the process, usually beginning during Stage 2, problem identification, and continuing into Stage 3, goal setting. Chapter 9, "Case Conceptualization: Understanding the Client's Concerns," explains this process and gives a basic, step-by-step guide that beginning clinicians can use to conceptualize client problems. In addition, in this chapter, you will be introduced to popular characters from literature and the media to help you develop your case conceptualization skills. We think you will enjoy and learn from this unique learning tool.

Chapter 10, "Treatment Planning," offers an overview of the treatment planning process, the next clinical tool discussed in Part III. The skills associated with treatment planning are needed to set goals for change and to decide what kind of counseling approach will be best. Thus, the focus of this chapter will be on (a) selecting achievable goals, (b) determining treatment modes, and (c) documenting the attainment of goals. Treatment planning is an outgrowth of diagnosis and case conceptualization and mainly occurs during Stage 3, goal setting. The success of counseling that will follow in Stage 4, work, is an outgrowth of successful treatment planning.

Chapter 11, "Case Management," the last chapter of Part III, examines the case management skills needed to monitor and document the professional helping process and to keep the relationship focused on the client's well-being. Thus, in this chapter, we will examine five elements of this important clinical tool: (a) documentation, (b) consultation, supervision, and collaboration, (c) communication with stakeholders, (d) business-related activities, and (e) caseload management. These case management skills are needed by every competent professional to monitor and safeguard the helping process.

Although not given a separate chapter, one other core area and clinical tool discussed in this part is theory. Theory is described briefly in Chapter 9 as an important tool when applying one's conceptual understanding of the client's problems. In this chapter, it is also noted that students will learn more about theory in a separate course in their training program. Finally, theory is also very briefly discussed in Chapter 10 as an important underpinning of the treatment planning process.

As with the earlier parts of the text, near the end of each chapter you will find a short section that discusses the importance of continuing to develop your skills throughout your career as a clinician.

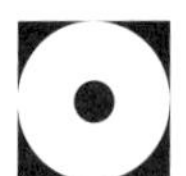

At this point, we recommend that you pause reading the text, turn to the DVD, and view all of the following sections:

Clinical Tools and Intake Interview Introduction

Intake Interview

Working Stage Interview

and

Termination Interview

CHAPTER 8

Diagnosis: Developing *DSM-IV-TR* Skills

An important part of the clinical assessment and appraisal process is skill in the use of mental health diagnosis. Diagnoses serve a number of purposes, including offering a shared language for communication among mental health professionals, being helpful when formulating case conceptualizations, and providing direction when developing treatment plans (see Chapters 9 and 10). Today, nearly all mental health professionals in the United States rely on the *DSM-IV-TR*, or the *Diagnostic and Statistical Manual of Mental Disorders, Fourth Edition, Text Revision* (American Psychiatric Association, 2000) as the main system for making a clinical diagnosis. Therefore, the ability to use the *DSM-IV-TR* is a required professional skill for all counselors and psychotherapists (Seligman, 2004).Whereas the natural helper has only pop-culture knowledge of diagnosis and knows little about its benefits, the professional counselor understands the reasons a diagnosis might be beneficial to clients as well as some of the drawbacks associated with its use.

In this chapter, we first introduce the *DSM-IV-TR* diagnostic system and explain what makes up a diagnosable mental disorder. Next, we explain the *DSM-IV-TR*'s multi-axial system for making a mental disorder diagnosis. This is followed by case illustrations to acquaint new clinicians with *DSM-IV-TR* diagnoses. Finally, we focus on how learning the diagnostic system is a developmental process and provide exercises to help new counselors become familiar with the *DSM-IV-TR*, the diagnoses, and its other contents. To supplement this chapter, Toolbox D provides a broader review of Axes I and II of the *DSM-IV-TR*.

The *DSM-IV-TR* Diagnostic System

The *Diagnostic and Statistical Manual (DSM)* was introduced by the American Psychiatric Association in collaboration with other mental health professional groups in 1952 and underwent revisions in 1964 (2nd edition), 1980 (3rd edition), 1987 (3rd edition, revised), 1994 (4th edition), and 2000 (4th edition, text revision). The current edition, *DSM-IV-TR*, contains about 300 separate diagnoses, is nearly

900 pages, weighs more than 4 pounds, and offers professionals some insight into many of the changes that will take place when *DSM-V* (5th edition) is published.

The advantage of the *DSM* system is that it is comprehensive enough to cover most types of concerns seen in a wide range of mental health settings, but a potential disadvantage is that negotiating the depth and wide range of this information is a formidable task for the new clinician. Therefore, new counselors will gain just a basic introduction to diagnoses in this textbook but will learn more and continue to develop diagnostic skills throughout their training.

In this section, we explain (a) the primary purpose of a diagnosis, (b) what comprises a mental disorder as defined by the *DSM-IV-TR*, (c) what is not a diagnosable mental disorder, (d) the importance of age, gender, socioeconomic status, and cultural considerations when making a diagnosis, and (e) how the *DSM-IV-TR* evolves along with professional advances and social change.

The Primary Purpose of a *DSM-IV-TR* Diagnosis

The primary purpose of *DSM-IV-TR* is to assist the clinician in describing and communicating client presentation and concerns, developing treatment plans, and determining the primary focus of counseling.

Describing and Communicating Client Presentation and Concerns

Perhaps the most important purpose of *DSM-IV-TR* is to help mental health professionals describe and communicate with other professionals who are familiar with the system. It is intended to enhance agreement and improve the sharing of information among clinicians about the client picture they are observing. The system is not intended to reflect any one theoretical orientation. Rather, *DSM-IV-TR* diagnoses are intended to be theory-neutral descriptions of behavior, thoughts, mood, physiology, functioning, and distress. Thus, using *DSM-IV-TR* categories and descriptors allows clinicians to describe clients and communicate with mental health colleagues while applying their own theoretical orientation and treatment plan.

Developing Treatment Plans

Although *DSM-IV-TR* diagnoses do not state a course of treatment to follow, they do provide information that is important and useful when planning treatment. For instance, for each disorder covered in the system, the *DSM-IV-TR* describes:

- the disorder's main features
- subtypes and variations in client presentations
- the typical pattern, course, or progression of symptoms
- how to differentiate the disorder from other similar ones

The *DSM-IV-TR* also provides findings about predisposing factors, complications, and associated medical and counseling problems when they are known. Clearly, based on the theoretical orientation of the clinician, this information can be critical in the development of treatment plans.

Determining the Primary Focus of Counseling

A diagnosis can help a clinician determine the primary focus of counseling. For example, a focus on a mood problem might be dealt with very differently from a focus on somatic complaints, and a focus on an adjustment problem is dealt with very differently from a focus on long-term life patterns, such as a personality disorder. Determining the focus can assist the clinician when deciding if certain interventions are called for, such as medical treatment and group psychotherapy, and social or institutional interventions, such as environmental adaptations in the community, school, or family.

What Is a *DSM-IV-TR* Mental Disorder?

The *DSM-IV-TR* system defines a mental disorder as a clinically significant pattern that occurs in an individual and is associated with present distress, impairment in one or more important areas of functioning, or significantly increased risk of distress or dysfunction (American Psychiatric Association [APA], 1994). Following from this definition, the *DSM* is a classification system of mental disorders that is based on sets of criteria made up of observable features. The job of the clinician is to find the best match between what the counselor observes the client to be experiencing and the criteria for the different clinically significant patterns conceptualized as mental disorders. This categorical, criterion-referenced approach stems from the traditional medical-scientific method of organizing, naming, and communicating information in as objective a fashion as possible (Schwitzer & Everett, 1997).

The *DSM-IV-TR* includes mental disorders of childhood and adulthood. It describes both time-limited difficulties, such as adjustment disorders, and more longstanding problems, such as personality disorders. The system covers a wide range of behavior, from substance abuse to sleep problems to grief reactions, and addresses characteristics of thought, mood, behavior, and physiology.

What Is Not a Diagnosable Mental Disorder?

Although critical in helping the clinician understand client problems, communicate about clients, and plan treatment, it is important to note that the *DSM-IV-TR* does not cover functional, normal, and ordered behavior or expected and culturally appropriate reactions to life events and developmental challenges.

Functional, Normal, and Ordered Behavior

One misperception beginning counselors sometimes have is that using clinical diagnoses, like those of the *DSM-IV-TR,* means that one must view all client concerns and interests from a strictly clinical, psychopathological viewpoint. In reality, the *DSM-IV-TR* system is only used to share information about a very small set of human behavior or experience—those conditions that meet the "mental disorder" definition. In fact, from a diagnosistic standpoint, most human behavior is functional, normal, and ordered rather than dysfunctional, abnormal, or disordered. Each *DSM-IV-TR* mental disorder is constructed to be a distinct pattern of difficulty that is currently causing the client distress, significant impairment in some area of day-to-day functioning, or increased risk of disability (APA, 1994; Schwitzer & Everett, 1997).

Expected and Culturally Appropriate Reactions

Client experiences that are regarded as expected reactions or culturally appropriate responses to life events are not diagnosable as mental disorders, even when they cause distress or dysfunction in the client's life. For example, while counseling may focus on the grief process following the loss of a loved one, a diagnosis of Major Depression usually is not made even when the person experiences major depression criteria such as extreme sadness, insomnia, or poor concentration during the first 2 months following the loss. Even significant disruptions in mood and functioning are agreed to be expected and culturally appropriate during the grief process.

Similarly, client concerns that are regarded as an expected, or culturally appropriate, phase of life developmental experiences are not diagnosed as mental disorders regardless of the distress or dysfunction they may cause in life. For example, identity confusion in adolescence, which is often associated with distress about long-term life goals, relationships, and values, is viewed as a normal, expected experience and therefore not diagnosed as a mental disorder.

Age, Gender, SES, and Cultural Differences in Making Diagnoses

The *DSM-IV-TR* was constructed with much greater attention to issues of age, gender, socioeconomic status (SES), and culture than were past editions. For example, age differences in symptoms often appear in *DSM-IV-TR,* such as the notation that Major Depression is associated with increased withdrawal in children, oversleeping in adolescents, and cognitive problems like memory loss in older adults.

Relevant gender-specific information about prevalence and symptoms is provided in *DSM-IV-TR*. For example, the counselor is alerted that bipolar disorders are equally common among men and women, unlike Major Depression, which is diagnosed more commonly among women, or Obsessive-Compulsive Disorder, which is diagnosed more commonly among men. Similarly, differences in prevalence according to socioeconomic status are described for some diagnoses.

Throughout the *DSM-IV-TR*, it is noted when clinicians tend to overdiagnose or misdiagnose certain disorders as a function of culture or age. For example, counselors are alerted that schizophrenia is sometimes diagnosed instead of Bipolar Disorder in non-White cultural groups and younger clients. Other cultural differences also are highlighted, such as the fact that clients from diverse backgrounds present depression in varying ways. For instance, somatic complaints, like headaches among Latinos and fatigue and weakness among Asians, are symptoms that are more likely to suggest depression in these cultural groups than in others.

The *DSM-IV-TR* also provides guidelines for describing the impact of a person's cultural context, such as the importance of recognizing an individual's cultural identity, cultural explanations of presenting complaints, and multicultural elements of the counselor–client relationship that might influence assessment and diagnosis.

Finally, the *DSM-IV-TR* includes an appendix of culture-specific client experiences not included elsewhere. For example, *nervios* is included as a common type of stress disorder among Latinos and includes symptoms of emotional distress, nervousness, tearfulness, and bodily complaints. And look at the term *koro*, also highlighted in the *DSM-IV-TR*: "A term, probably of Malaysian origin, that refers to an episode of sudden and intense anxiety that the penis (or in females, the vulva and nipples) will recede into the body and possibly cause death . . ." (APA, 2000, p. 900).

Diagnosis, Professional Advances, and Social Change

The diagnoses in the earlier editions of the *DSM* were based on the opinions of a group of national experts in particular areas. This is called the "expert consensus" method. In contrast, today, diagnoses in the *DSM-IV-TR* are based on 150 literature reviews, 40 reanalyses of already existing clinical data, and the contributions of 60 different professional organizations, which provided the members of multiple task forces, work groups, and field teams that evaluated the diagnoses in each area of expertise. Diagnoses are generally added, subtracted, or changed in the *DSM* when research is available to support such revisions. Thus, the *DSM-IV-TR* is best thought of as a work in progress rather than a static, never-changing codification.

The *DSM*'s historical management of the issue of sexual orientation illustrates the system's responsiveness to changing professional and social viewpoints. In *DSM-II*, "homosexuality" was classified as a mental disorder in keeping with the professional and social standards of the time. However, based on a change by the expert consensus method, the disorder was replaced by "Sexual Orientation Disorder" in later printings of the *DSM-II* and then by "Ego-dystonic Homosexuality" in *DSM-III*. These diagnoses were made only if the individual was experiencing distress or impairment in functioning related to same-sex orientation. This diagnosis then was removed from a later revision of the *DSM-III* (*DSM-III-R*) and from the *DSM-IV*. Instead, "persistent and marked distress about sexual orientation" is now provided as one of several examples of situations in which the counselor may want to indicate that this issue is the main focus of counseling, and it would be listed under the diagnosis "Sexual Disorder Not Otherwise Specified."

Other examples of how changes in society and the profession abound in *DSM-IV-TR*. For example, important changes have occurred in recent editions in the diagnoses of substance-related disorders, attention-deficit hyperactivity disorder (ADHD) and several other childhood disorders, and eating disorders. Mental health professionals must use lifelong continuing education and professional development to stay up-to-date about the edition of the diagnostic system that currently is in use.

Understanding the Multi-Axial Diagnostic System of *DSM-IV-TR*

The phrase "multi-axial diagnosis" can cause confusion and intimidation for beginning clinicians. Thus, in this section, we first offer a brief overview of the multi-axial diagnostic system and follow this with a more detailed examination of each of the five "axes" that are a part of the system.

The *DSM-IV-TR* uses five different axes, or mechanisms for gathering data. These axes help the counselor record information about clients' experiences, describe clients' presentation or way of being, and develop treatment plans. Because there are five axes, professionals making a diagnosis are viewing their clients holistically, or from several points of view (Seligman, 2004). The five different axes are as follows:

Axis I: Clinical Disorders and Other Conditions That May Be a Focus of Clinical Attention. This includes all childhood and adult mental disorders with the exception of personality disorders and mental retardation. It also includes problem areas that are not considered mental disorders, called "other areas that may be a focus of clinical attention."

Axis II: Personality Disorders and Mental Retardation. This is reserved for recording two specific groups of diagnoses—Personality Disorders and Mental Retardation—both of which are longstanding, entrenched, rigid, and typically, lifelong conditions.

Axis III: General Medical Conditions. This axis provides a place to list medical problems and physical complaints (e.g., chronic pain, thyroid disorder) that might be associated with the client's counseling concerns.

Axis IV: Psychosocial and Environmental Problems. Axis IV provides a place to list external, social, relational, or environmental problems (e.g., poverty, recent divorce) that might be associated with the client's counseling concerns.

Axis V: Global Assessment of Functioning, or GAF Scale. This scale ranges from 1 to 100 and is used by the clinician to estimate the client's overall functioning in everyday life (see page 184).

A fully prepared, formal *DSM-IV-TR* diagnosis provides complete information about the client's experiences on all five axes. The following illustrates such a diagnosis:

Axis I: Major Depressive Disorder, Single Episode, Moderate
Axis II: No diagnosis
Axis III: Chronic back pain
Axis IV: Threat of job loss
Axis V: GAF = 45

In this example, the diagnosis describes a client who is experiencing symptoms of a moderate Major Depression, including significantly low mood for at least 2 weeks, plus associated features such as poor appetite and sleep and loss of pleasure (Axis I); shows no signs of any long-term personality disorder symptoms (Axis II); has difficulties with chronic back pain—a general medical condition (Axis III); is in threat of job loss—a psychosocial stressor (Axis IV); and has several "serious" symptoms such as periodic thoughts about suicide (Axis V). Additional examples of fully prepared diagnoses appear in the *DSM-IV-TR* (see APA, 2000). A detailed examination of each axis follows.

Axis I and Axis II: The Disorders

Axis I and Axis II provide the most important mental health information about the client's presentation. An Axis I diagnosis indicates the client's main areas of clinical concern and is used to record all disorders, problems, and counseling foci with the exception of the Axis II disorders, which include the personality disorders and mental retardation.

Axis I: Clinical Disorders and Other Conditions That May Be a Focus of Clinical Attention[1]

It is on Axis I that the clinician answers the questions: "Does the client show signs and symptoms of any of the fifteen major classes of Axis I mental disorders?" and "Are there conditions other than clinical syndromes that should be a focus of clinical attention?" (LaBruzza & Mendez-Villarrubia, 1994, p. 86). When more than one Axis I disorder is present, they all are recorded on Axis I; however, the primary diagnosis is indicated by listing it first.

DSM-IV-TR's interchapter organization is designed to help the clinician use the system. First to appear in *DSM-IV-TR* are disorders of childhood (this includes the Axis II disorder of mental retardation). This is followed by four "red flag" or "rule out" chapters and then by the commonly diagnosed mood and anxiety disorders. Next comes a series of classes of disorders that have shared symptom features. Next in *DSM-IV-TR* are the adjustment disorders, the personality disorders (Axis II), and then other conditions that might be a focus of counseling.

Axis I diagnoses are made by matching the client's experiences with the symptom criterion list corresponding to the diagnosis. The text includes 15 individual Axis I diagnostic classes, with each class described in a separate chapter. Each diagnostic class is a collection of diagnoses that share natural similarities. For example, all of the mood disorders (e.g., depression, bipolar disorder, seasonal affective disorder) appear together in onc chapter. Similarly, substance-related disorders (e.g., alcohol abuse, cocaine dependence, withdrawal) can all be found in one chapter.

A typical starting point when formulating an Axis I diagnosis is to determine which diagnostic class, or chapter, seems to hold the best tentative match with the client's presentation. For instance, are the signs and symptoms mainly suggestive of a mood problem (Mood Disorders chapter); anxiety, a phobia, or posttraumatic stress (Anxiety Disorders chapter); sleep problem (Sleep Disorders chapter); sexual desire or performance problem (Sexual and Gender Identity Disorders chapter); or anorexia, bulimia, or other eating problem (Eating Disorders chapter)? In other

[1] For a more in-depth analysis of Axis I and Axis II diagnoses, see Toolbox D.

words, the clinician first asks, "Can I narrow down the client's primary concerns from all fifteen classes of Axis I disorders to one likely chapter (or diagnostic class)?" The following briefly defines the Axis I diagnoses as they are ordered in *DSM-IV-TR*.

DISORDERS USUALLY DIAGNOSED IN CHILDHOOD In an effort to offer somewhat of a developmental focus, the first Axis I chapter in the text contains disorders that usually are diagnosed before age 18, in "infancy, childhood, or adolescence" (APA, 1994, p. 37). Although the disorders in this section are generally found in childhood, at times individuals are not diagnosed with the disorder until they are adults. Particularly important for school counselors, the disorders include learning disorders, motor skills disorders, communication disorders, pervasive developmental disorders, attention-deficit and disruptive behavior disorders, feeding and eating disorders of infancy or early childhood, tic disorders, elimination disorders, and other disorders of infancy, childhood, or adolescence.

THE FOUR RED FLAG CHAPTERS Next in *DSM-IV-TR*, we find four "red flag" chapters that contain critical conditions that should be considered first, identified, or ruled out by the clinician (Schwitzer & Everett, 1997). When the client is experiencing a condition in any of these chapters, this condition usually takes priority in treatment planning. These issues tend to be overarching, systemic, powerful, impairing, debilitating, and typically must be addressed before going on to the remaining classes of disorders.

The first red flag chapter describes delirium (disturbances in consciousness), dementia (multiple cognitive deficits), amnestic disorders (disturbances in memory), and other severe cognitive disturbances that most likely take priority in a person's life when they are present and will require medical treatment. The next red flag chapter describes mental disorders related to specific medical problems (called *general medical conditions*) that, in turn, require medical treatment. Next appears a chapter describing substance use disorders (abuse, dependence) and substance-induced disorders (intoxication, withdrawal, mood, sleep, or sexual problems associated with substance use). The last red flag chapter contains schizophrenia and other psychotic disorders.

COMMON OUTPATIENT DISORDERS Following the four red flag chapters are two chapters containing the most commonly used diagnostic classes, particularly in outpatient settings: Mood Disorders and Anxiety Disorders (Seligman, 2004). The Mood Disorders chapter contains two main types of disorders: Depressive disorders, characterized by low mood, loss of interest or pleasure, and associated features; and Bipolar Disorders, characterized by manic episodes of abnormally "elevated, expansive, or irritable mood" (APA, 1994, p. 328). The Anxiety Disorders chapter contains clinical problems of stress and anxiety, including panic disorders and agoraphobia; social phobias and specific phobias of animals, places, and so on; obsessive-compulsive and generalized anxiety disorders, in which anxious mood, thoughts, or behaviors invade many areas of the person's life; and acute stress disorder and posttraumatic stress disorder, which bring anxiety plus a "reexperiencing" of catastrophic or life-threatening events (see Exercise 8.1).

EXERCISE 8.1 **Practice Making Mood and Anxiety Disorder Diagnoses**

Refer to the *DSM-IV-TR* to answer each of the following questions. Don't worry if it takes a while to find the answers. And ask a classmate, colleague, or instructor for suggestions if needed.

1. Your new client has been diagnosed with "Major Depressive Disorder, Recurrent, with Melancholic Features." Locate the Mood Disorders and answer the following:
   a. For her symptoms to be diagnosed in this manner, what is the minimum number of times she has experienced a Major Depressive episode?
   b. What is the minimum length of time for each episode to last?
   c. Which depressive symptoms *must* she have experienced during the episodes?
   d. Might the depressive symptoms have been caused by alcohol abuse?
2. Your new client has been experiencing anxiety symptoms ever since his involvement in a life-threatening car accident. He has felt dazed and hypervigilant. Locate the Anxiety Disorders and answer the following:
   a. If the symptoms have been present for less than a month, what diagnosis is likely?
   b. If the symptoms have been present for more than a month, what diagnosis is likely?
   c. What are some of the ways he may be reexperiencing the event?
   d. What are some of the ways he may be avoiding stimuli related to the event?

Answers appear at the end of the chapter.

DISORDERS ORGANIZED BY SHARED SIMILARITIES Following the common diagnostic chapters are seven chapters that are organized by similarity of symptoms, also referred to as shared phenomenology of features (Schwitzer & Everett, 1997). These include the Somatoform Disorders, which share the common feature of physical symptoms suggesting a medical problem with a psychological element; Factitious Disorders, which share the common feature of intentionally producing or feigning physical or psychological symptoms to create for the client a "sick role"; Dissociative Disorders, which share the common feature of disruption in usually sound consciousness, memory, identity, or perceptions; Sexual and Gender Identity Disorders which share features in the area of sexual behavior; Eating Disorders, which share features in the area of eating behavior; Sleep Disorders, which share features in the area of sleep behavior; and Impulse-Control Disorders Not Classified Elsewhere, which share features in the area of impulsive behavior, such as problems with gambling or stealing.

ADJUSTMENT DISORDERS The Adjustment Disorders, the next chapter in *DSM-IV-TR*, have in common clinically significant emotional or behavioral symptoms that occur in response to an identifiable psychosocial or environmental stressor. Coming later in the text, this chapter is used after the red flag, common outpatient disorders, and disorders of shared symptomatology chapters have been considered and eliminated (or "ruled out"). When symptoms are clinically significant but are not severe enough to warrant any of the diagnoses appearing earlier in the text, and when the symptoms are in response to significant life stressors, then the clinician moves to consider the diagnosis of Adjustment Disorder (see Exercise 8.2).

EXERCISE 8.2 Practice Understanding Axis I Disorders

Refer to the *DSM-IV-TR* to answer each of the following questions. Ask a classmate, colleague, or instructor for suggestions if needed.

1. Your new client's symptoms have been diagnosed as Adjustment Disorder With Depressed Mood following a job loss.
   a. How recently did the job loss occur?
   b. Her unemployment and symptoms both continue for more than 6 months. How does this affect the diagnosis of her symptoms?
2. Locate the Mood Disorders and Adjustment Disorders.
   What are the distinctions among the diagnoses of Major Depressive Disorder, Dysthymia, Substance-Induced Depressive Disorder, and Adjustment Disorder With Depressed Mood?
3. Locate the Anxiety Disorders and Adjustment Disorders.
   What are the distinctions among the diagnoses of Panic Disorder, Generalized Anxiety Disorder, and Adjustment Disorder With Anxiety?

Answers appear at the end of the chapter.

THE "OTHER CONDITIONS" CHAPTER The section called Other Conditions That May Be a Focus of Clinical Attention appears after all Axis I and Axis II diagnoses. This section lists various issues, problems, areas of growth and development, and other counseling themes and topics that may be a focus of treatment but are not causing enough clinically significant symptoms or distress to warrant a mental disorder diagnosis. Included here are such items as Problems of Abuse or Neglect, Relational Problems (Parent-Child, Sibling), Academic, Occupational, Religious or Spiritual, and Phase of Life Problems. Also given are notations to indicate "No Diagnosis" and "Diagnosis Deferred." These items appear at the end of the text as a convenience to help describe, on Axis I, all of the aspects of the client's concerns. Despite the fact that these problems are listed on Axis I, they are not considered mental disorders that are diagnosable (see Exercise 8.3).

EXERCISE 8.3 Practice Making "Other Conditions" Diagnoses

Refer to the *DSM-IV-TR* to answer the following question. Ask a classmate, colleague, or instructor for suggestions if needed.

1. Where would you begin the assessment and diagnostic process if your client's main concern is his normal adjustment to the many changes being brought on by retirement?

Answer appears at the end of the chapter.

Axis II: Mental Retardation and Personality Disorders

Axis II answers the questions:

> *Does the client evidence any long-term pattern of maladaptive character traits that cause significant impairment or distress?", "Does the client [show signs and symptoms that] meet criteria for any of the ten specified* DSM-IV *personality disorders?", and "Is there evidence of mental retardation [or borderline intellectual functioning]?"* (LaBruzza & Mendez-Villarrubia, 1994, p. 86)

As noted, an Axis II diagnosis makes a statement about the presence of a personality disorder, important personality features, mental retardation, or borderline intellectual functioning. Mental retardation is a lifelong condition, stable over time, characterized by significantly subaverage intellectual functioning, accompanied by limited functioning in adapting to everyday life demands (APA, 1994). Personality disorders are sets of features that characteristically first appear in adolescence or young adulthood; are stable over time; comprise enduring, pervasive, inflexible patterns of behavior and inner experience, which are different from social-cultural or developmental expectations; and cause distress or dysfunction. Let's examine both of these categories.

MENTAL RETARDATION Mental Retardation is the first mental disorder presented in the *DSM-IV-TR* and can be found in the text's first diagnostic class, or chapter, entitled Disorders Usually First Diagnosed in Infancy, Childhood, or Adolescence. The narrative description includes diagnostic features, severity subtypes, recording procedures for making the Axis II diagnosis, associated features and disorders, specific culture, age, and gender features, prevalence, course, family patterns, and differential diagnoses. The exact criteria and recording procedures for making the Mental Retardation diagnosis are provided in a set-off box.

There are three criteria for Mental Retardation (APA, 1994): (a) significantly subaverage intellectual functioning, demonstrated by an IQ score of about 70 or lower on a professionally administered IQ test, (b) deficits or impairments in everyday adaptive functioning in at least two areas, such as: self-care, home living, social skills, academic skills, work, leisure, health, or safety, and (c) onset of the disorder before age 18 years.

There are five subtypes of Mental Retardation: Mild, Moderate, Severe, Profound, and Severity Unspecified. These reflect the level of severity of impairment according to intelligence test scores. For example, the Axis II diagnosis for a person with a tested IQ level of between 50 and 70, with impairment in at least two areas of everyday functioning, would be:

Axis II: 317 Mild Mental Retardation

Finally, "Borderline Intellectual Functioning" is indicated on Axis II when the focus of clinical attention is associated with the intellectual functioning of a client whose IQ score falls in the 71–84 range. This condition can be found in the chapter of the text entitled, Other Conditions That May Be a Focus of Clinical Attention, and is not considered a formal diagnosis.

PERSONALITY DISORDERS The Personality Disorders are presented in the last chapter of diagnosable mental disorders in the *DSM-IV-TR.* The narrative description includes diagnostic features, recording procedures for making the Axis II diagnosis, associated features and disorders, specific culture, age, and gender features, prevalence, course, family patterns, and differential diagnoses. General criteria for making a personality disorder diagnosis are provided. Following the discussion of general criteria, the exact criteria for each Personality Disorder are described in narrative form and then set off in a criterion box.

The main criterion of the Personality Disorder diagnosis is the presence of "an enduring pattern of inner experience and behavior that deviates markedly from the expectations of the individual's culture" (APA, 1994, p. 633), manifest in two or more of the following areas: cognition (the ways the person perceives and interprets self, others, and events), affect (range, intensity, lability, and appropriateness of emotional responses to self, others, and events), interpersonal functioning (effectiveness and appropriateness when relating to others), and impulse control (adequate and appropriate control of impulsive thoughts and behaviors). The enduring personality pattern must be inflexible, pervasive across many different personal and social situations, and must cause "significant functional impairment or subjective stress" (APA, 1994, p. 633).

The *DSM-IV-TR* includes mental diagnoses for 11 different personality disorders. As a convenience and to help in making a diagnosis, personality disorders are grouped together into three sets, called "clusters," on the basis of similarity and to help in diagnosis. The three clusters include Odd-Eccentric, Dramatic-Emotional, and Anxious-Fearful. There is a residual category for Personality Disorders Not Otherwise Specified.

> *Cluster A: Odd-Eccentric*
> The three personality disorders in this cluster are each characterized by the appearance of odd or eccentric behavior. Included are the Paranoid Personality Disorder, Schizoid Personality Disorder, and Schizotypal Personality Disorder. Individuals experiencing these disorders appear strangely suspicious of others (Paranoid), oddly detached from social relationships (Schizoid), or bizarre in their beliefs and actions (Schizotypal).
>
> *Cluster B: Dramatic-Emotional*
> The four personality disorders in this cluster are each characterized by the appearance of dramatic interpersonal relationship behavior. Sometimes this is referred to as "acting out" behavior in relationships (LaBruzza & Mendez-Villarrubia, 1994, p. 397). Included are the Antisocial Personality Disorder, Borderline Personality Disorder, Histrionic Personality Disorder, and Narcissistic Personality Disorder. In their relationships with others, individuals experiencing these disorders show disregard for others (Antisocial), frantic fluctuations and impulsivity (Borderline), excessive emotion and attention seeking (Histrionic), or grandiosity and need for admiration (Narcissistic).
>
> *Cluster C: Anxious-Fearful*
> The three personality disorders in this cluster are each characterized by behavior guided by anxiety or fears. Included here are Avoidant Personality Disorder, Dependent Personalty Disorder, and Obsessive-Compulsive Personality Disorder. Individuals experiencing these disorders fear criticism and rejection by others and therefore avoid significant interpersonal relationships (Avoidant); fear separation from others and therefore are unduly dependent, submissive, or clinging in their relationships (Dependent); or fear loss of control and therefore are preoccupied with order, perfection, and personal and interpersonal control (Obsessive-Compulsive).

Personality Disorder Not Otherwise Specified
This final category includes personality disorders that show patterns causing distress or dysfunction; are enduring, inflexible, and pervasive across many different personal and social situations; but do not meet the full criteria for any of the 10 preceding specific personality disorders. An example is the presence of features of several different specific personality disorders in combination that do not meet the full criteria for any one disorder but cause social or occupational impairment (APA, 1994).

Personality disorders are recorded on Axis II in the following manner:

Axis II: 301.83 Borderline Personality Disorder

Intrachapter Organization of Axes I and II

Once the clinician has narrowed the diagnostic formulation to the most likely diagnostic class, he or she should contrast the several specific disorders within the chapter to find the best match with the client's presentation. This requires a familiarity with each chapter of the *DSM-IV-TR*. To assist the clinician, each chapter is organized almost identically and includes information about diagnostic features, subtypes and specifiers, recording procedures, associated features, other information significant to the disorder (issues related to culture, age, gender, prevalence, course, and familial patterns), and differential diagnosis.

DIAGNOSTIC FEATURES Diagnostic criteria required for each disorder are thoroughly discussed in narrative form, sometimes illustrated by behavioral examples, and summarized in bullet or list form in a set-off, highlighted box. Specific directions for making a diagnosis are set off in each box. The clinician must read carefully to learn whether all criteria must be met before a diagnosis is given or whether the diagnosis can be made by meeting some of the criteria (e.g., two of five). Similarly, information about frequency of symptoms (e.g., occurs at least twice per week) and about minimum duration (e.g., present at least 1 month) must be followed when making the diagnosis. By comparison, the diagnostic features information provided in the narrative form preceding the set-off box is more extensive and explains or expands on the set-off criteria list found in each box.

SUBTYPES AND SPECIFIERS When a diagnosis carries with it subtypes (e.g., schizophrenia, paranoid type), or specific distinctions are made according to narrow differences in symptoms or duration or severity (e.g., mild, moderate, or severe), these subtypes and specifiers are described thoroughly in narrative form and then summarized in the highlighted box that contains the diagnostic criterion set (see Exercise 8.4).

EXERCISE 8.4 **Learning about Specifiers**

Refer to the *DSM-IV-TR*.

1. Name some of the most common types of specifiers found in the *DSM-IV-TR*.

Answer appears at the end of the chapter.

RECORDING PROCEDURES Usually two types of recording procedure are given: one for subtypes and specifiers and one for writing out the numerical code that accompanies the diagnosis. First, directions are given for using the subtypes and specifiers when they are a part of a diagnosis. In the earlier example, the diagnosis of "Major Depressive Disorder" is completed by adding the *subtype*, "Single Episode," and the severity *specifier*, "Moderate":

Axis I: Major Depressive Disorder, Single Episode, Moderate

Second, directions are given for writing out the numerical code, which is shorthand for the Axis I and Axis II diagnoses. The numerical codes in the *DSM-IV-TR* come from the *International Classification of Diseases, Tenth Revision, Clinical Modification (ICD-10-CM)*. The numerical code is a quick way to indicate a diagnosis and is used by many institutional and governmental organizations, billing systems and databases, and others. It is not necessary to memorize or overly focus on learning the numerical codes. The codes are given with the name of the disorder throughout the *DSM-IV-TR* and can be easily looked up in the text. In the earlier example, adding the numerical coding would result in the following for Axes I and II:

Axis I: 296.22 Major Depressive Disorder, Single Episode, Moderate
Axis II: V71.09 No diagnosis

ASSOCIATED FEATURES Associated features are clinical features that are not part of the diagnostic criteria for a mental disorder but may frequently occur in association with the disorder. For example, depressive symptoms such as low mood, social withdrawal, and irritability may accompany (or be associated with) a severe eating disorder, such as anorexia nervosa. The presence of associated features can help the clinician more confidently and accurately make a diagnosis. Although associated features can enhance assessment, they are not listed in the criteria set that is set off in box form for each mental disorder because they are not required as a part of the diagnosis.

OTHER INFORMATION SIGNIFICANT TO DISORDERS The *DSM-IV-TR* also offers information concerning issues related to culture, age, gender, prevalence, course of illness, and familial patterns. This information, when known, is discussed in the narrative and can help the clinician more confidently and accurately make a diagnosis. Although this information can enhance assessment, it is not listed in the set-off criteria set box because it is not part of the actual diagnosis.

DIFFERENTIAL DIAGNOSIS Differential diagnoses are competing diagnoses the clinician should consider before settling on a particular disorder. These are listed for every disorder and help the clinician avoid overlooking other possible mental disorders the client might be experiencing. Differential diagnoses are presented in the narrative description for each diagnosis. In many cases, other diagnoses to be considered are also set off in the criterion list box.

In summary, diagnostic features and subtypes and specifiers combine in each chapter to fully describe each mental disorder. Recording procedures give directions for making a correct formally written diagnosis and for using the numerical coding procedures when needed. Associated information and "other" information is there to assist clinicians with the assessment process. Differential diagnoses remind the clinician of possible alternative diagnoses that may be worth considering. The end result is a formal *DSM-IV-TR* diagnosis (see Exercise 8.5).

EXERCISE 8.5 **Practice Making Axis I and Axis II Diagnoses**

Using the manual, complete the following *DSM-IV-TR* "scavenger hunt." Don't worry if it takes a while to find the answers. If need be, ask a classmate, colleague, or instructor for suggestions. Where would you begin the assessment and diagnosis process if your client's main concern is:

1. His firm untrue belief that his wife is cheating on him with many other men, in spite of all evidence to the contrary and what everyone else thinks.
2. Dysphoric mood, fatigue, and insomnia after a period of cocaine use.
3. Recurrently pulling out her hair.
4. Distress caused by the inflexible need for emotional displays and to be the center of attention, present in most social situations, beginning in college, and present continuously throughout adulthood.
5. His inability to achieve an erection in spite of good physical health.
6. Irresistible attacks of sleeping, occurring daily, not due to a medical problem or substance use.

Answers appear at the end of the chapter.

Axis III: General Medical Conditions

On Axis III, physical and medical problems, especially those that might be associated with the person's mental health concerns, are recorded. It is on Axis III that the clinician answers the questions: "Are there any physical signs and symptoms present?", "Does the client have a documented history of any injuries or medical disorders?", and "Could a general medical condition be causing the clinical problems noted on Axis I?" (LaBruzza & Mendez-Villarrubia, 1994, p. 86–87).

In addition to information about physical and medical problems, Axis III is where you can record any prescribed medications the client is taking and whether those medications may have psychological or psychiatric side effects. Also, Axis III allows you to record information about the client's use of any illicit or "street" drugs that may have medical consequences.

Clinicians working in psychiatric inpatient settings, hospital and medical settings, and certain other clinical settings may be required to provide formal general medical condition diagnoses on Axis III. Formal medical diagnoses on Axis III are accompanied by the appropriate, corresponding *International Classification of Disease, Tenth Revision, Clinical Modification (ICD-10-CM)* code. For example, a formally prepared entry for Axis III indicating the client was suffering from an actively problematic HIV infection would appear as follows:

Axis III: 042 HIV infection, causing specified acute infections

A formally prepared entry for Axis III indicating the client was suffering from asthma would be as follows:

Axis III: 493.20 Asthma, chronic obstructive

For convenience, a large number of the common general medical conditions and their *ICD-10-CM* codes are provided in Appendix G of the *DSM-IV-TR.*

By comparison, most counselors and psychotherapists who are outpatient clinicians working in agency, school, or independent practice settings typically record medical signs and symptoms informally in their own working diagnostic notes. Examples of informal recordings on Axis III typical of outpatient clinicians are:

Axis III: HIV-positive, causing infections

and

Axis III: Asthma

Axis III adds an important dimension to diagnosis and treatment planning as it broadens the understanding of clients by addressing medical and physical issues that may be influencing their symptoms.

Axis IV: Psychosocial and Environmental Problems

Axis IV records psychosocial problems and problems with the social environment, especially those that might be associated with the person's mental health concerns. It is on Axis IV that the clinician answers the questions: "What psychosocial or environmental problems is the client facing?", "What stressors are currently taxing the client's ability to cope?", and "How is the client meeting such basic needs as survival, food, shelter, clothing, safety, education, employment, friendship, affection, social interaction, and self-esteem?" (LaBruzza & Mendez-Villarrubia, 1994, p. 87). Further, since crises in a person's life often involve a problem or failure in the person's support network, it is on Axis IV that the clinician answers the question: "What is the client's social support system and how well is it functioning?" (LaBruzza & Mendez-Villarrubia 1994, p. 87).

Common stressors that are often recorded on Axis IV include losses, positive and negative life changes, and anniversaries of emotionally significant events (LaBruzza, 1994). Common environmental and psychosocial problems often recorded include living in poverty, experiencing parental neglect, divorce, and being incarcerated (Seligman, 2004).

In some settings, a checklist-style form is used to record all of the psychosocial and environmental stressors experienced by a client. When using such a form, the clinician first identifies the relevant categories of problems and then indicates the specific client issues (APA, 2000). Categories typically used for Axis IV problems are: "Problems with primary support group, problems related to the social environment, educational problems, occupational problems, housing problems, economic problems, problems with access to health care services, problems related to interaction with the legal system/crime, and other psychosocial and environmental problems" (APA, 2000, pp. 31–32). For example, an Axis IV recording using the categories and issues, as on a checklist, would appear as follows:

Axis IV: Problems with primary support group—disruption of family by divorce

and

Axis IV: Housing problems—unsafe neighborhood

When a checklist of problem categories is not used, the clinician simply lists the specific client problems on Axis IV in descriptive professional language, such as:

Axis IV: Disruption of family by parents' divorce

and

Axis IV: Unsafe neighborhood

Like Axis III, Axis IV offers us additional insight into those areas in a client's life that are causing additional stress and are influencing the client's problems.

Axis V: Global Assessment of Functioning

On Axis V, otherwise known as the Global Assessment of Functioning (GAF) Scale, the clinician estimates in a single numerical rating the client's current functioning (Table 8.1). It is on the GAF Scale that the clinician answers the questions: "How well is the client currently functioning in the psychological, social, and occupational [or academic] aspects of his or her life?", "How severe are the current symptoms of the disorder?", and namely, "What score would the client receive on the GAF scale?" (LaBruzza & Mendez-Villarubia, 1994, p. 87).

TABLE 8.1 **Global Assessment of Functioning Scale (GAF)**

Code	(**Note:** Use intermediate codes when appropriate, e.g., 45, 68, 72)
100–91	**Superior functioning in a wide range of activities, life's problems never seemto get out of hand, is sought out by others because of his or her many positive qualities. No symptoms.**
90–81	**Absent or minimal symptoms** (e.g., mild anxiety before an exam), **good functioning in all areas, interested and involved in a wide range of activities, socially effective, generally satisfied with life, no more than everyday problems or concerns** (e.g., an occasional argument with family members).
80–71	**If symptoms are present, they are transient and expectable reactions to psychosocial stressors** (e.g., difficulty concentrating after family argument); **no more than slight impairment in social, occupational, or school functioning** (e.g., temporarily falling behind in schoolwork).
70–61	**Some mild symptoms** (e.g., depressed mood and mild insomnia) **OR some difficulty in social, occupational, or school functioning** (e.g., occasional truancy, or theft within the household), **but generally functioning pretty well, has some meaningful inter-personal relationships.**

(*continued*)

TABLE 8.1 *(continued)*

60–51	**Moderate symptoms** (e.g., flat affect and circumstantial speech, occasional panic attacks) **OR some difficulty in social, occupational, or school functioning** (e.g., few friends, conflicts with peers or co-workers).
50–41	**Serious symptoms** (e.g., suicidal ideation, severe obsessional rituals, frequent shoplifting) **OR any serious impairment in social occupational, or school functioning** (e.g., no friends, unable to keep a job).
40–31	**Some impairment in reality testing or communication** (e.g., speech is at times illogical, obscure, or irrelevant) **OR major impairment in several areas, such as work or school family relations, judgment, thinking, or mood** (e.g., depressed man avoids friends, neglects family, and is unable to work; child frequently beats up younger children, is defiant at home, and is failing at school).
30–21	**Behavior is considerably influenced by delusions or hallucinations OR serious impairment in communication or judgment** (e.g., sometimes incoherent, acts grossly inappropriately, suicidal preoccupation) **OR inability to function in almost all areas** (e.g., stays in bed all day; no job, home, or friends).
20–11	**Some danger of hurting self or others** (e.g., suicide attempts without clear expectation of death: frequently violent; manic excitement) **OR occasionally fails to maintain minimal personal hygiene** (e.g., smears feces) **OR gross impairment in communication** (e.g., largely incoherent or mute).
10–1	**Persistent danger of severely hurting self or others** (e.g., recurrent violence) **OR persistent inability to maintain minimal personal hygiene OR serious suicidal act with clear expectation of death.**
0	Inadequate information

Source: American Psychological Association (APA), *DSM-IV-TR*, 2000, p. 34. Reprinted by permission.

Higher numbers on the GAF Scale reflect better functioning, and the lowest numbers reflect individuals with severe symptoms and very poor functioning. Clients doing fairly well with some meaningful interpersonal symptoms and only mild symptoms typically are indicated by a GAF score of 61 or above. Intermediate client functioning may fall in the moderate symptom range of 51 to 60 or the serious symptom range of 41 to 50. Clients evidencing impaired reality testing or major impairment in several areas are indicated by a score of 40 or below (LaBruzza, 1994). According to Seligman (2004), clients seen in outpatient settings, presenting concerns such as moderate Mood Disorders and Anxiety Disorders, typically fall in the 50–70 range on the Global Assessment of Functioning (GAF).

The GAF score recorded on Axis V is followed by an indicator of the time frame described. For example, the GAF score could be recorded for "Current" functioning, "Highest in past year," "At intake," "At admission," "At termination," "At discharge," "At Counseling Session 3," or some other relevant time frame. Further, recording two GAF scores for two different points in time sometimes is used to describe client change. For example, an Axis V recording of "GAF = 65 (Current), GAF = 85 (Highest in past year)" indicates a person who has been functioning very well, with no or minimal symptoms or problems, but who currently is experiencing a mild decline in functioning and mild symptoms or problems. Similarly, an Axis V recording of

"GAF = 50 (At intake), GAF = 71 (At termination)" signifies a person, at intake, with serious symptoms, such as suicidal ideation and impairment at work or elsewhere, and who is now finishing counseling and experiencing only transient symptoms, mostly in response to life stressors (see Exercise 8.6).

EXERCISE 8.6 **Practice Using the GAF Scale**

New counselors must master the use of the Global Assessment of Functioning Scale (GAF) to provide reliable diagnostic entries on Axis V. Here are two case illustrations. Read the illustrations and use the GAF Scale to determine your rating of the client's functioning.

Illustration 1: Shaneeka is a 14-year-old girl who is the only child currently living with her parents. She is a good student and is known as an outgoing child. Five months ago, her maternal grandfather, who had been living with the family for 10 years, died. Shaneeka's mother has had difficulty with the loss of her father and is quite depressed, but will not seek professional help. Three months ago, Shaneeka's school performance began to drop because of stomach pain and feeling distracted. It was recommended that she speak with the school counselor about her present situation.

Shaneeka's previous functioning has been quite high; she has been a good student and was interpersonally outgoing. Correspondingly, the GAF score best describing her earlier functioning falls in the 81–90 range, indicating that her mental health symptoms were absent and her functioning was good in all areas. Recently, she has experienced some decline in functioning.

Currently, she is experiencing only mild symptoms, characteristic of a GAF score of 61 or above. Although the current symptoms are causing some difficulty in functioning at school, they appear to be relatively mild (in the 61–70 range). Although her symptoms might be explained or expected in light of the loss of her grandfather and her mother's grief reaction, her symptoms are not transient, as would be symptoms that fall in the 71–80 range; they have been present for 3 months. Further, there is no mention of moderately severe depression symptoms or any additional troubles at school, with peers, or family, which would be suggestive of the 51–60 range. Taken together, the best GAF score for Shaneeka is:

Axis V: GAF = ___ (Current), GAF = ___ (Highest in past year)

Illustration 2: Mary is a 31-year-old married woman who is a clerical worker with three children. Her problems began about 6 months ago, after her husband had an affair with a female neighbor. Since that time, Mary has experienced increasing fears and suspicious thoughts that have been described as paranoid ideation. During the last 2 months, her job performance has deteriorated. She recently started withdrawing from friends but continues her role as mother without obvious difficulty. She is not suicidal. She has had lifelong mild anxiety and insomnia. Her work record is good.

Mary's previous functioning in work, as a parent, and in other roles apparently has been good; however, much of the time, she has struggled with some mild symptoms of anxiety and insomnia. Correspondingly, the GAF score best describing her earlier functioning falls in the 61–70 range: some mild symptoms, but generally functioning pretty well, with some meaningful interpersonal relationships. Recently, she has experienced a significant decline in functioning and increase in distress. Currently, she is experiencing moderate or serious symptoms beyond "mild," characteristic of a GAF score below 61.

Although the symptoms are causing difficulty in functioning at work, so far the symptoms have not interfered with her role as mother, so she is not experiencing major impairment in several areas, such as work and family relations, which would be characteristic of a GAF score in the 31–40 range. Although the symptoms are causing distress and impairing her occupational functioning, so far she has not experienced more serious symptoms such as suicidal ideation or engaging in severe ritual behavior (characteristic of a GAF score in the 41–40 range). The moderate difficulties she is experiencing appear to be characteristic of the 51–60 range of the GAF. Taken together, the best GAF score for Mary is:

Axis V: GAF = ___ (Current), GAF = ___ (Highest in past year)

Answers appear at the end of the chapter.

DSM-IV-TR Diagnosis: Two Case Illustrations

Now that we have introduced all five axes that make up a *DSM-IV-TR* diagnosis, let's take a look at two short case illustrations. This will give you a better idea of what a diagnosis using all five axes looks like. First, we return to Sienna, our client presented in Chapter 2, and then we introduce a new client, Janine.

CASE ILLUSTRATION 8.1 *DSM-IV-TR* Diagnosis: Sienna

As you may recall from Chapter 2, Sienna is a 23-year-old college student who came to the counseling center presenting moderate, persistent depression; problems with her mother; relationship problems with her boyfriend, roommate, and others; and career indecision and identity confusion.

Axis I:	Adjustment Disorder with Depressed Mood
	V61.20 Parent–Child Relational Problem
Axis II:	No diagnosis
Axis III:	None
Axis IV:	Problems with primary support group
Axis V:	GAF = 61 (At intake)

On Axis I, Sienna seems to be presenting emotional and behavioral symptoms (her low mood and other indicators of mild to moderate depression) in response to identifiable stressors (transition to college, dealing with current relationships and adult life demands, and difficulties with the changing relationship with her mother), suggesting an Adjustment Disorder with Depressed Mood rather than a diagnosis of a Mood Disorder such as Major Depression. Sienna's difficulties with her changing relationship with her mother seem significant enough to warrant a separate listing as one important focus of counseling, so we also included "Parent–Child Relational Problem" on Axis I.

She presents no indicators that she is experiencing a Personality Disorder, so "No Diagnosis" is recorded on Axis II. Similarly, no known medical problems have been discussed, so "None" is recorded on Axis III. Her main psychosocial stressors seem related to her relationships in the college environment, and so "Problems with primary support group" is listed on Axis IV. Finally, the fact that Sienna is experiencing some mild symptoms, including mood problems, and some disruption in functioning, including academic and career concerns, but still is functioning pretty well overall, with some meaningful relationships and continued academic efforts, all is summarized by a GAF score = 61 on Axis V.

We will learn more about Sienna in the chapters that follow.

CASE ILLUSTRATION 8.2 *DSM-IV-TR* Diagnosis: Janine

Now let's meet a new client, Janine. Here we will present basic information about Janine's presenting concerns and make a tentative diagnosis of her symptoms. In Chapters 9, 10, and 11, we will revisit both Sienna and Janine.

Janine is a 48-year-old woman who came to a community mental health center in a rural county. Like Sienna, Janine was experiencing problems with low mood and depression. She reported loss of appetite, loss of interest in seeing other people or taking part in hobbies or other activities, some difficulty concentrating, and some trouble with short-term memory.

Janine is unemployed, having been recently laid off from her job of 15 years due to a plant closing. She was also recently diagnosed with adult-onset diabetes. Her family includes her male romantic partner, with whom she is living, her father and brother, who live nearby in the same small town, and an adult son from an earlier marriage, who lives out of state.

Axis I:	Major Depressive Disorder, Single Episode, Mild
Axis II:	No diagnosis
Axis III:	Diabetes
Axis IV:	Poverty, Unemployment
Axis V:	GAF = 51 (At intake)

On Axis I, Janine seems to be presenting all of the symptoms of a Major Depressive Episode: depressed mood most of the day, nearly every day, for more than 2 weeks; little interest or pleasure in activities; troubles with appetite, sleeping, memory, and concentrating; fatigue; and problematic feelings of low self-worth. She reports no previous episodes of depression, no overwhelming suicidal ideation, and she is still functioning moderately well day to day. Considering her various symptoms, her intake worker noted on Axis I a diagnosis of "Major Depressive Disorder, Single Episode, Mild."

She presents no indicators that she is experiencing a Personality Disorder, so "No Diagnosis" is recorded on Axis II. The fact that she was recently diagnosed with a medical problem, diabetes, is recorded on Axis III. The fact that she is confronted with the psychosocial and environmental stressors of "Poverty" and "Unemployment" is recorded on Axis IV. Finally, the fact that Janine is experiencing moderate symptoms, including mood problems and moderate impairment in her everyday functioning, is summarized by a GAF score = 51 on Axis V.

We will learn more about Janine in upcoming chapters.

Practicing Making a Diagnosis

Making a diagnosis using *DSM-IV-TR* can be an arduous process and takes much practice. Although *DSM-IV-TR* is a thorough text, the amount of information can be daunting, and making a diagnosis is a process that is learned over time.

Exercise 8.7 enables you to begin to practice making diagnoses. Examine these two cases, and, by reviewing *DSM-IV-TR*, decide what diagnosis you would make using all five axes. Check your answers with those at the end of this chapter. Then, when you have time, continue to develop your own cases and attempt to determine the diagnoses that fit those cases.

EXERCISE 8.7 **Practice Making Diagnoses Using All Five Axes**

Using the *DSM-IV-TR*, work individually or in small groups to form your own complete five-axis diagnostic impressions for the following practice cases. Compare your results with other individuals or small groups.

Practice Case 1

Willie is a 24-year-old African American woman who has been assigned to your caseload at the local community counseling center. When seen at intake, Willie appears thin and tired, and she describes herself as feeling "worn out." She speaks slowly, describes feeling "down" most of the time and having very little energy. Recently, Willie left her husband of 2 years, taking her 18-month-old son with her. Right now, she is living with her parents and plans to search for an apartment of her own, once she has the energy to do so. Willie reports that she left her husband because, since the birth of their son, her husband has been moody, they have argued "constantly," and on several occasions now, her husband has hit her in the stomach. She is afraid that the physical fights might escalate and that her husband might eventually start hurting the baby.

Willie has been separated from her husband for 6 weeks and reports feeling depressed the whole time. She says she has not slept much or had much appetite during this time period. She cannot ever remember feeling "down" like this before; in fact, she says that before these marital troubles, she had been pretty happy, had always been pretty good at school, and now has a good job as a school nurse and is sort of worried about her change in mood. Willie says she has diabetes, but reports that the diabetes is under control. Her family doctor has assured her that her current mood change is not a result of insulin problems.

Right now, her work doesn't hold much interest for her, though, and not much makes her feel good. Some days, she calls in sick because she "doesn't have the energy to face it." Although she "would never do it" because of her young son, the thought of ending it all crosses her mind sometimes, especially late at night. Every now and then, she has a beer with her father to relax a little while the baby sleeps.

Axis I:
Axis II:
Axis III:
Axis IV:
Axis V:

Practice Case 2

Hal is a 42-year-old White man who has been referred to your private practice by his primary care physician. Hal recently was diagnosed HIV+, and his doctor is concerned about how he is reacting to the news. In her referral note, she comments that Hal is experiencing anxiety, but she is hesitant to prescribe sedatives right now and hopes you can assist him. Hal himself says he is upset because he has always been able to "handle life's curves" in the past. He describes himself as previously being a stable, calm person who is usually the supportive one in his friendships and intimate relationships. In fact, it is his partner who usually relies on him for emotional grounding.

By comparison, Hal says that a few days after receiving the news of his diagnosis, he became gradually more worried, had butterflies in his stomach most of the time, felt nervous, and even had terrible dreams about awful things happening to him in some sort of hospital room. So far, he has managed to stay focused enough at his job managing a music store to continue his work. However, when he reads stories related to AIDS in the music trade papers or hears certain sentimental songs, he retreats to his office with feelings of "sort of dread, like panic, and shortness of breath—but they quickly pass."

In spite of his symptoms, Hal has tried to "keep up with my part of my relationship," sees friends regularly, and continues his volunteer work. Still, he is seeking relief from his "nerves" so he can better focus on dealing with his medical concerns.

Axis I:
Axis II:
Axis III:
Axis IV:
Axis V:

Answers appear at the end of the chapter.

LEARNING TO BE A DIAGNOSTICIAN: An Ongoing Process

The *DSM-IV-TR* can seem unwieldy, complex, cumbersome, and just plain too big to ever master. New clinicians usually have an uncomfortable outsider's feeling of "not knowing the language." That's why the objective of this chapter has been to provide an introduction to *DSM-IV-TR* and its multi-axial diagnostic system. You will have opportunities to develop skills and competence making actual diagnoses later on, in future coursework, supervised field placements, and other more advanced training. Your goal at this point in your development should be just to become familiar with the system.

Most clinicians will not need to become overly familiar with all sections of the *DSM-IV-TR*. A more manageable plan is to master the few classifications you will see most often in your professional setting. For example, school counselors might limit their expertise mostly to childhood disorders. Emergency services workers might become most familiar with the chapters dealing with psychotic presentations and substance-related disorders. Community counselors and independent practitioners might mainly concentrate on Mood, Anxiety, or Adjustment Disorders, depending on their practice.

As you continue on your journey as a clinician, you will increasingly become more familiar with *DSM-IV-TR*. And just when you begin to settle back and relax in confidence, *DSM-V* will be published, then *DSM-VI*, and so on. The more we learn, the more there is to learn. So relax, let your fingers do the walking, and begin learning your way around the *DSM-IV-TR*. But be prepared—around the corner for all of us is *DSM-V*.

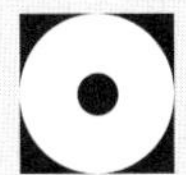

At this point, we recommend that you pause reading, return to the DVD, and take another look at the sections entitled:

Intake Interview.

While viewing this segment, pay particular attention to issues related to diagnosis.

Chapter Summary

This chapter introduced the diagnosis of mental disorders using the *DSM-IV-TR*. First, we offered an overview of the *DSM-IV-TR*. We noted that the primary purpose of a *DSM-IV-TR* diagnosis is to describe and communicate client presentation and concerns, to help in developing treatment plans, and to assist in the determination of the primary focus of counseling. We defined the term *mental disorder* and noted that the *DSM* is a classification system based on sets of criteria made of observable features. We pointed out that mental disorders are not functional, normal, ordered behaviors or expected and culturally appropriate reactions to life. We highlighted the fact that *DSM-IV-TR* has paid more attention to age, gender, socioeconomic status, and cultural differences than past editions. We also demonstrated how *DSM-IV-TR* has changed over the years as a function of professional advances and social change. Finally, we discussed the rigorous process *DSM* goes through in the change process.

The next part of the chapter examined the multi-axial diagnosis of *DSM-IV-TR*. We explained the purpose, recording procedures, and domain of each of the five axes. In our discussion of Axis I, Clinical Disorders and Other Conditions That May Be a Focus of Clinical Attention, we explained the order of the chapters that are used when making an Axis I diagnosis, including the disorders of childhood, the four "red flag" chapters (delirium, dementia, amnestic, and other cognitive disorders; mental disorders related to medical problems; substance use and induced disorders; and schizophrenia and other psychotic disorders), the two chapters that represent the common outpatient disorders (mood and anxiety disorders), the seven chapters of disorders organized by shared similarities (somatoform, factitious, dissociative, sexual and gender identity, eating, sleep, and impulse control disorders), the adjustment disorders, and the other conditions that may be a focus of clinical attention, such as relationship problems and phase of life problems. We noted that items in this last chapter are listed on Axis I but are not considered diagnosable mental disorders.

In our discussion of Axis II, we explained the recording of diagnoses of mental Retardation and Personality Disorders. We reviewed the criteria and subtypes of mental retardation (Mild, Moderate, Severe, Profound, and Severity Unspecified), and the criteria and clusters of personality disorders (Odd-Eccentric, Dramatic-Emotional, and Anxious-Fearful). We pointed out that both mental retardation and personality disorders are longstanding, entrenched, rigid, and typically, lifelong conditions.

Next, we explained that the *DSM-IV-TR's* intrachapter organization, or the material provided inside each chapter, when available, provides additional insight about a disorder. This information includes diagnostic features, subtypes and specifiers, recording procedures, associated features, other information significant to disorders (e.g., specific culture, age, gender, prevalence, course, and familial pattern), and differential diagnosis.

Turning to Axis III, we discussed physical and medical problems, prescribed medication, and street drugs that are recorded here. We also distinguished the formal recording of medical diagnosis that is often used in inpatient settings versus the informal usage often found in outpatient settings. We next discussed the psychosocial and environmental problems that are recorded on Axis IV and explained how to record stressors on this axis. We then discussed Axis V, explaining the Global Assessment of Functioning (GAF) Scale. We noted that GAF scores with higher numbers indicate better functioning, and the lowest numbers reflect individuals with severe symptoms and poor functioning. We also explained how to indicate the time frame when using a GAF score.

Near the end of the chapter we presented two case examples and then two practice cases, which demonstrated common mental disorder diagnoses in counseling settings. We concluded the chapter by discussing the fact that learning about diagnosis is an ongoing process that involves knowing the current diagnostic system and being prepared for changes in the future. We noted that all clinicians must be familiar with current changes and trends in diagnosis.

Answers to Chapter 8 Exercises

EXERCISE 8.1 Practice Making Mood and Anxiety Disorder Diagnoses

1. Your new client has been diagnosed with "Major Depressive Disorder, Recurrent, With Melancholic Features."

a. Two or more episodes—diagnostic criteria for Major Depressive Disorder (*DSM-IV-TR*, p. 375)

b. Duration at least 2 weeks—criteria for Major Depressive Episode (p. 356)

c. At least one symptom must be (1) Depressed Mood or (2) Loss of interest or pleasure—criteria for Major Depressive Episode (p. 356)

d. No. According to exclusionary criteria for differential diagnoses, for the Major Depressive Disorder diagnosis, the symptoms cannot be due to physiological effects of a substance—criteria for Major Depressive Episode (p. 356)

2. Your new client has been experiencing anxiety symptoms ever since his involvement in a life-threatening car accident.

a. Acute Stress Disorder—Criterion G. Disturbance lasts 2 days–4 weeks (p. 471)

b. Posttraumatic Stress Disorder—Criterion E. Disturbance lasts more than 1 month (p. 467). Duration of symptoms is the main distinction between acute stress disorder and posttraumatic stress disorder. Acute Stress Disorder indicates reactions to a recent traumatic event that could potentially develop into Posttraumatic Stress Disorder.

c. Intrusive distressing recollections; distressing dreams or nightmares; feeling as if the event is recurring; psychological distress or physiological reactivity to event cues—Criterion B (p. 467)

d. Efforts to avoid thoughts and conversation about event; efforts to avoid places and people arousing recollections; inability to recall aspects of event; etc.—Criterion C (p. 467)

EXERCISE 8.2 Practice Understanding Axis I Disorders

1. Your new client has been diagnosed with adjustment disorder with depressed mood following a job loss.

a. Less than 3 months ago – Diagnostic Criterion A for Adjustment Disorder (p. 683)

b. Specify "Chronic" in place of "Acute" – Diagnostic criteria set for Adjustment Disorder (p. 683)

c. Axis IV Psychosocial Stressors and Environmental Problems – diagnostic instructions (pp. 31–32)

d. Suggests moderate symptoms, moderate difficulty in social functioning, recorded on Axis V, Global Assessment of Functioning—diagnostic instructions (pp. 32–34)

2. What are the distinctions among the diagnoses of Major Depressive Disorder, Dysthymia, Substance-Induced Depressive Disorder, and Adjustment Disorder With Depressed Mood? See the Decision Tree for Differential Diagnosis of Mood Disorders, Appendix A (pp. 752–753). Major Depressive Disorder and Dysthymia differ by symptom set, severity, chronicity, and severity. Major Depressive Disorder is characterized by either a single episode or recurring episodes in which depressed mood is present for most of the day, every day. Dysthymic Disorder is characterized by chronic moderately low mood, present for at least 2 years (1 year in adolescents). A Substance-Induced Depressive Disorder is the result of the individual's use of a street drug, medication, or exposure to a toxin that is etiologically related to the depression symptoms. A diagnosis of Adjustment Disorder With Depressed Mood might have many symptoms similar to the mood disorders but is of moderate to lower severity and is a psychological response to an identifiable stressor, beginning within 3 months of the onset of the stressor and persisting no more than 6 months after the stressor terminates.

3. What are the distinctions among the diagnoses of Panic Disorder, Generalized Anxiety Disorder, and Adjustment Disorder With Anxiety? See the Decision Tree for Differential Diagnoses of Anxiety Disorders, Appendix B (pp. 754–755). Although Panic Disorder and Generalized Anxiety Disorder both may be characterized by a period of excessive anxiety and worry, they are differentiated by the focus of the individual's concern. An individual with Panic Disorder experiences recurrent unexpected Panic

(continued)

EXERCISE 8.2 *(continued)*

Attacks, followed by at least 1 month of concern about having another attack. By comparison, a diagnosis of Generalized Anxiety Disorder is characterized by excessive anxiety and worry, lasting at least 6 months, about a number of different events and situations. An individual with Adjustment Disorder With Anxiety may experience some of the emotional and behavioral symptoms of panic and anxiety disorders, but the symptoms are of moderate or lower severity and are in response to an identifiable stressor.

EXERCISE 8.3 **Practice Making "Other Conditions" Diagnoses**

1. Your client is dealing with normal adjustment to retirement. Diagnostic Class: No diagnostic class since main feature is problem of how to deal with a normal life adjustment; Section of *DSM-IV-TR*: Other Conditions That May Be a Focus of Clinical Attention; Found under: Additional Conditions; Focus of Clinical Attention: Phase of Life Problem, recorded on Axis I (p. 742).

EXERCISE 8.4 **Learning about Specifiers**

1. Some common types of specifiers: *Severity:* Mild, Moderate, Severe; In Partial Remission, In Full Remission; *Course Specifiers:* Different course specifiers are provided for various mental disorders (e.g., Early Onset, Late Onset, With Onset during Intoxication, Acute, or Chronic); *Subtypes:* Different subtypes are provided for various mental disorders (e.g., Bulimia Nervosa, Purging Type; Bulimia Nervosa, Non-Purging Type).

EXERCISE 8.5 **Practice Making Axis I and Axis II Diagnoses**

***DSM-IV-TR* "Scavenger Hunt"**

1. Diagnostic Class: Schizophrenia and Other Psychotic Disorders; Main Feature: Nonbizarre Delusion; Clinical Disorder: Delusional Disorder; Type: Jealous Type (pp. 323–329)
2. Diagnostic Class: Substance-Related Disorders; Found under Substance-Induced; Substance Withdrawal; Clinical Disorder: Cocaine Withdrawal (pp. 201–209)
3. Diagnostic Class: Impulse-Control Disorders Not Elsewhere Classified; Main Feature: Recurrently pulling out hair; Clinical Disorder: Trichotillomania (pp. 674–677)
4. Diagnostic Class: Personality Disorders; Main Feature of Class: Inflexible pattern of behavior, in multiple social contexts, onset in young adulthood, enduring in adulthood; Distinguishing Feature: Emotional displays, etc.; Axis II Diagnosis: Histrionic Personality Disorder (p. 711–714)
5. Diagnostic Class: Sexual and Gender Identity Disorders; Found under Sexual Dysfunctions; Dealing with excitement phase of sexual response cycle; Main Feature: Erectile Dysfunction; Clinical Disorder: Male Erectile Disorder (p. 545–547)
6. Diagnostic Class: Sleep Disorders; Found under: Primary Sleep Disorders, Dyssomnias; Main Feature: Sleeping attacks while awake; Clinical Disorder: Narcolepsy (p. 609–615)

EXERCISE 8.6 **Practice Using the GAF Scale**

Axis V: GAF = 65 (Current), GAF = 85 (Highest in past year)

Axis V: GAF = 51 (Current), GAF = 61 (Highest in past year)

EXERCISE 8.7 **Practice Making Diagnoses Using All Five Axes**

Practice Case 1

Diagnostic Impressions

Axis I:	Major Depressive Disorder, Single Episode, Moderate
Axis II:	No Diagnosis
Axis III:	Diabetes
Axis IV:	Problems with primary support group—Marital Separation
Axis V:	GAF = 52 (Current)

Discussion

Axis I. Clinical disorders and other conditions that may be a focus of counseling are recorded on Axis I. Willie's level of distress and dysfunction warrant a mental disorder diagnosis, going beyond a nondiagnosable condition such as "relationship problem." Her distress mainly occurs in the area of mood but seems to have begun with her marital discord and separation. Therefore, two possible classes of disorders seem likely to characterize her difficulties: a Mood Disorder or an Adjustment Disorder.

Although the onset of her difficulties coincides with her marital stresses, the severity of her problems is beyond that characterized by a simple Adjustment Disorder. Instead, her low mood, low energy, poor sleep and appetite, and passing thoughts of suicide—present for more than the required 2-week duration for the diagnosis—all fit the description of a Major Depressive Disorder. Further, her only substance use appears to be an occasional alcoholic drink. By her recollection, this is her first and only episode, so the diagnosis of her symptoms is "Major Depressive Disorder, Single Episode."

Her symptoms are causing significant disruption, but she is not actively suicidal and, for the most part, finds the energy to perform daily functions in her work and parenting roles, and she has a future plan to search for her own apartment; therefore, we described her depression as "Moderate."

Axis II. Willie does not report, or show in the interview, any signs of a longstanding inflexible pattern of interpersonal or intrapersonal difficulty, so no diagnosis of personality disorder is warranted. Similarly, she works as a school nurse and is of normal intelligence, so no diagnosis of mental retardation is required.

Axis III. Medical problems are recorded on Axis III. Willie reports having diabetes and this is recorded on Axis III. Given her disrupted eating and sleeping patterns, it may be important to assist Willie to monitor her management of her medical problems—even if not the main focus of counseling

Axis IV. Psychosocial and environment stressors are recorded on this axis. For Willie, the main social stressor is marital separation, which, for convenience, we distinguish as a problem with primary support group.

Axis V. A Global Assessment of Functioning characterizing the client's overall daily functioning is recorded on Axis V. Willie is experiencing moderate symptoms, with moderate difficulty in occupational functioning at times, suggesting a middle GAF score in the 50s. She reports occasional passing thoughts of suicide and unrelieved depressive symptoms, suggesting a GAF score = 52 at the time of the intake.

Practice Case 2

Diagnostic Impressions

Axis I:	Adjustment Disorder With Anxious Mood, Acute
Axis II:	No Diagnosis
Axis III:	HIV Infection
Axis IV:	Recently diagnosed HIV+
Axis V:	GAF = 60

Discussion

Axis I. Hal's distress and dysfunction mainly occur in the area of anxiety and are clearly associated with a disturbing life event. There appear to be two possible classes of disorders that might characterize his difficulties: an Anxiety Disorder or an Adjustment Disorder.

In addition, if the reactions are culturally expectable, appropriate, and with low severity, "no diagnosis on Axis I" or a nondiagnosable focus of clinical attention might be considered. However, Hal's symptoms—including disruptions at work, nightmares, feelings of dread, and persistent unrelieved feelings of anxiety—appear severe enough to warrant a diagnosis.

Although his symptoms are primarily anxious in nature, none of the Anxiety Disorders are a good fit. For example, although a person with Posttraumatic Stress Disorder might have nightmares, these would be recollections of a traumatic event; Hal is not reexperiencing a trauma through his dreams. Similarly, although a person with Generalized Anxiety Disorder experiences persistent daily worry, the worry is about multiple life situations; Hal's worries are confined to his HIV+ diagnosis.

In turn, his symptoms are causing enough distress and dysfunction, in response to a major life stressor, to meet the criteria for an "Adjustment Disorder." The symptoms began shortly after his diagnosis, meeting the Adjustment Disorder criteria. The symptoms are anxiety related. They have been present less than 6 months and therefore are specified as "Acute."

Axis II. Hal does not report, or show in the interview, any signs of a longstanding inflexible pattern of interpersonal or intrapersonal difficulty, so no diagnosis of personality disorder is warranted. Similarly, he works as a music store manager and is of normal intelligence, so no diagnosis of mental retardation is required.

Axis III. Hal has recently been diagnosed with an HIV infection, and this is recorded on Axis III. Here, the HIV+ diagnosis is particularly relevant to the focus of counseling.

Axis IV. For Hal, the main psychosocial stressor is his knowledge of his recent diagnosis, and this is recorded on Axis IV.

Axis V. Hal is experiencing significant symptoms in the mild difficulty range, with some difficulty in occupational functioning at times and persistent anxiety symptoms, suggesting a GAF score in the very low 60s. He reports occasional nightmares and occupational interference, with occasional panic attacks, suggesting a GAF score = 60 at the time of the intake.

CHAPTER 9

Case Conceptualization: Understanding the Client's Concerns

This chapter examines the clinical tool of case conceptualization, a key part of the clinical assessment and appraisal process. Case conceptualization picks up where descriptive diagnosis leaves off and includes an examination of the client's presenting problem, related problems, root causes, and factors currently keeping the problem going. It gives the clinician a bridge between knowing what the client's concerns are and deciding what to do about them. It allows the clinician to understand a client's needs, through his or her unique theoretical perspective, and subsequently apply appropriate counseling skills and treatment strategies. Whereas natural helpers have little understanding of the case conceptualization process, professional counselors use case conceptualization to help focus on client needs and eventual treatment plans.

In this chapter, we first define and explain what case conceptualization is. We discuss the purpose of conceptualization and why new counselors sometimes feel overwhelmed when learning conceptual skills. Next, we introduce a specific, step-by-step method that new counselors can use in the conceptualization process. We include case illustrations and practice exercises throughout the chapter to acquaint you with case conceptualization. Finally, we focus on how learning case conceptualization skills is an ongoing developmental process.

Understanding Case Conceptualization

Effective mental health treatment depends on using a valid framework to assess, appraise, and make sense of client needs (Hinkle, 1994; Seligman, 2004). Conceptual skills provide clinicians with a rationale for their approach to treatment (Seligman, 2004). Further, with today's emphasis on brief counseling approaches (Budman & Gurman, 1983, 1988; Gelso & Johnson, 1983) and eclectic models of treatment

(Mahalick, 1990; Norcross & Prochanska, 1982; Smith, 1982), quick client assessment, conceptualization, and treatment planning have become essential. In fact, exploring client concerns, developing a conceptualization, specifying goals, and building a treatment plan generally are completed in the first few sessions in most counseling models today (Burlingame & Fuhriman, 1987; Neukrug, 2002). Case conceptualization and related intervention skills are so important that our ethical codes require clinicians to be competent in using them, and learning them has become one key task of clinical training (Ellis & Dell, 1986; Loganbill, Hardy, & Delworth, 1982).

Defining Case Conceptualization

When we asked novice counselors—new clinicians who had some experience with clients but were just beginning their clinical career—how they defined "case conceptualization," here is what they said:

- "Case conceptualization is how you understand the issue or problem presented by a client."
- "The overall approach to assessing the client's situation."
- "Getting a picture of what is going on for the client, where he or she wants to go, and how to get there."
- "What the counselor sees as the client's situation—the counselor's impression of what the client needs."
- "An overall assessment of a client's condition, situation, state, or needs."
- "Using theory to fit together the client's issues, presenting problem, background, and possible interventions."

These new counselors agreed that conceptualization involves "picking apart the important details of a case" to gain a "comprehensive understanding of a client and his or her needs." They felt that case conceptualization was part of the whole clinical assessment process—that conceptualizing the client's needs is based on "a broad view of a client's case, including diagnosis, history, test results, goals, etc." They also believed that although case conceptualization takes into account "the *client's* perspective of his or her needs and desires for assistance," ultimately it is "the *clinician's* understanding of the client's needs and the *clinician's* ideas of how to serve the client" that drive case conceptualization. Those are good definitions that are in line with how we define case conceptualization. We see case conceptualization as a clinical thought process that includes the following three theoretical or conceptual elements:

1. Observing, assessing, and measuring client behaviors, thoughts, feelings, and physiological features
2. Using these observations, assessments, and measurements to find patterns and themes in the client's concerns
3. As a function of the clinician's theoretical orientation, using the patterns and themes to interpret, explain, or make clinical judgments about the etiological factors (underlying or root causes) and sustaining factors (features keeping the problem going) associated with the person's concerns

Ultimately, the case conceptualization process is used to address, reduce, manage, or resolve the client's unwanted problems by developing a plan to tackle the problems directly or by working on the etiological and sustaining factors that are keeping the problems going. (The treatment planning aspect of case conceptualization will be discussed in Chapter 10.)

Case Conceptualization: Some Examples

To give you a better picture of what case conceptualization is all about, it might be helpful to see a couple of examples. For our first illustration, let's return to our client, Sienna, who was introduced in Chapter 2. After reviewing the information presented in Chapter 2, page 16, take a look at Case Illustration 9.1. As you read this illustration, consider the "clinical thinking" process that is taking place.

CASE ILLUSTRATION 9.1 Introduction to Case Conceptualization: Sienna

What follows is an explanation of Sienna's difficulties using a case conceptualization model that includes the elements just noted. A mention of treatment planning, which will be covered in Chapter 10, concludes this illustration. As you will remember from Chapter 2, Sienna is a 23-year-old college student who came to the counseling center presenting moderate, persistent depression.

Element 1: Observe, assess, and measure client behaviors, thoughts, feelings, and physiological features:
When the counselor more fully explored all of Sienna's areas of difficulty, a number of important problems emerged: symptoms of depression, including low mood, troubles with sleep, appetite, concentration, and energy level; difficulties in relationships with several important people in her life, including feeling dependent on her boyfriend, having conflict with her mother, and feeling powerless with her roommate; and young adult independence and identity problems, including unclear academic goals, career indecision, multicultural adjustment questions, and concerns about being independent.

Element 2: Find patterns and themes by using observations, assessments, and measurements:
First, the counselor grouped together all of Sienna's moderate depression symptoms—depressed mood, melancholic rumination, sleep disruption, poor concentration, low motivation, and so on. Second, Sienna's dependent relationship issues, conflictual family ties, passive romantic role, and powerlessness with her roommate were organized together into a theme of "relationship dependence issues." Third, a theme of "identity confusion" was formed from her unclear academic goals, career indecision, cultural questions, and anxiety about life planning.

Element 3: Use the patterns and themes that are found to interpret, explain, or make clinical judgments about the person's concerns: Here the counselor uses his or her own theoretical perspective to come up with theoretical explanations of Sienna's concerns to decide on the best focus for their counseling work together and the best strategy for treatment.

For example, using a humanistic (or person-centered) perspective, Sienna's (a) depression, (b) relationship dependence, and (c) general anxiety about life choices might come together to lead to theoretical inferences of low self-esteem or poorly developed self-empowerment. Further, according to the humanistic perspective, it might be inferred that her poor self-esteem was rooted more deeply in feelings of having a "flaw"—the sense that "something is terribly wrong with me"—that come from experiences during her development.

Alternatively, for a clinician using a psychodynamic perspective, Sienna's three symptom groups might be conceptually related to "autonomy" difficulties (fears of becoming a fully functioning adult independent who is emotionally independent of her family). Further, according to the psychodynamic perspective, it might be inferred that her autonomy difficulties are tied to fears of "disintegration" ("I will be overwhelmed by my own independence") or fears of "abandonment" ("I will lose my family relationships if I am successful").

And using a cognitive-behavioral perspective, Sienna's passivity in relationships and her avoidance of making important life decisions might be explained theoretically by "negative self-talk" (undermining, catastrophic self-statements) and having learned ineffective interpersonal behaviors.

Treatment Planning: Determine a treatment plan to address, reduce, manage, or resolve the client's unwanted problems: As we will see in the next chapter, the clinician's theoretical perspective and the way the client's case is conceptualized will lead to a decision about the goals to be accomplished in counseling and a conceptually driven plan for treatment to reach those goals.

Notice that when implementing the first element of observing, assessing, and measuring, the counselor goes beyond Sienna's presenting problem of low mood to explore other signs of depression and to find out if additional client concerns and symptoms were present. That is how the clinician discovers that Sienna also is having troubles with her mother, boyfriend, and roommate and some problems making key life decisions. When finding themes and patterns (Element 2), the counselor organizes Sienna's different issues so they fit together into three areas of concerns: depression, relationship problems, and young adult identity problems. Then, by applying the patterns and themes to the clinician's theory of counseling (Element 3), the clinician comes to understand and explain what is causing Sienna's difficulties. In our example, we give alternative theoretical interpretations based on three possible orientations: humanistic, psychodynamic, and cognitive-behavioral. All of these elements lead toward a treatment plan specifically designed for the client.

EXERCISE 9.1 **What Theoretical Approach Is Best?**

Although you may not have fully formed your own theoretical perspective, as best as you can, compare the humanistic, psychodynamic, and cognitive-behavioral perspectives to understanding Sienna's symptoms by answering the following questions:

1. What do the three perspectives have in common when explaining Sienna's concerns? How do they differ?
2. Which do you think does the best job of capturing, interpreting, and getting to the causes of her concerns?
3. Which will lead to the best plan of action for working with Sienna to reach her goals?
4. Which seems closest to your own viewpoint at this early stage in your training?

Consider these questions and then meet in dyads or small groups to discuss them.

For our second example, let's return to our client, Janine, who was introduced in Chapter 8. As you will recall, Janine is a client who came to a mental health center for help with depression. Once again, as you read this second illustration, consider the "clinical thinking" process involved in case conceptualization.

CASE ILLUSTRATION 9.2 Introduction to Case Conceptualization: Janine

In this example, our client is Janine, a 48-year-old woman who came to a community mental health center in a rural county. Like Sienna, Janine was experiencing problems with low mood and depression. She reported loss of appetite, loss of interest in seeing other people or taking part in hobbies or other activities, some difficulty concentrating, and some trouble with short-term memory. Janine was unemployed, having been recently laid off from her job of 15 years due to a plant closing. She was also recently diagnosed with adult-onset diabetes. Her family includes her male romantic partner, with whom she is living, her father and brother, who live nearby in the same small town, and an adult son from an earlier marriage, who lives out of state.

What follows is an explanation of Janine's difficulties using a case conceptualization model that includes the three elements noted earlier. Treatment planning, which will be covered in Chapter 10, concludes this illustration.

Element 1: Observe, assess, and measure client behaviors, thoughts, feelings, and physiological features:

As with Sienna, Janine sought counseling for feelings of depression. When the clinician more fully explored Janine's areas of difficulty, a number of important problems emerged: symptoms of depression, including daily low mood and tearfulness, social isolation, loss of interest in once enjoyable activities, loss of appetite, difficulty with concentration and short-term memory, and lack of energy; a poor relationship with her father, rarely speaking with him, and conflicts in her relationship with her brother; and although she writes and phones her son, she rarely receives any response from him. She also has dealt with the stresses that result from poverty, which she has experienced most of her life.

Element 2: Find patterns and themes by using observations, assessments, and measurements:
Janine's clinician grouped all of her presenting problems and symptoms into two logical themes. First, Janine's daily feelings of depression and sadness, social isolation, loss of appetite, lack of energy, loss interest in once enjoyable activities, and difficulty with concentration and short-term memory were grouped together as symptoms of a depressive disorder. Second, a theme of "family conflict" was formed from her three different problematic relationships with her father, brother, and son.

Element 3: Use the patterns and themes that are found to interpret, explain, or make clinical judgments about the person's concerns:
The clinician used a cognitive theoretical perspective to make inferences about Janine's areas of difficulty. From a cognitive perspective, the counselor linked Janine's low mood and the nature of her relationship conflicts to a negative view of self, negative interpretations of life experiences, and negative projections about the future. Part of Janine's belief system is that she will never be able to enjoy her life and do the things she could previously. The counselor believes this "faulty thinking" has led to the current depressive episode and some of her other difficulties.

Treatment Planning: Determine a treatment plan to address, reduce, manage, or resolve the client's unwanted problems:
As we will see in the next chapter, the clinician's theoretical perspective and the way the client's case is conceptualized lead to a decision about the goals to be accomplished in counseling and a conceptually driven plan for treatment to reach those goals. Janine's counselor used a cognitive perspective to set treatment goals and build a treatment plan. The clinician sees the cause of Janine's mood problems to be her negative view of self, her experiences, and her view of the future. Correspondingly, the counselor's plan is to assist Janine to develop healthy cognitive patterns and beliefs about self and the world that will lead to alleviation of her depressive symptoms.

Notice that when implementing the first element of observing, assessing, and measuring, the counselor goes beyond Janine's presenting problem of low mood to explore other signs of depression and to find out if additional client concerns and symptoms were present. That is how the clinician discovers Janine's psychosocial stressors, including recent unemployment and a recent medical diagnosis of adult-onset diabetes, and finds out something about her family relationship conflicts. Next, notice how the counselor organizes Janine's many symptoms into two areas of concerns: a depressive disorder and family relationship conflicts. Then, see how the clinician's theory of counseling is used to understand the patterns and themes causing Janine's difficulties. Finally, all of this is brought together in a treatment plan that can be designed to address the identified issues. In this example, the counselor used a cognitive theoretical perspective (see Exercise 9.2).

EXERCISE 9.2 **How Comfortable Are You with Clinical Thinking?**

As you can see in Janine's case, the counselor's interpretation, or conceptualization, of the client's needs has a direct impact on what kind of service is delivered. The responsibility for clinical thinking, which includes assessing, diagnosing, and conceptualizing the client's needs to set treatment goals and build an effective treatment plan, is an important clinical duty. It can feel exciting and intellectually charged, or it can feel like an awesome responsibility and overwhelming. Some counselors feel negatively about, or at odds with, the clinical need to "analyze" the client's concerns. To see where you fit into this part of the path from natural helper to professional counselor, consider these questions and then meet in pairs or small groups to discuss your answers.

1. What immediate feelings, thoughts, or reactions do you have when you think about being in the clinical role of case conceptualizer and treatment planner?
2. What will interest or excite you about this part of being a professional helper?
3. What concerns do you have?
4. What ethical considerations or reservations do you have?

Feeling Overwhelmed by Case Conceptualization

As you may have already discovered, the pressure to form an understanding of the client's needs, select a counseling focus, and design a treatment plan can be challenging. In fact, if you are like many new counselors, reading over illustrations like the ones just presented can leave you feeling quite overwhelmed by the "thinking" part of being a counselor. But you are not alone in feeling this way. Beginning clinicians often experience ambiguity and confusion as they work with each new client to develop their own reliable framework for doing case conceptualization (Loganbill, et al., 1982; Martin, Slemon, Hiebert, Hallberg, & Cummings, 1989). It is not surprising that new clinicians tend to lack confidence in their abilities at case conceptualization (Glidewell & Livert, 1992). In fact, Robbins and Zinni (1988) found that many counseling students felt they lacked the conceptual skills needed in their training sites. Contrast this with more experienced clinicians who tend to have one trusted, abstract, general theoretical framework that they are able to systematically apply to the task of conceptualizing the different problems presented by each new client.

To help you feel more confident in your case conceptualization skills, in the remainder of this chapter we provide a step-by-step method designed to assist counselors in developing consistent, rational frameworks for client conceptualization. This method, known as the *inverted pyramid* (Schwitzer, 1996, 1997), offers you a specific plan to identify and understand client concerns.

Inverted Pyramid Method of Case Conceptualization

The purpose of the inverted pyramid method (Schwitzer, 1996, 1997) is to give students and beginning clinicians a specific four-step plan that can be used to identify and understand client concerns. In addition, the inverted pyramid gives you a way

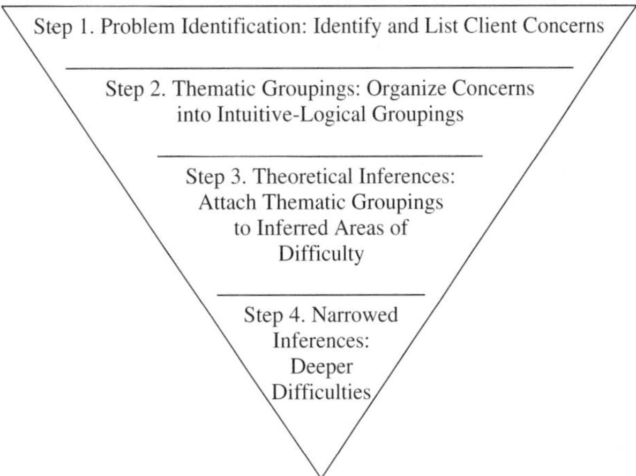

Figure 9.1 Inverted Pyramid Method of Case Conceptualization: Four Steps

to discuss clinical cases with your instructors, clinical supervisors, and treatment team members when you begin getting practical experience. This inverted pyramid plan uses four steps in clinical problem formulation:

1. Broadly identifying client difficulties and symptomatic behavior
2. Organizing client difficulties and symptomatic behavior into logical groupings or constellations
3. Tying symptom groups into deeper theoretical, interpretive, or causal inferences
4. Narrowing these causal influences to the even deeper difficulties in development or adjustment

The process of widely identifying client concerns and narrowing them down to their deeper causes is pictured diagrammatically as a funnel, or inverted pyramid. The completed pyramid presents horizontally and vertically organized information about client thoughts, affects, behaviors, relationships, developmental themes, and adjustment patterns.

The four steps of the method provide a process that can be followed to develop a coherent, theory-driven conceptual understanding of client symptoms, their function or importance, and their developmental roots. In turn, the completed process and accompanying diagram provide a guide to the selection of treatment focus and goals. The focus and goals you select may be verified and potentially addressed, or revised, over the course of psychotherapy (Patton & Robbins, 1982; Schwitzer, 1996). The four steps and the pyramid pattern are shown in Figure 9.1.

Step 1. Problem Identification: Identify and List Client Concerns

In the first step of the pyramid approach, wide latitude is used to identify the client's presenting concerns, associated concerns, and relevant aspects of the person's adjustment, development, or functioning. One need not apply a special theory at this point; instead, in this early information-gathering stage, a "wide net" is cast as you gather the information you will need later to conceptualize the client's concerns and needs (Dumont, 1993). Casting a wide net allows you to understand the client's presenting problem in more detail (e.g., depression) or to find out about related problems, sometimes called "associated concerns" or "collateral concerns" (e.g., career indecision and family conflicts).

Exploring the Presenting Problem

As we discussed in Chapter 1, the clinician usually begins the interview with inquiries about the client's reasons for seeking assistance. Specifically, information should be collected about four aspects of the client's presenting problem:

1. client behaviors (e.g., problematic relationships, eating difficulties, school problems, avoidance)
2. client thoughts (self-statements, ruminations, fantasies)
3. client affect (low mood, anxiety, irritation and anger, guilt)
4. physiology of the client (sleep, appetite, or sexual drive problems; fatigue; anxiety reactions)

Exploring Additional Areas of Concern

The clinician next inquires about the person's functioning in more general areas (Baker & Siryk, 1984), such as:

1. adjustment to school, work, or other major life roles or areas of functioning (managing college academic demands, good job performance, etc.)
2. social adjustment (family roles and relationships, romantic relationships, work and leisure group interactions, etc.)
3. personal-emotional adjustment (behavior, thoughts, affect, physiology in areas beyond the presenting problem)

Specific Inquiries about Parental and Family Relationships

Next, the clinician follows with specific inquiries about parental and family relationships. A brief developmental history is collected, including information about the client's previous experiences with school and/or work, peer/social relationships, family, and moods and thoughts.

Thoughts, Feelings, and Behaviors during the Session

Some clinicians collect additional notes about the client's thoughts, feelings, and behavior right in the interview session. They observe and describe the client's way of understanding the world, how he or she expresses feelings, and the kinds of behaviors exhibited during the session.

BOX 9.1

Summary of Step 1. Problem Identification: Identify and List Client Concerns

A. PRESENTING PROBLEM
   1. Behavior
   2. Thoughts
   3. Feelings
   4. Physiology

B. ADDITIONAL AREAS OF CONCERN
   1. Work, School, and Other Major Life Roles or Areas of Functioning
   2. Social Adjustment
   3. Personal-Emotional Adjustment

C. FAMILY AND DEVELOPMENTAL HISTORY
   1. Parental and Family Relationships and History
   2. Previous School and Work Experiences
   3. Previous Peer and Social Experiences

D. IN-SESSION OBSERVATIONS AND NOTES RELATED TO BEHAVIORS, THOUGHTS, AND FEELINGS DURING THE INTERVIEW

E. CLINICAL INQUIRIES
   1. Medical Problems
   2. Medical and Psychiatric Drug Prescriptions
   3. Past Psychotherapy Experiences and Hospitalizations
   4. Substance Use
   5. Suicidality and Other Harmful Thoughts, Feelings, and Impulses

F. PSYCHOLOGICAL ASSESSMENT
   1. Problem Checklists
   2. General Personality Inventories
   3. Measures of Specific Clinical Problems
   4. Mental Status Exam

Routine Inquiries Concerning Health-Related Issues

The clinician, during this step, should makes routine clinical inquiries about medical problems, prescriptions, previous therapy experiences, substance use, suicidal or homicidal ideation, or past history of harm to self or others.

Use of Psychological Assessments

Next, clients often complete general psychological assessments. These may include problem checklists, general personality inventories such as the MMPI or California Personality Inventory, or assessment instruments that measure specific clinical problems, such as the Beck Depression Inventory or the Eating Disorder Inventory. In addition, as discussed in Chapter 6, a mental status exam, which is the assessment of the client's appearance and behavior, emotional state, thought components, and cognitive functioning, is often used to assist the clinician in making judgments about the client's adjustment (Polanski & Hinkle, 2000).

Step 1, problem identification, is outlined in Box 9.1. Ideally, an exhaustive listing is compiled of any and all information that may be useful and descriptive when thinking clinically about the client's needs. A shorthand statement to summarize the inverted pyramid method of case conceptualization's first step is: "Intake, testing, assessment: Casting a wide net."

Step 2. Thematic Groupings: Organize Concerns into Intuitive-Logical Constellations

The second step of the process is to organize all of the client problems and symptoms, identified during Step 1, into intuitively logical groupings or constellations. This step is configural; that is, the goal is to group together (or "configure") client problems that seem to serve similar functions in the client's life, seem to operate in similar ways, or affect the client in similar ways. Rather than adhering to theoretical assumptions, in this second step, the idea is to more intuitively or holistically identify the common denominators among wide-ranging client data, according to the way they affect the client's everyday life, the meaning they have for the client, or the function they seem to fill.

At Step 2, the clinician relies on his or her clinical judgment to begin organizing the client's issues in a way that makes the most sense. This is an important part of the conceptualization process because it will help the clinician begin to make a judgment about what the focus of counseling should be and what treatment plan is called for to help the client.

Different Ways of Intuitive-Logical Clinical Thinking

As we mentioned earlier, in Step 2 the clinician uses intuitive-logical clinical judgment, rather than a rigid theoretical orientation, to begin organizing symptoms according to sensible common denominators. Four different intuitive-logical ways of clinical thinking commonly used by clinicians include the (a) descriptive-diagnosis approach, (b) clinical targets approach, (c) areas of dysfunction approach, and (d) intrapsychic approach.

DESCRIPTIVE-DIAGNOSIS APPROACH (LOOK FOR DISORDERS) In this approach, clinicians organize the client's adjustment, development, distress, or dysfunction into groupings according to the way varying symptoms are pieces of the same disorder or diagnosis (e.g., putting all of the symptoms together to show a depressive disorder such as major depression). Here the clinician's logical-intuitive clinical thinking is moving toward inferences, interpretations, treatment focus, and treatment planning based on the eventual diagnosis or disorder identified (Schwitzer & Everett, 1997). Clinicians might use *DSM-IV-TR* when applying this approach.

CLINICAL TARGETS APPROACH (LOOK AT THOUGHTS, FEELINGS, BEHAVIORS, AND PHYSIOLOGY) In this approach, clinicians organize the different aspects of the client's adjustment, development, distress, or dysfunction into four domains that include irrational thoughts (thoughts), distressing mood (feelings), dysfunctional and maladaptive actions (behaviors), and problematic physical aspects (physiology). Here the clinician's logical-intuitive thinking is moving toward inferences, interpretations, treatment focus, and treatment planning based on these four areas.

AREAS OF DYSFUNCTION APPROACH (LOOK FOR LIFE ROLES AND THEMES) Some clinicians organize groupings according to their effect on the client's everyday life.

BOX 9.2

Summary of Step 2. Thematic Groupings: Organizing Concerns into Intuitive-Logical Constellations

Here the clinician uses intuitive-logical clinical judgment to begin organizing symptoms according to sensible common denominators. Four different approaches are commonly used:

A. *DESCRIPTIVE-DIAGNOSIS APPROACH:* Sorting together the different pieces of information about client's adjustment, development, distress, or dysfunction to show larger clinical problems as reflected through a diagnosis.

B. *CLINICAL TARGETS APPROACH:* Sorting client information according to the basic division of behavior, thoughts, feelings, and physiology.

C. *AREAS OF DYSFUNCTION APPROACH:* Sorting together areas of dysfunction according to important life situations, life themes, or life roles and skills.

D. *INTRAPSYCHIC APPROACH:* Sorting together the different pieces of information about client's adjustment, development, distress, or dysfunction to show clinical patterns in the ways life events are associated with the person's personal experience and identity.

For instance, the clinician might look for common denominators according to (a) important life situations, such as problems at work, in one's marriage, or in one's neighborhood or social organization, (b) important life themes, such as problems in relationships with others, problems making decisions, or problems controlling anger, and (c) important life roles or skills, such as problems in parenting, deciding on a career, or moving into adulthood. This approach to organizing client issues examines the client's adjustment, development, distress, or dysfunction by common denominators according to problematic themes of everyday life.

INTRAPSYCHIC APPROACH (LOOK FOR INTRAPERSONAL LIFE THEMES) In comparison with the areas of dysfunction approach, which looks for common denominators according to areas of *external* life functioning, some counselors organize groupings according to their effects on *internal* or *intrapersonal* functioning. This approach to organizing client issues divides the different pieces of the client's adjustment, development, distress, or dysfunction by common denominators according to the intrapsychic roles they play. This usually means arranging the material uncovered in Step 1 according to how it helps the person, internally, to keep up their self-esteem or sense of self, keep their personality intact, and handle psychoemotional threats to their psychological well-being. Here the counselor's logical-intuitive clinical thinking is moving toward inferences, interpretations, treatment focus, and treatment planning that will be based on understanding and resolving the ways in which external, impinging life events affect the person's personal experience, identity, actions, and functioning (May, 1988).

Step 2, thematic groupings, is outlined in Box 9.2. A shorthand statement to summarize the inverted pyramid method of case conceptualization's second step is: "Intuitive-logical clinical thinking: Grouping symptoms by similarities and themes."

BOX 9.3
Summary of Step 3. Theoretical Inferences: Attach Thematic Groupings to Inferred Areas of Difficulty

The clinician's theory is used to narrow in on possible treatment issues.

A. Apply the clinician's theoretical perspective.

B. Tentatively match thematic groups or constellations with clinician's theoretical approach.

C. Previous symptom constellations are combined to reflect deeper or causal aspects of client's problems.

D. Narrowing of diagram reflects smaller unifying, central, explanatory, causal, or underlying themes.

E. Refined themes are potential foci of treatment.

Step 3. Theoretical Inferences: Attach Thematic Groupings to Inferred Areas of Difficulty

In contrast to Steps 1 and 2, where the clinician uses intuitive-logical clinical thinking to identify and begin organizing client concerns, Steps 3 and 4 are theoretical in that they apply the clinician's formal theoretical perspective to what he or she has learned about the client. In Step 3, an attempt is made to tentatively match the thematic groupings or constellations developed in the previous steps to areas of difficulty according to the counselor's theoretical perspective. It is here that the previously identified symptom constellations are refined to reflect inferences about deeper aspects or causal roots of the client's difficulties.

This refinement is reflected by placement of this step deeper on the pyramid diagram. The narrowing diagram emphasizes the organization of client-problem constellations into a still smaller number of themes that are unifying, central, explanatory, causal, or underlying in nature. In turn, the refined themes are more theoretically meaningful in providing counseling. These themes become one set of potential foci for treatment. A shorthand way to summarize the inverted pyramid method of case conceptualization's third step is: "Using theory: Inferring areas of difficulty." (see Box 9.3.)

Step 4. Narrowed Inferences: Deeper Client Difficulties

Applying the same theoretical orientation used in Step 3, in Step 4 the clinician forms still-deeper, more encompassing, or more central, causal themes, when they are present. These themes are distilled further into existential, fundamental, or underlying questions of life and death (suicidal and homicidal thoughts and meaning-of-life issues), deep-rooted shame or rage, extreme loss of identity, fragile personality structures, or other deep concerns.

Working all the way down the pyramid through Steps 3 and 4 should help beginning counselors methodically apply their own theoretical framework to even

BOX 9.4
Summary of Step 4. Narrowed Inferences: Deeper Client Difficulties

The clinician's theory continues to be used to address deeper issues:

A. Apply same theoretical orientation used in Step 3.

B. Connect thoughts, feelings, behaviors, and other experiences identified in the topmost portions to deeper dynamics.

C. Form still-deeper, more encompassing, or more central, causal themes, when present (e.g., existential, fundamental, or underlying questions of life and death).

D. Not all client problems are rooted in deep dynamics; in that case, this part of the pyramid may be left unfilled.

BOX 9.5
The Use of Theory to Infer Areas of Client Difficulty and Deeper Difficulties

A counselor uses the same theoretical orientation at Steps 3 and 4 to infer, interpret, or explain the client symptoms and themes observed in Steps 1 and 2. To make these sort of inferences about underlying difficulties and root causes (Step 3) and even deeper roots or deepest difficulties (Step 4), the counselor must decide on a theoretical approach and apply it.

For new counselors, this usually raises the questions, "But which theory should I use?" and "Which theory is the best?" In part, the "best" theory is one that is well-suited to the client's characteristics. The best theory also is one that has been proven effective with the sort of symptoms and problems the client is experiencing.

The best theory also depends on the counselor. Every clinician must explore and decide on a theoretical orientation (or a small handful of approaches) that he or she feels most comfortable using, has the most confidence in, and can competently use. In part, the best theory is the one that is a good match with our own characteristics, attitudes, skills, and beliefs.

There are many theories and approaches to doing counseling. Some of them are illustrated in the case examples and practice cases found in this textbook. The most common today are psychodynamic, humanistic, behavioral, cognitive, and brief solution focused.

You will be learning about these and other approaches in great detail during your coursework and supervised field placements. But in the meantime, here is a short description of the five most commonly used approaches (Corey, 2005; Gladding, 2001; Seligman, 2001):

PSYCHODYNAMIC

The psychodynamic approach assumes that a client's difficulties in some way reflect or repeat earlier issues in the person's family of origin. Clinicians who use this approach believe that, by addressing both the current issues and symptoms and its origins in developmental family experiences, the client's presenting concerns can be resolved and the person can become better able to deal with similar problems when they arise in the future. Treatment emphasizes looking at conscious and unconscious thoughts and feelings and uses such techniques as interpretation, transference, and analysis. Brief models of psychodynamic therapy focus on the client's most important concerns. This approach places great emphasis on Steps 3 and 4 of the inverted pyramid.

(*continued*)

BOX 9.5 (*continued*)

HUMANISTIC
The humanistic approach, also called the client-centered or person-centered approach, assumes that client difficulties should be dealt with mainly in the present. Counselors using this approach believe that for the most part, the client, not the counselor, should direct the focus of the counseling process. The counselor's role is to be active but as nondirective as possible. Treatment emphasizes communicating empathy, emotional congruence, and acceptance. It deemphasizes elaborate interventions, interpretations, or analysis, in favor of creating an empathic, congruent, accepting interpersonal environment, in which the client explores concerns and finds his or her own answers. This approach places equal emphasis on all four steps of the inverted pyramid.

BEHAVIORAL
The behavioral approach assumes that client difficulties are mainly the result of faulty learning and faulty behavioral conditioning. Clinicians using this approach focus mainly on modifying and changing a person's actions—or behaviors. When used in combination with a cognitive approach, a cognitive-behavioral approach focuses on both changing thoughts and modifying actions. Treatment is structured—stressing behavioral learning strategies, reconditioning and counterconditioning, systematic desensitization, modeling, social learning, and reinforcement. This approach places the most emphasis on Step 3 of the inverted pyramid.

COGNITIVE
The cognitive approach assumes that client difficulties are mainly the result of faulty thinking (or cognition). Clinicians using this approach focus mainly on modifying a person's thought processes so they no longer overgeneralize or use distorted, dysfunctional thought patterns. This approach often is used in combination with behavioral methods, forming the cognitive-behavioral approach. Treatment is relatively structured—stressing exercises and activities to replace dysfunctional cognitions with those that are more accurate and realistic, enabling clients to deal more effectively with present and future difficulties. This approach places the most emphasis on Step 3 of the inverted pyramid.

BRIEF SOLUTION FOCUSED
The brief solution focused approach is largely grounded in behavioral, cognitive, and cognitive-behavioral treatment methods. This approach assumes the goals of counseling are to address and solve current problems in client's thoughts, behaviors, mood, and physiology. Clinicians using this approach assist clients to expect and pursue positive change. Treatment is semistructured, focuses on presenting concerns, and combines an eclectic mix of techniques aimed at producing change as efficiently as possible. This approach mainly emphasizes the symptoms and themes of Steps 1 and 2 of the inverted pyramid; however, brief solutions may be directed at deeper causes found in Steps 3 and 4 to produce symptom relief and client change.

the most threatening, scariest, darkest, most disruptive and despairing client difficulties. These steps are especially intended to help new counselors recognize the connections between the less overwhelming, more "surface," more accessible, easy-to-identify symptoms seen in Steps 1 and 2 with theoretical inferences about client problems and with deeper questions about self, sense of isolation, and issues of despair in Steps 3 and 4 (Mahoney, 1991). In other words, when the pyramid is complete, the counselor should be able to see on paper how the thoughts, feelings, behaviors, and other experiences identified in the topmost portions of the pyramid are related to (or rooted in) deep dynamics (see Boxes 9.4 and 9.5).

Of course, not all client problems are rooted in deep dynamics. When no theoretical inference is needed at Step 4, this part of the pyramid may be left unfilled. However, it is the clinician's job during case conceptualization to explore whether deep issues are present, and if they are, it is the clinician's task during treatment planning to determine whether they should be addressed. A shorthand statement to summarize the inverted pyramid method of case conceptualization's fourth step is: "Using theory: Inferring the deepest areas of difficulties."

Applying the Inverted Pyramid Method: Another Look at Sienna and Janine

We began this chapter by defining case conceptualization and then illustrating the conceptualization of two case examples: Sienna and Janine. Now that we have explained the four-step inverted pyramid method, let's take another look at our two case examples and apply the pyramid approach (Case Illustrations 9.3 and 9.4).

Step 1: Problem Identification

Although Sienna at first discussed her symptoms mostly in terms of depression, the counselor developed a wider, inclusive list of all the symptomatic concerns that could be identified.

Step 2: Thematic Groupings

Sienna's various concerns were sorted and group together into three themes according to common denominators:

1. *Moderate Depression Symptoms:* Sienna's depressed mood, melancholic rumination, sleep and concentration troubles, and so on.
2. *Relationship/Dependence Difficulties*: Sienna's dependence, conflicts, and difficulties in three important relationships, including her boyfriend, mother, and roommate.
3. *Identity Confusion:* Sienna's academic and career indecision and forestalled life planning and multicultural identity questions.

Step 3: Theoretical Inferences

In the third step, symptom groupings or themes are attached to general theoretical inferences. Although numerous illustrations could be offered from differing theoretical perspectives, here are examples of three common theoretical perspectives: humanistic, psychodynamic, and cognitive-behavioral. Of course, an eclectic or integrative approach, which mixes or integrates more than one pure theory, also could be used.

1. *Humanistic:* Sienna's depression, relationship dependence and conflict avoidance, and fears of establishing an independent adult identity might lead to theoretical inferences of low self-esteem.
2. *Psychodynamic:* Here Sienna's symptom groups might be conceptually related to autonomy difficulties.
3. *Cognitive-Behavioral:* Sienna's dependence and passivity might lead to inferences about damaging, catastrophic self-statements and learned avoidance.

CASE ILLUSTRATION 9.3 Applying the Inverted Pyramid Method to Sienna

The figure below illustrates case conceptualization using the inverted pyramid method. As we recall from case illustrations 2.1 and 8.1, Sienna initially sought counseling for the problem of persistent, moderate depression. The figure and discussion that follow should help you see how the clinician applies the four steps of the inverted pyramid to form a conceptualization of Sienna's concerns.

Step 1. Problem Identification: Identify and List Client Concerns

Low mood – Obsessive worry – Sleep trouble – Poor appetite – Poor concentration – Problems with boyfriend – Conflicts with mother – Unassertive with roommate – Career indecision – Multicultural questions – Anxiety about independence – Low energy – Unclear academic goals

Step 2. Thematic Groupings: Organize Concerns into Logical Constellations

(1) Moderate depression (2) Relationship/Dependence problems (3) Identity confusion

Step 3. Theoretical Inferences: Attach Thematic Groupings to Inferred Areas of Diffculty

Fragile self-esteem (humanistic perspective)
or
Autonomy conflicts (psychodynamic perspective)
or
Catastrophizing and learned avoidance (cognitive-behavioral perspective)

Step 4. Narrowed Inferences: Deeper Difficulties

Undeveloped self-worth/"Fatal flaw" (humanistic perspective)
or
Abandonment/Disintegration (psychodynamic perspective)
or
No suicidal threat; no deeper inferences seen (cognitive-behavioral perspective)

Step 4: Deeper Theoretical Inferences

In Step 4, the client's difficulties are further explained by deeper inferences underlying her adjustment difficulties and symptom patterns. The clinician continues using the same theoretical approach used in Step 3.

1. *Humanistic:* Here it might be inferred that Sienna's fragile self-esteem was rooted more deeply in feelings of having a "fatal flaw"—the sense that "something is terribly wrong with me"—and in turn, her passing thoughts of suicide.
2. *Psychodynamic:* Sienna's ambivalence about adult autonomy might be conceptually tied to fears of disintegration ("I will be overwhelmed by my independence") or abandonment ("I will lose my family relationships if I am successful") that at times are expressed or dealt with through melancholy thinking about the alternative of suicide.
3. *Cognitive-Behavioral:* In Sienna's case, once the clinician ruled out the risk of suicidal action, no deeper theoretical inferences were required because the Step 3 inferences captured the roots of the client's difficulties from the cognitive-behavioral perspective.

Step 1: Problem Identification

In the first step of the inverted pyramid, a comprehensive list of Janine's presenting and associated problems was derived.

Step 2: Thematic Groupings

Janine's various symptoms were sorted into two logical constellations.

1. *Depression:* Her daily feelings of depression and sadness, social isolation, loss of appetite, and other symptoms were sorted under the heading of depression. It was also decided that her recent unemployment and diagnosis of adult-onset diabetes fit in this category as psychosocial stressors related to her depression.
2. *Family Conflict:* The second constellation is family conflict, which includes the poor relationships Janine has with her son, father, and brother.

Step 3: Theoretical Inferences

In the third step, symptom groupings or themes were attached to general theoretical inferences. Using a cognitive theoretical perspective, the counselor inferred that Janine's depression and other difficulties were rooted in faulty thinking. More specifically, several elements of faulty thinking were inferred: (a) negative view of self, (b) negative interpretations of life experiences, and (c) negative projections about the future.

Step 4: Deeper Theoretical Inferences

In Step 4, the counselor continued the conceptual process using the cognitive theoretical perspective. From this perspective, the different elements of Janine's faulty thinking, and the depression and other difficulties they are causing, are rooted in a deeper, significant, overall faulty negative worldview. This includes

CASE ILLUSTRATION 9.4 Applying the Inverted Pyramid Method to Janine

The figure below illustrates case conceptualization using the inverted pyramid method. As we recall from Case Illustration 8.2, Janine initially came into the community mental health center and, like Sienna, was concerned about symptoms of depression. The figure and discussion that follow should help you see how the clinician applies the four steps of the inverted pyramid to form a conceptualization of Janine's concerns.

Step 1. Problem Identification: Identify and List Client Concerns

Daily feelings of depression – Tearful when discussing depressive symptoms – Social isolation – Loss of interest in once enjoyable activities – Loss of appetite – Poor relationships with son, father, and brother – Lack of energy – Difficulty with concentration and short-term memory Recent unemployment – Recent adult-onset diabetes diagnosis

Step 2: Thematic Groupings: Organize Concerns into Logical Constellations

(1) Depression
(2) Family conflict

Step 3. Theoretical Inferences: Attach Thematic Groupings to Inferred Areas of Difficulty

(Three areas of inferred difficulty using a cognitive theoretical perspective)
(1) Negative view of self
(2) Negative interpretations of experiences
(3) Negative projections about future

Step 4. Narrowed Inferences: Deeper Difficulties

(Deeper cognitive distortion using cognitive approach)
Deepest faulty belief:
"I don't believe I will ever enjoy life and do the things I could do before."

Janine's pessimistic, depressive, faulty beliefs that she will never be well again, will never be able to resolve her difficulties, will never be able to enjoy life again, and will never be able to do the things she could do previously.

Using Popular Characters to Increase Familiarity with Case Conceptualization

Case conceptualization is complex. By understanding theoretically just where the problem really lies, good case conceptualizations provide the bridge between diagnosis (describing the problem) and treatment planning (building a plan to bring about change). But mastering this "thinking" part of being a professional counselor can be a challenging, if not a daunting, task. First, it requires time and experience and becoming much more familiar with how case conceptualization is done, and then, it requires "practice, practice, and more practice!"

Using "cases" drawn from historical figures and popular characters has been one well-established method of practicing and demonstrating formulation skills. Training programs commonly use fictional characters and popular movie characters to illustrate client dynamics and psychopathology (Greenberg, 1993; Schwitzer et al., 2005). You will find this way of practicing case conceptualization useful for several reasons (Schwitzer et al., 2005).

First, you won't have any trouble locating a practice "caseload." If you are not yet working in a site with a real counseling-client caseload, popular characters give you an easily available, ample supply of practice cases. You can also look for characters who are more culturally diverse, cover more phases of the life span, and present a wider range of presenting concerns than you might see among real-life clients in your training site.

Second, you will avoid the ethical problem of working within the limits of your existing competence (see American Counseling Association, 1995; APA, 2003; National Association of Social Workers, 1999). You can use popular culture clients to strengthen your conceptual skills without having to worry about the effects of your work on an actual person's well-being.

Third, practice cases get around the ethical issues related to confidentiality. Ethical considerations have an impact on when and with whom actual client cases can be discussed for training and professional development purposes (e.g., ACA, 1995, Section B.5.a.). But practice cases can be discussed freely in class and with instructors, colleagues, supervisors, and peers.

Fourth, you don't need to be skilled at conducting an interview to begin practicing case conceptualization. When working with real clients, the chance to work on case formulation skills is somewhat dependent on the counselor's existing skills at information gathering and conducting an intake (APA, 2000; Loganbill et al., 1982; Martin et al., 1989). Further, with real clients, information can become available only slowly, over a long time period during the course of counseling; some clients may be less able or less willing to share all of the information useful for practicing case conceptualization skills; and practicing these skills may not be suited to all real-life clients in all real-life clinical settings. By comparison, when you use fictional characters as practice cases, all the available information appears more quickly for your use.

Four Practice Clients

Following are four examples that demonstrate the four-step inverted pyramid method of case conceptualization. The cases were selected by four novice counselors and include the heroine of a novel (Scarlett O'Hara), a biographical character (Maya Angelou's Marguerite), someone drawn from a children's fairy tale (Hansel), and a movie character (Snow White's Wicked Queen). Each case provides an introduction to the character, a case summary, and then a completed four-step case formulation. As you read the examples, you will see how four beginning clinicians, each with a different theoretical perspective, prepared cases using the inverted pyramid method. We have included three female characters and one male character, of which one client is African American and the others are White. Three are adults and one is a child.

PRACTICE CLIENT 9.1

Scarlett O'Hara

INTRODUCING THE CHARACTER

Scarlett O'Hara, drawn from the novel *Gone with the Wind* (Mitchell, 1964), cannot be fully understood except against the backdrop of the time period that shaped her—the South and all of its customs around the time of the Civil War. Concerned mostly about social status and perceptions, Scarlett marries her first husband not out of love, but for self-serving purposes. Following his death and flouting the societal norms of the time, Scarlett reenters the social scene of the South. After the fall of Atlanta, Scarlett flees to Tara, her family's plantation where she grew up. Here she finds her mother dead, sisters dying of typhoid, and father out of his mind with grief. It is up to Scarlett to make decisions, keep starvation at bay, and prevent the whole family from being thrown out of their home. She marries again not for love, but for money that she desperately needs. When her husband is killed, Scarlett agrees to marry Rhett Butler but has little chance for happiness since she still idealizes the first unrequited love of her life, Ashley. Lack of honesty takes its toll on the marriage, and Rhett states he no longer loves her and is leaving. The book ends with Scarlett declaring she will win him back.

CLIENT SUMMARY

Scarlett came in to the counseling center seeking help dealing with stress in her marriage and grief over the death of a close friend. She described herself as being "out of step" with the rest of society and said she feels restless and uncertain of what the future holds.

Scarlett reports various symptoms of stress and describes a recurring nightmare of being lost in a foggy landscape, being pursued, and running to find a "safe haven." She says she has been experiencing stress symptoms and nightmares ever since fleeing Atlanta when the city was overtaken during the war. She has never before sought counseling.

CASE CONCEPTUALIZATION USING THE INVERTED PYRAMID METHOD

Step 1. Problem Identification: Identify and List Client Concerns

Unhappy marriage, recurring nightmares of being in danger, grief, mood volatility, feeling misunderstood and unaccepted by most people, lack of direction for the future, and lack of satisfaction with life achievements.

Step 2. Thematic Groupings: Organize Concerns into Logical Constellations

Symptoms were organized into three thematic groups:

1. *Loss and Grief*: combining death of close friend, loss of husband's love, recurring nightmare of being lost and in danger
2. *Loss of Self-Confidence:* combining her lack of direction for future, dissatisfaction with past achievements, both incongruent with her actual success, surviving, and thriving after events that would have brought down many of her peers
3. *Lack of Social Adjustment:* combining her feelings of being misunderstood and unaccepted by peers, frequent mood instability when facing stressful situations

Step 3. Theoretical Inferences: Attach Thematic Groupings to Inferred Areas of Difficulty

The counselor used existential and psychology of women (feminist psychology) theoretical perspectives. From an existential-feminist psychology perspective, it was inferred that the client comes from a social system that discourages independent thinking and autonomy in women. Etiology and sustaining factors are inferred to include two underlying existential and social construct themes:

1. *Problematic Gender-Role Expectations*, leading to fragile feelings about self (loss of self-confidence, lack of social adjustment) when going outside the unfair, narrow bounds of approved behavior
2. *Need to Engage in Meaning-Making* regarding choices made to survive the war and reconstruction

Step 4. Narrowed Inferences: Deeper Difficulties

The counselor continued with an integration of existential and psychology of women theoretical perspectives. It was inferred that a still-deeper underlying etiological theme is guilt over remaining alive and powerful when many "who did the right thing" did not survive.

REFLECTION AND DISCUSSION

Once you have read through the counselor's conceptual formulation, practice by drawing the completed inverted pyramid figure with the information and formulation provided by the counselor in the practice case. Next, make a few written notes about your reactions to the conceptualization. With what elements do you agree or have questions? What are your thoughts about the theoretical perspectives the counselor selected? Finally, discuss your reactions in pairs, triads, small groups, or as a class.

PRACTICE CLIENT 9.2

Maya Angelou's Marguerite Johnson

INTRODUCING THE CHARACTER

Marguerite Johnson is the main character of Maya Angelou's (1969) autobiographical novel, *I Know Why the Caged Bird Sings*. Angelou presents Marguerite as a studious, intelligent, high-functioning adolescent girl. The book tells of numerous early traumas. For instance, at age 3, Marguerite and her 4-year-old brother were sent away by their parents to live with their grandmother—an early experience of rejection that seemed to shape Marguerite's subsequent behavior and affect. At age 8, Marguerite returns to her mother and is sexually assaulted by her mother's boyfriend, who himself dies suspiciously soon after. Marguerite becomes withdrawn, sullen, and silent. Later, now living with her father, she was stabbed during a confrontation with the father's girlfriend. At age 16, Marguerite's adolescent sexual awakening and desire for normal female experiences result in pregnancy and a son who becomes a source of pride and life purpose.

CLIENT SUMMARY

Marguerite came in to counseling to address feelings about being abandoned by her mother and father. She also wanted to discuss issues revolving around sexual abuse she experienced as a child. Her current pattern is to avoid intense issues and emotions, and she sometimes acts on feelings in a passive-aggressive manner.

Marguerite reports that she has experienced problems and problem behaviors throughout her childhood and adolescence, including repressing feelings of anger, resentment, betrayal, compensation, pregnancy, sexual abuse, intense guilt, not speaking out loud for a long period during childhood, truancy, and avoiding deep personal relationships.

CASE CONCEPTUALIZATION USING THE INVERTED PYRAMID METHOD

Step 1. Problem Identification: Identify and List Client Concerns

Denial of difficult feelings, compensation, teen pregnancy, survival of childhood sexual abuse, (excessive) guilt, escapism, childhood history of discontinued speech, socially withdrawn, loose parental attachments, truancy, avoidance of confrontation, and self-blame.

Step 2. Thematic Groupings: Organize Concerns into Logical Constellations

Symptoms were organized into three thematic groups:

1. *Avoidance of Conflict and Hurt:* combining being nonconfrontational, self-blame, denial, etc.
2. *Inability to Form Close Relationships:* combining effects of childhood difficulties, weak attachments, etc.
3. *Isolating Self from the World:* combining childhood silence, social withdrawal, truancy

Step 3. Theoretical Inferences: Attach Thematic Groupings to Inferred Areas of Difficulty

The counselor used a contemporary psychodynamic theoretical perspective and inferred that Marguerite was using basic defenses for self-cure and self-protection. According to this perspective, etiology and sustaining factors included four underlying themes:

1. *Repression:* "I can't handle my painful emotions, like those I feel toward my parents and others who hurt me, so I'll push them out of my mind."
2. *Denial:* "Instead of recognizing how bad the rape experience was, I believe it felt good and Mr. Freeman was just showing me love when he touched me."
3. *Reaction Formation:* "I treat my mother kindly and with respect because she is beautiful and wonderful, and I do not have any reasons deep down to be enraged."
4. *Sublimation:* "Instead of being angry, I will put my energy into my studies and socially acceptable pursuits."

Step 4. Narrowed Inferences: Deeper Difficulties

The counselor continued with a psychodynamic theoretical perspective. It was inferred that a still-deeper underlying etiological theme sustaining Marguerite's difficulties is a fundamental fear of abandonment ("I am worthless and do not deserve to love, so if I'm not careful, or show who I really am, everyone will leave me").

REFLECTION AND DISCUSSION

Once you have read through the counselor's conceptual formulation, practice by drawing the completed inverted pyramid figure with the information and formulation provided by the counselor in the practice case. Next, make a few written notes about your reactions to the conceptualization. With what elements do you agree or have questions? What are your thoughts about the theoretical perspective the counselor selected? Finally, discuss your reactions in pairs, triads, small groups, or as a class.

PRACTICE CLIENT 9.3

Hansel

INTRODUCING THE CHARACTER

In the Grimm Brothers' fairy tale (Marshall, 1990), Hansel and his sister, Gretel, are the children of a poor woodcutter and his wife. The wife contrives to reduce the number of hungry mouths in the home by abandoning the two children in the forest. Stranded and hungry, they wander deep into the forest and discover a cottage made of cake, bread, and candy. Soon after the starving children begin eating away at the house, they discover it is owned by an evil hag. The children undergo a traumatic event when the hag attempts to fatten them up and then cook them in an oven for a meal of her own. The children contrive to escape and return to the protection of the father, whose wife has passed away during the children's absence.

Clinical conjecture suggests that Hansel's difficulties are not yet over. Once home, he begins having recurring nightmares, avoids going into the woods to gather firewood, and has difficulty concentrating on his usual games. His distressing behaviors seem to heighten when his father decides to help the children build a seasonal gingerbread house. As Gretel constructs the house, Hansel becomes visibly agitated, rocks back and forth in his seat, and later smashes the gingerbread house to pieces. Hansel's father contacts the village counselor.

CLIENT SUMMARY

Hansel's father sought assistance after Hansel became overwhelmed with anxiety and smashed a family gingerbread house. The father also reports that Hansel has become less involved with family activities and is having nightmares and difficulty concentrating. Hansel's behavior changes have been present about 4 months and began shortly after his return from an outing in which he and his sister were left in the woods, became lost, and narrowly escaped being eaten by an evil hag.

CASE CONCEPTUALIZATION USING THE INVERTED PYRAMID METHOD

Step 1. Problem Identification: Identify and List Client Concerns

Exposure to threatened death and trauma, previous malnutrition, abandonment by parental figures, disturbing dreams, repetitive play and intense distress when exposed to reminders of the trauma, avoidance of places (e.g., woods), inability to recall elements of the trauma (the hag's demise), diminished interest in family activities, difficulty concentrating, angry outbursts, and difficulty staying asleep.

Step 2. Thematic Groupings: Organize Concerns into Logical Constellations

Symptoms were organized into three thematic groups:

1. *Feeling Unsafe, Anxious, and Alone:* combining intense distress, avoiding places, etc.
2. *Unconscious Reenactment of Trauma:* combining disturbing dreams, inability to recall elements of the truama, repetitive play with toy oven

3. *Retreat from Feelings of Anger:* combining denial of abandonment by parents, being overcome by angry outbursts when retreat from anger gives way

Step 3. Theoretical Inferences: Attach Thematic Groupings to Inferred Areas of Difficulty

The counselor used an eclectic theoretical approach that combined the humanistic perspective with child counseling/play therapy perspectives. It was inferred that Hansel's exposure to trauma and death (of the hag) led to three problematic types of self-doubts about his adjustment to the world:

1. *Feeling scared and alone*
2. *Believing "I am a bad person for what happened"*
3. *Feeling "I am afraid I have no one to turn to and nowhere safe to go"*

Step 4. Narrowed Inferences: Deeper Difficulties

The counselor continued with the eclectic approach combining a humanistic theoretical perspective with methods that are appropriate for counseling with children. It was inferred that a still-deeper underlying etiological theme is a fear of imminent death or destruction.

REFLECTION AND DISCUSSION

Once you have read through the counselor's conceptual formulation, practice by drawing the completed inverted pyramid figure with the information and formulation provided by the counselor in the practice case. Next, make a few written notes about your reactions to the conceptualization. With what elements do you agree or have questions? What are your thoughts about the theoretical perspective the counselor selected? Finally, discuss your reactions in pairs, triads, small groups, or as a class.

PRACTICE CLIENT 9.4

Wicked Queen

INTRODUCING THE CHARACTER

The Wicked Queen in the Disney movie version of the Grimm's fairy tale *Snow White and the Seven Dwarfs* (Grimm, 1972; Hollis & Sibley, 1987) brings to life the malicious stepmother stereotype. The Wicked Queen, stepmother of Snow White, the title character in the fairy tale, is a jealous woman who uses magic to evil ends. The Queen is extremely insecure and is so threatened by Snow White (a princess who presumably is next in line for the throne) that she forces her to wear rags and assigns her to toil as a scullery maid in the castle. When the vain Wicked Queen consults her magic mirror to confirm her beauty, only to have the mirror tell her that Snow White is the most beautiful woman in the land, the envious Queen pursues evil plots to do away with Snow White. It is significant that the Wicked Queen does not have any meaningful relationships with any characters in *Snow White*. In fact, she seems to view other characters as either impediments to be gotten rid of (Snow White) or as a means to an end.

CLIENT SUMMARY

The Wicked Queen was referred by Doc for treatment of auditory and visual hallucinations. The Queen sees the image of another person's face in her "magic" mirror, which she reports speaks to her about her relative appearance to that of other girls and women in the kingdom. Doc also shared the impression that the Wicked Queen appears evil, extremely vain, and self-absorbed. According to Doc, there is a concern that the Wicked Queen may not be receptive to mental health treatment.

The Wicked Queen says that her magic mirror began speaking to her after the death of her husband. She is isolated and reports no close interpersonal relationships. She takes great pride in her appearance and role as ruler of her country. The Queen has a history of lying and misrepresenting herself and is alleged to have poisoned Snow White and possibly others, although this could not be proved. Based on Department of Social Services reports, it is believed that the Wicked Queen's earlier behavior met *DSM-IV-TR* diagnostic criteria for childhood onset of conduct disorder.

CASE CONCEPTUALIZATION USING THE INVERTED PYRAMID METHOD

Step 1. Problem Identification: Identify and List Client Concerns

Visual and auditory hallucinations; poor self-esteem; paranoia related to appearance; lack of meaningful interpersonal relationships; poor self-image; deceitfulness; poor impulse control; criminal behavior (attempted murder); lack of remorse; history of conduct disorder in childhood; history of abuse and abandonment; preoccupation with looks; need for affirmation of beauty; jealousy; grandiosity; vindictiveness; growing up in impoverished family; abandoned at age 2 by parents; raised by grandmother, who placed overemphasis on physical appearance and was convinced that her granddaughter's beauty would provide a way out of poverty; parental history of alcohol dependence; parental history of mental illness.

Step 2. Thematic Groupings: Organize Concerns into Logical Constellations

Symptoms were organized into five groups:

1. *Hallucinations:* combining visual and auditory hallucinations
2. *History of Abuse and Abandonment:* combining parental alcohol dependence and mental illness, abandonment, grandmother issues
3. *Antisocial Behaviors:* combining deceitfulness, criminal behavior, vindictiveness, poor impulse control, conduct disorder history
4. *Poor Self-Image:* combining lack of meaningful relationships, poor self-image, need for affirmation
5. *Narcissism:* combining paranoia related to appearance, preoccupation with looks, jealousy, grandiosity

Step 3. Theoretical Inferences: Attach Thematic Groupings to Inferred Areas of Difficulty

The counselor used a humanistic theoretical perspective and inferred that the Wicked Queen's poor self-image, antisocial behavior, and narcissism were related to her developmental family experiences of abuse and abandonment, which together formed two etiological themes:

1. *Fragile Self-Esteem*
2. *Difficulty Forming Relationships*

A referral also was made for a psychiatric consultation to assess the hallucinations.

Step 4. Narrowed Inferences: Deeper Difficulties

The counselor continued with the humanistic perspective and inferred that underlying the two themes of fragile self-esteem and difficulty forming relationships was a still-deeper etiological theme: *Undeveloped Self-Worth*.

REFLECTION AND DISCUSSION

Once you have read through the counselor's conceptual formulation, practice by drawing the completed inverted pyramid figure with the information and formulation provided by the counselor in the practice case. Next, make a few written notes about your reactions to the conceptualization. With what elements do you agree or have questions? What are your thoughts about the theoretical perspective the counselor selected? Finally, discuss your reactions in pairs, triads, small groups, or as a class.

Additional Questions and Exercises Using Popular Characters

Practice cases using popular characters often raise unique clinical issues for consideration. Exercises 9.3 and 9.4 offer additional questions to consider when using such characters.

EXERCISE 9.3 **Afterthoughts about Chapter 9 Practice Cases**

For each of the following questions, first consider your own responses and then discuss in class your responses in small or large groups:

1. Scarlett's identity questions, relationship problems, and other issues were conceptualized from a feminist psychology theoretical perspective that emphasized the influences of society on her symptoms. How does this compare with other theoretical perspectives that place less emphasis on societal influences and greater emphasis on individual functioning? What theoretical approach might you select as Scarlett's psychotherapist? How would you use the four-step model to conceptualize her case?
2. The case of Angelou's Marguerite was conceptualized from a brief psychodynamic theoretical perspective. However, questions have been raised in recent years about the use of various theoretical orientations with culturally diverse caseloads. For example, some clinicians debate the relative value of "White middle-class" psychoanalytic approaches for culturally different clientele. What have you learned about matching approaches with client characteristics? What theoretical approach might you select as Marguerite's counselor? How would you use the four-step model to conceptualize her case?
3. Hansel illustrated the use of case conceptualization with clients who are children. What special considerations do you think are needed when assessing and conceptualizing the needs of child clients?
4. Selecting the Wicked Queen as a popular character practice case raises issues related to stereotyping (in this case, of stepmothers) and awareness of cultural context (here, whether talking to mirrors is culturally appropriate and expectable behavior in the cultural context of fairy-tale kingdoms). How can you use popular characters to gain a better perspective on your own "blind spots" to stereotyping and awareness of culture? What other popular characters come to mind that might be useful practice clients for considering such issues?

EXERCISE 9.4 **Additional Practice Using Popular Character Clients**

If you don't yet have a full-fledged real-life caseload of your own with which to practice case conceptualization, select one or more popular character clients from literature or fiction writing, biography, television, movies, or another media. First, write a brief introduction to the character that brings out the most important elements of the person's life. Second, write a brief case summary that presents the character as a counseling client. Third, formulate a start-to-finish inverted pyramid method case conceptualization. Share your efforts, discuss your work, and get feedback. With enough advance practice, when you begin to have your own real-life client caseload, you should feel more comfortable and confident and you will have a little more experience to get going!

LEARNING CASE CONCEPTUALIZATION: An Ongoing Process

Case conceptualization is a critical clinical tool. Eventually, as you become a more experienced clinician, you will find your own preferred theoretical orientation, and you will develop your own reliable system for conceptualizing client needs. At that point, when you meet a new client, you will have in mind a theoretical plan for picking apart the important details of a case to gain a comprehensive understanding of a client and his or her needs. However, it takes quite a lot of classroom instruction, practice doing case conceptualization, and clinical experience with a wide range of clients to reach such an advanced stage.

In the meantime, case conceptualization can seem like a difficult puzzle to solve. Until you have your own caseload, the best place to start is with popular character practice clients. Continue to work on the four-step method with many different characters. Share your work with instructors, peers, and supervisors to learn from their feedback.

You also should look for opportunities to join case conferences, case staffings, and grand rounds at such places as training clinics, college or community counseling centers, field placements sites, jobs, or professional development opportunities (e.g., conferences). Become exposed to the case formulations of as many different experienced professionals as you can.

In addition, begin taking a close look at the different theories of counseling and psychotherapy you have started to study. Notice which theories seem to fit well with your own clinical characteristics, and consider which approaches are best designed for the sort of clients you would like to work with and the type of setting at which you expect to be employed. Finally, bring what you have learned in this chapter with you as we take a look at treatment planning and case management in the chapters that follow.

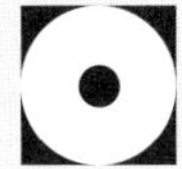

At this point, we recommend that you pause reading, turn to the DVD, and take another look at the sections entitled:

Intake Interview.

While viewing this segment, pay particular attention to issues related to case conceptualization.

Chapter Summary

This chapter introduced the clinical tool of case conceptualization. First, we offered definitions of case conceptualization. We noted that case conceptualization involves three elements, including (a) observing, assessing, and measuring client behaviors, thoughts, feelings, and physiological features; (b) using these observations, assessments, and measurements to find patterns and themes in the client's concerns; and (c) as a function of the theoretical orientation of the clinician, using the patterns and themes found to interpret, explain, or make clinical judgments about the etiological factors and sustaining factors associated with the person's concerns. We also pointed out that although the client's perspective of his or her needs should be taken into account, case conceptualization ultimately is the clinician's understanding of the client's needs and the clinician's ideas of how to serve the client.

Next, we presented a four-step model called the inverted pyramid method for doing case conceptualization. We said that the inverted pyramid method gives novice counselors a reliable step-by-step process for conceptualizing each new client's situation. We also presented the inverted pyramid diagram, which illustrates the process of distilling widely collected client information into narrower and deeper explanations. We explained the four steps in the following ways.

Step 1, problem identification, involves identifying and listing client concerns. Here counselors cast a "wide net" when collecting information about client behaviors, thoughts, feelings, and physiology. Clinicians use the intake interview, problem checklists, and psychological measures to collect information at Step 1.

Step 2, thematic groupings, involves organizing the client's concerns into intuitive-logical groups according to themes. We compared four different types of clinical thinking that counselors use at Step 2: (a) the descriptive-diagnosis approach, organizing groupings according to the way different symptoms are elements of the same disorder; (b) the clinical targets approach, organizing groupings according to the basic division of thoughts, feelings, behaviors, and physiology; (c) the areas of dysfunction approach, organizing groupings according to their effect on the client's everyday life; and (d) the intrapsychic approach, organizing groupings according to their effects on the client's internal, or intrapsychic, functioning.

Steps 3 and 4 are "theoretical." They are inferential, interpretive, or explanatory. Whereas in Steps 1 and 2 the clinician uses intuitive-logical thinking to identify and begin organizing client concerns, in Steps 3 and 4 the clinician applies a more formal theoretical perspective to what he or she has learned about the client. In Step 3, theoretical inferences, thematic groupings or constellations developed in the previous steps are matched to inferred areas of difficulty according to the counselor's theoretical perspective. In Step 4, narrowing inferences, the counselor goes further theoretically to infer the deepest, most causal roots of the client's concerns. Working all the way down the inverted pyramid through Step 4 helps beginning counselors develop a full, deep conception of the client's functioning.

We presented two case illustrations to demonstrate the inverted pyramid method of case conceptualization: the case of Sienna, whom we first met in Chapter 2, and the case of Janine, whom we met in Chapter 8. We will revisit these clients in the chapters that follow.

Near the end of the chapter, we introduced an approach to practicing case conceptualization that uses popular characters drawn from literature and fiction, biographies, television and movies, and other media. Showing how this can be done, we used four case examples drawn from literature and the movies, including the cases of Scarlett O'Hara, Maya Angelou's Marguerite, the fairy-tale character Hansel, and Snow White's Wicked Queen.

Next, we suggested that you practice case conceptualization by choosing and working with your own popular character clients. We noted that practicing case conceptual skills in this manner avoids some of the pitfalls sometimes encountered with real-life clients. For instance, we noted that when using popular characters, you won't have any trouble locating a practice caseload. Second, you will avoid the ethical problem of working within the limits of your existing competence. Third, practice cases get around the ethical issues related to confidentiality. Fourth, you don't need to be skilled at conducting an interview to begin practicing case conceptualization. And finally, with real clients, information can become available only slowly, but with fictional characters, all the available information appears more quickly for your use.

We concluded the chapter by discussing the fact that learning case conceptualization is an ongoing process. We suggested that readers continue to practice with fictional cases to improve their comfort, confidence, and familiarity with case conceptualization before working with real-life clients. We also recommended gaining as much exposure as possible to case conceptualization in actual settings and suggested that readers begin learning as much as possible about different theoretical perspectives.

CHAPTER 10

Treatment Planning: Building a Plan for Change

Once the clinician has identified the client's concerns through thoughtful listening, information gathering, and diagnosis, and after the clinician has carefully applied the case conceptualization process, treatment planning is ready to begin. Whereas the professional counselor has an intentional, well-designed plan for directing the change process toward desired outcomes, the natural helper generally "shoots from the hip" when making suggestions for an individual. Occasionally, shooting from the hip can be helpful, but unfortunately, such unplanned responses sometimes can be degrading or harmful to the person.

In this chapter, we first define and explain what treatment planning is. We discuss the purpose of treatment planning and how a good treatment plan is beneficial to our work with clients. We also discuss how a well-documented treatment plan is beneficial to the clinician. Next, we introduce specific steps for building a basic, generic treatment plan: selecting achievable goals, determining what the treatment will be, and establishing how change will be measured. We include case illustrations and practice exercises throughout the chapter to acquaint you with treatment planning. Finally, we discuss the ongoing process of learning how to build treatment plans.

Understanding Treatment Planning

Defining Treatment Planning

Treatment planning is action oriented and goal directed. It moves from knowing what the client's concerns are to deciding what to do about them. Treatment planning provides a "road map" for reaching the desired clinical outcomes and is the tool by which clinicians put their case conceptualization and theoretical perspective into action.

As in the previous chapter, we asked our group of novice counselors—new clinicians just beginning their clinical careers—how they would define treatment planning. Here is what they said:

- "Treatment planning is goal setting and agenda setting."
- "Developing a plan with objectives, strategies, and goals for working with a client in therapy."
- "A written plan of problems, objectives, goals; type of therapeutic interventions; service provider and timetable for bringing about change."
- "Developing an approach to treatment and services based on the client's wants and needs."
- "A process by which the counselor plans out the goals of therapy and how to go about achieving those goals in an estimated number of sessions."

These new counselors agreed that treatment planning provides the therapist and client with a game plan for reducing or eliminating disruptive symptoms that are impeding the client's ability to reach positive mental health and outlines the steps to be taken in helping the client to reach wellness or acceptable coping skills. These responses provide a good snapshot of what treatment planning is all about. Along the same lines as these beginning counselors, an experienced clinician has offered us the following widely accepted definition of treatment planning:

> *[Treatment planning is] plotting out the counseling process so that both counselor and client have a road map that delineates how they will proceed from their point of origin (the client's presenting concerns and underlying difficulties) to their destination, alleviation of troubling and dysfunctional symptoms and patterns, and establishment of improved coping mechanisms and self-esteem.* (Seligman, 1993, p. 288; 1996, p. 157)

In defining treatment planning for this text, we take the position that it is a vital aspect of mental healthcare delivery (Jongsma & Peterson, 2003; Seligman, 1993, 2004). We view competent clinicians as those who move methodically from assessment and case conceptualization to the formulation and implementation of the treatment plan (Jongsma & Peterson, 2003; Schwitzer & Everett, 1997). Thus, our definition of treatment planning includes three aspects: (a) selecting achievable goals, (b) determining treatment modes, and (c) documenting the attainment of goals.

Selecting Achievable Goals

Treatment plans give the therapeutic work structure and direction (Seligman, 2004) by focusing on choosing specific objectives that lead to intervention strategies (Jongsma & Peterson, 2003). It includes selecting achievable goals for change from among the presenting concerns, associated concerns, etiological factors, and/or sustaining factors that are causing the client distress or dysfunction. Clients and practitioners benefit from a clear, written treatment plan that includes specific goals because it reminds both to think of counseling in terms of therapeutic outcomes instead of waiting for a vague sense of when the client feels as if he or she has improved (Jongsma & Peterson, 2003).

Determining Treatment Modes

Treatment plans include a broad array of activities, or treatment modes. The clinician must make decisions about who will be the service provider (e.g., setting, specific staff), what treatment formats will be employed (e.g., individual, group, couples, family, medication), what therapeutic approach will be used (e.g., person-centered, psychodynamic, cognitive-behavioral), which specific interventions will be employed, and what the duration of the counseling relationship is expected to be. Of course, since issues can change or emerge throughout the helping relationship, and because the clinician gets better insight into the appropriateness and effectiveness of the interventions selected once they are implemented, the treatment plan should be viewed as a road map that will be reviewed and possibly updated periodically (Jongsma & Peterson, 2003). A carefully designed treatment plan, based on research findings and the counselor's clinical knowledge about treatment effectiveness, should increase the likelihood of successfully reaching the desired counseling outcomes (Seligman, 2004).

Documenting the Attainment of Goals

Treatment plans provide documentation of treatment (Jongsma & Peterson, 2003) and, along with posttreatment evaluations, give the counselor a tool to substantiate the work being done (Seligman, 2004). Being able to confirm the efficacy of one's work is important for two reasons in the world of professional counseling. First, collecting payments or funding from third-party payers such as insurance companies, HMOs, and government sources typically is dependent on being able to show what goals were set, what interventions were used, what milestones were reached along the way, and whether the goals were ultimately accomplished. Second, in the current climate of increased patient and client litigation, liability is an important professional concern. Here a treatment plan that documents the process and progress of our work with clients can provide one solid defense against exaggerated or false claims or other types of malpractice suits (Jongsma & Peterson, 2003; Seligman, 2004).

Case Illustrations: Sienna and Janine

To give you a better picture of what treatment planning involves, it is helpful to once again return to our two case examples of Sienna and Janine, who were introduced earlier and discussed in Chapter 9 when we examined case conceptualization. First, we offer an abbreviated treatment plan for Sienna and for Janine, and later in the chapter, after we detail the treatment planning process, we expand on our treatment plans.

For our first illustration, let's return to our client Sienna. Take a moment to reacquaint yourself with the discussions about Sienna presented in Chapters 2 and 9. Then, read Case Illustration 10.1 and try to gain a general picture of what treatment planning comprises.

CASE ILLUSTRATION 10.1 Introduction to Treatment Planning: Sienna

As seen in Chapter 2, Sienna is a 23-year-old college student who came into the counseling center presenting moderate and persistent depression. Sienna also has been dealing with relationship and dependence problems with her boyfriend, mother, and others and with problems achieving adult independence and identity (review the case conceptualization presented in Chapter 9).

A. SELECTING ACHIEVABLE GOALS FOR CHANGE

Sienna sought counseling to reduce her feelings of depression. When the counselor more fully explored all of Sienna's areas of difficulty, three logical themes were conceptualized: (a) her depressed mood, worry, sleep trouble, poor appetite, poor concentration, and low energy; (b) dependence problems and conflicts in important relationships; and (c) identity confusion.

The treatment plan developed was to address Sienna's symptoms of depression and her dependence in relationships. Specific goals written in the treatment plan included:*

- Alleviate Sienna's depressed mood and have her return to her previous level of effective functioning
- Decrease Sienna's level of dependence and conflict in her relationships with her mother and with her boyfriend

B. DETERMINING TREATMENT MODES (E.G., SERVICE PROVIDER, TREATMENT FORMAT, THERAPEUTIC APPROACH, THERAPEUTIC INTERVENTIONS, AND DURATION OF COUNSELING)

According to the case conceptualization from a humanistic perspective, Sienna's themes were seen to be rooted in low self-esteem, an underdeveloped sense of self-worth, and diffusion of identity. Correspondingly, the treatment of choice would be individual counseling using humanistic (or person-centered) interventions. Specifically, the plan would be to "develop improved self-esteem and increased self-worth, which would lead to alleviation of depressive symptoms, alleviation of dependence in important relationships, and an increased sense of identity (knowing who she is)."

To do this, the counselor would:

- See the client 1 hour weekly for person-centered counseling
- Develop a nurturing supportive environment where Sienna could feel free to honestly assess her current level of functioning
- Promote client insight through the use of person-centered skills (e.g., empathy, unconditional regard, genuineness)
- Encourage the client to record her thoughts, feelings, and behaviors and examine her role in significant relationships

(*continued*)

(*continued*)

C. DOCUMENTING ATTAINMENT OF GOALS

The goal of developing healthy feelings of self-worth and accurate perceptions of self that lead to the alleviation of depressive symptoms, the alleviation of dependence in relationships, and an increased sense of identity would be measured by:

- The client's self-reported success in replacing negative feelings related to poor self-esteem with positive feelings of self-worth
- The client's self-reported success in alleviating depressive symptoms
- The client's self-reported success in reducing dependence needs and conflict
- A decreased score on a test of depression and an increased score on a test of self-esteem
- Overall improvement as reported by the client and viewed by the clinician as measured on the GAF Scale

* Identity confusion was seen as partly developmental, and it was felt it might be alleviated by addressing the first two goals. If not, it can be added to the treatment plan later.

Notice that in the first step, although Sienna presents depressive symptoms, relationship dependence, and identity confusion, the counselor determines that the main treatment goals will be to reduce or eliminate the symptoms of depression and to reduce or eliminate the relationship conflicts and dependence and has selected not to directly address the identity confusion issues at this point. Next, notice that the counselor, guided by a specific theoretical orientation and case conceptualization, determines that humanistic psychotherapy will be utilized to address the fragile self-esteem and underdeveloped self-worth believed to be "causing" the depression and maintaining the client's relationship-dependence problems. This is followed by the counselor determining that change will be assessed by observations of the client in their sessions together, by client record and self-reports, by positive changes in GAF scores (return to Chapter 8, if needed, to review the GAF), and by pre–post changes in mood and behavior as measured by psychological testing. Now try Exercise 10.1.

EXERCISE 10.1 **Developing Your Treatment Plan for Sienna**

Sienna's treatment plan gives just a cursory illustration of the treatment planning process. At this point, we certainly don't expect you to have a complete understanding of how to build a treatment plan. However, as an exercise, think about what goals you would set for Sienna and what therapeutic approach you might use if you were her counselor. Specifically, consider the following questions and then discuss them in small groups.

1. What areas of difficulty do you believe would be most important to address?
2. What would be your goals for change?
3. What conceptual approach and which interventions would you plan to employ to help Sienna change?

For our second example, let's return to our community counseling client Janine, who was introduced in Chapter 8 and discussed in the previous chapter. Here again, as you read through this second illustration, consider what treatment planning might involve. Take a moment to reacquaint yourself with the discussion of Janine presented in Chapters 8 and 9 and then read Case Illustration 10.2.

CASE ILLUSTRATION 10.2 Introduction to Treatment Planning: Janine

As seen in Chapter 9, Janine is a 48-year-old White woman who came into a rural community mental health center. Like Sienna, Janine was experiencing low mood and other symptoms of depression. Janine has also been dealing with unemployment and a recent diagnosis of adult-onset diabetes (review the case conceptualization presented in chapter 9).

A. SELECTING ACHIEVABLE GOALS FOR CHANGE

Janine sought counseling to eliminate her feelings of depression. When the counselor more fully explored all of Janine's areas of difficulty, two logical themes were conceptualized: (a) her feelings of depression and sadness, social isolation, loss of appetite, lack of energy, loss of interest in pleasurable activities, difficulty concentrating, and short-term memory problems—all of which fit with symptoms of a depressive disorder; and (b) problematic relationships with her father, brother, and son—or collectively, family conflicts.

The treatment plan developed was to first address Janine's symptoms of a depressive disorder. Although important, reducing the family conflicts and psychosocial stressors were not immediate goals of counseling, as the depression was seen as an overriding problem that needed to be addressed prior to these other issues. These other issues can be addressed in a modified treatment plan or in the future. Specifically, the goal that was selected was to:

- Alleviate depressed mood and return to previous level of effective functioning

B. DETERMINING TREATMENT MODES (E.G., SERVICE PROVIDER, TREATMENT FORMAT, THERAPEUTIC APPROACH, THERAPEUTIC INTERVENTIONS, AND DURATION OF COUNSELING)

According to the case conceptualization, from a cognitive perspective, the therapist linked Janine's low mood to a negative view of self, negative interpretations of life experiences, and negative beliefs about the future.

Correspondingly, the treatment of choice would be individual psychotherapy using cognitive interventions. Specifically, the plan would be to:

- Develop healthy cognitive patterns and beliefs about self and the world that lead to the alleviation of depressive symptoms

(continued)

(continued)
To do this, the counselor would:

- See the client for individual counseling 1 hour weekly
- Assist the client in analyzing her cognitive self-talk to assess dysfunctional thinking
- Assist the client in replacing negative and self-defeating talk with realistic and positive cognitive messages
- Meet with a psychiatrist for possible antidepressant medication as an adjunct to therapy

C. DOCUMENTING ATTAINMENT OF GOALS
The goal of developing healthy cognitive patterns and beliefs about self and the world that lead to alleviation of depressive symptoms, achieved through assessing and changing negative self-talk, would be measured by:

- The client's self-reported success in learning to replace self-defeating thoughts with positive thoughts
- The clinician's observation of the client's success in learning to replace self-defeating thoughts with positive thoughts
- Alleviation of depressive symptoms, as measured by observation and psychological testing
- Increased GAF score
- Decrease in antidepressant medication dosage if prescribed

Notice that in the first step, although Janine presents (a) a depressive disorder, (b) family conflicts, and (c) psychosocial stressors of unemployment, medical diagnosis of diabetes, and lifelong problems with poverty, the counselor determines that the primary treatment goal will be to reduce or eliminate the symptoms of depression. Next, guided by a specific theoretical orientation and case conceptualization, the counselor determines that cognitive therapy will be utilized to address the faulty thinking believed to be "causing" the depression. Then, the counselor states change will be assessed by: observations of the client, pre–post changes in mood as measured by testing, increased GAF scores, and decreased medication dosage. Now try Exercises 10.2 and 10.3.

EXERCISE 10.2 **Developing Your Treatment Plan for Janine**

Janine's treatment plan gives just a cursory illustration of the treatment planning process. At this point, we certainly don't expect you to have a complete understanding of how to build a treatment plan. However, as an exercise, think about what goals you would set for Janine and what therapeutic approach you might use if you were her counselor. Specifically, consider the following questions and then discuss them in small groups.

1. What areas of difficulty do you believe would be most important to address?
2. What would be your goals for change?
3. What conceptual approach and which interventions would you plan to employ to help Janine change?

Exercise 10.3 **How Comfortable Are You with Professional Decision Making?**

The responsibility for clinical decision making and treatment planning—deciding on goals, interventions, and indicators of change—is an important clinical responsibility. It can feel empowering and professionally exciting, it can feel like an overwhelming responsibility for the welfare of another person, and some counselors feel negatively, or at odds, with the clinical need to map out such a specific behavioral plan for treatment. To see where you fit into this part of the path from natural helper to professional counselor, consider the following questions. First, make some mental or written notes answering each of these questions as completely as you can and then discuss your responses in pairs or small groups.

1. What immediate feelings, thoughts, reactions do you have when you think about being in the clinical role of treatment planner?
2. What will interest or excite you about this part of being a professional helper?
3. What concerns do you have?
4. What ethical considerations or reservations do you have?

Building a Treatment Plan

> *The process of developing a treatment plan involves a logical series of steps that build on each other much like constructing a house.* (Jongsma & Peterson, 2003, p. 4)

The foundation of the treatment plan is assessment, appraisal, and conceptualization of the client's concerns, and this foundation leads to the selection of achievable goals for change. After goals are chosen, the clinician, in consultation with the client, will determine what treatment or interventions will be used. The final logical step, then, is to establish exactly how change will be measured—in other words, to establish how you and the client (and other interested parties) will know that the goals have been accomplished. Although there are a variety of paper-and-pencil formats used in clinical treatment planning, all formats in today's world of professional counseling focus on three steps: selecting achievable goals for change, determining the treatment, and establishing how change will be measured. Expanding on the discussion earlier in this chapter, what follows is a step-by-step process for building a treatment plan.

Step 1: Selecting Achievable Goals for Change

An accurate understanding of the client's needs is required before a decision can be made about which problems to address. This requires effective work by the clinician in the earliest stages of the helping relationship. During Stage 1, rapport and trust building, the clinician must establish good rapport and begin listening carefully to understand the client's presenting concerns.

During Stage 2, problem identification, the clinician must accurately identify and describe the client's broader set of needs. This includes accurately assessing not only the client's presenting concerns (e.g., feelings of worry and anxiety) but also associated concerns (e.g., social difficulties, work problems), etiological factors leading to the concerns (e.g., punitive, critical family experiences while growing up), and sustaining factors maintaining the concerns (e.g., poor self-esteem, self-defeating thinking, verbally abusive boss). Further, the clinician must gain an accurate appraisal of the client's level of distress and/or dysfunction resulting from the various concerns. Diagnosis is used to define and describe the client's difficulties, and case conceptualization is used to understand and tie together the presenting and associated concerns and etiological and sustaining factors.

During Stage 3, goal setting and treatment planning, the clinician selects achievable goals for change. It is an outgrowth of all previous clinical activity in Stages 1 and 2. This process involves selecting the problems to address, assessing the urgency and dysfunction of the problem, using case conceptualization, assessing client motivation for change, understanding the impact of real-world influences on setting realistic goals, and using behaviorally measurable goals.

SELECT THE PROBLEMS Although the client may discuss a variety of issues during the early assessment stages, the clinician must sort out the most significant problems to be the targets of counseling. Usually, a primary concern will be identified, along with several secondary or other concerns. An effective treatment plan can only address a few selected concerns, or it will lose its effectiveness (Jongsma & Peterson, 2003). The clinician must prioritize the issues for which the client is seeking help to select treatment that will address the client's greatest needs.

URGENCY AND DYSFUNCTION The first consideration when selecting problems to be addressed is the magnitude of the person's difficulties (Seligman, 2004). Issues causing the most concern—that is, those that cause the greatest psychoemotional distress or the most disruption in everyday functioning—typically require more immediate attention. Some issues receive priority and require immediate attention, such as suicidality and other forms of self-harm (e.g., anorexia or compulsive self-mutilation); potential for harm to others; the diagnostic "red flag" problems of delirium, dementia, amnestic and other cognitive disorders, and mental disorders due to a general medical condition; schizophrenia and other psychotic disorders; substance abuse; and any other problem causing substantial distress or disruption.

CASE CONCEPTUALIZATION The next consideration in problem selection is case conceptualization. The clinician must use his or her professional judgment to decide whether the most important targets for treatment involve (a) individual symptoms or concerns, such as those recorded in Step 1 of the inverted pyramid method of case conceptualization (e.g., sleep problem, concentration problem; see Chapter 9); (b) groups or constellations of symptoms, such as those represented by a *DSM-IV-TR* diagnosis (e.g., all the symptoms of posttraumatic stress disorder) or those recorded in Step 2 of the inverted pyramid method of case conceptualization (e.g., a client's anger management problems at home, at work, and elsewhere—all addressed together; see Chapter 9); or (c) inferred difficulties such as "poor self-esteem" or "faulty thinking" as noted in Step 3 of the inverted pyramid method (see Chapter 9). Any of these targets—specific symptoms, groups of symptoms, or inferred difficulties—may be written into a treatment plan as the defined problem for which change is expected.

CLIENT MOTIVATION Although treatment planning requires the clinician to take on the role of trained expert, the clinician must actively collaborate with the client in selecting the focus of counseling to achieve his or her commitment to the change process. Clients may be self-referred, referred by family or others close to them, or mandated to counseling by the courts or another authority. The client's motivation to take part in counseling and cooperate with treatment during the work stage depends largely on whether he or she believes the treatment will address his or her greatest needs and will resolve the problems of greatest interest. The client's collaboration is required when deciding which symptoms, symptom groups, or inferred difficulties will become the defined problems according to the treatment plan.

REAL-WORLD INFLUENCES The problems selected must lead to achievable goals that are realistic and reasonable within all of the constraints of the helping relationship and are appropriate for the agency or counseling setting. For example, school counselors typically should not set goals that require intensive personal psychotherapy to achieve. Similarly, outpatient therapists should not set goals requiring extensive longer term therapy if the client can only make a commitment for a few sessions (Robbins & Zinni, 1988). Both client and counselor should understand the real-world constraints of the relationship when determining what problems will be the focus of treatment.

BEHAVIORALLY MEASURABLE GOALS A specific operational (or behavioral) definition is required for each problem that is identified for inclusion in the treatment plan. The exact symptom pattern, as it is experienced by the individual client, should be described in clear, precise language. For example, a client's problem with anger management could be described as follows (Jongsma & Peterson, 2003): "overreactive hostility to insignificant irritants, use of abusive language, and history of explosive aggressive outbursts out of proportion to any precipitating stressors leading to assaultive acts or destruction of property" (p. 16).

In turn, the goals for change also should be written in clear, exact, operational, behavioral language. This description will be used to assess whether the expected change has been achieved at the end of counseling. For example, the end goal for a client with an anger management problem could be written behaviorally as follows (Jongsma & Peterson, 2003): "Decrease overall intensity and frequency of angry feelings, and increase ability to recognize and appropriately express angry feelings as they occur" (p. 16). It takes practice and experience to write clear, specific, behaviorally explained problems and goals when treatment planning (see Box 10.1).

Step 2: Determining the Treatment

Prioritizing and selecting the problems to be addressed and deciding on clear, operational, measurable goals for change form the foundation of the treatment plan. Determining what the treatment will be naturally follows. In this step, three questions must be answered: Who will be the service provider? What treatment formats will be employed? What interventions will be used? In addition, the treatment approach must be stated in behavioral terms.

BOX 10.1

Summary of Step 1: Selecting Achievable Goals for Change

The clinician collaborates with the client to select achievable goals for change from among the presenting concerns, associated concerns, etiological factors, and/or sustaining factors that are causing the client distress or dysfunction.

SELECT THE PROBLEMS TO BE ADDRESSED
Prioritize the issues for which the client is seeking help to select treatment that will address the client's greatest needs.

URGENCY AND DYSFUNCTION
Consider the urgency and amount of dysfunction when choosing goals. The following in particular should be addressed:

- issues of suicidality and other forms of self-harm or potential for harm of others
- the diagnostic red flag problems of delirium, dementia, amnestic and other cognitive disorders, mental disorders due to a general medical condition, and schizophrenia and other psychotic disorders
- substance-related concerns
- any other problem causing substantial distress or disruption

CASE CONCEPTUALIZATION
Use your case conceptualization and theoretical orientation to choose goals.

- individual symptoms or concerns, such as those recorded in Step 1 of the inverted pyramid method of case conceptualization
- symptom groupings, such as those represented by *DSM-IV-TR* diagnoses or those recorded in Step 2 of the inverted pyramid
- inferred difficulties, such as those recorded in Steps 3 and 4 of the inverted pyramid

CLIENT MOTIVATION
Consider whether client believes the treatment will address his or her greatest needs and will resolve the problems of greatest interest.

REAL-WORLD INFLUENCES
Choose realistic goals.

- appropriate for the agency or counseling setting
- achievable within existing session limits

BEHAVIORALLY MEASURABLE GOALS
Choose goals that can be clearly defined and measured.

- exact symptom pattern should be described in clear, precise language
- goals for change also should be written in clear, exact, operational, behavioral language
- these descriptions will be used to assess whether the expected change has been achieved

SERVICE PROVIDER In determining the service provider, the clinician must consider what would be the most appropriate counseling setting, which types of mental health professionals are best suited to the client's needs, and whether an outside referral is indicated.

Setting

Deciding who will be the service provider begins with determining which agency or counseling setting is best suited to address the client's needs. Some general settings include inpatient hospitalization, marriage and family counseling centers, outpatient mental health settings, private practices, schools, college counseling centers, and so forth. Other settings include more specialized centers designed for special populations such as the needs of women, children, low socioeconomic clients, and so on. Still other settings provide services tailored to specific issues: suicide crisis centers; centers for depression or anxiety; clinics for sleep disorders, eating disorders, and so forth. When designing the treatment plan, the clinician must be sure that the counseling setting can provide the "therapeutic repertoire" needed to meet the client's greatest needs (Jongsma & Peterson, 2003, p. 6; Seligman, 2004).

Mental Health Professional

Deciding who will be the service provider also means determining which type of mental health professional is best equipped to address the client's needs. Some problems can be addressed within the repertoire of generalist professional counselors or psychotherapists. Other problems may be better suited to the unique family systems training of licensed family counselors, clinical social workers, or the doctoral-level education of clinical psychologists. Specialized services such as psychological testing and assessment may require the work of a licensed professional with expertise in testing, such as a psychologist. Similarly, diagnosis and appraisal for medication may require the services of a psychiatrist. Further, individual staff's training, clinical experience level, areas of expertise, clinical repertoire, and professional dynamics must be considered when assigning clients to a specific clinician's caseload.

Outside Noncounseling Referral

Some client issues are better suited for referral to service providers outside the counseling arena. For example, concerns associated with physical health, poverty, unemployment, environmental problems, legal-criminal problems, financial and debt issues, custody issues, and religious doctrine questions may be more effectively addressed by referral to health services, social services, legal services, financial counseling, child protection services, clergy, or other noncounseling services.

TREATMENT FORMATS There are a number of treatment formats that can be used when working with clients, and the clinician must decide which would be most efficacious for positive client outcomes. Often, the decision about treatment format is made concurrently with choosing the service provider. Common outpatient treatment formats include individual counseling or psychotherapy; structured workshops, support groups, specialized counseling groups, and group psychotherapy; and couples, marital, and family counseling. Crisis or emergency services, or other support services, also may be required for those involved in outpatient therapy. Other specialized counseling formats, such as career counseling, academic counseling, and so on, might be required for some clients, while psychological assessment, psychiatric intervention, and medication also are commonly needed by clients. When inpatient services are required for substance treatment or serious mental disorders, the following is often employed: individual, family, and group therapy; assessment; medication intervention; and milieu therapy (combining different approaches within the inpatient environment).

INTERVENTIONS The treatment plan specifies exactly what type of "work" will take place during the work stage of counseling relationship. Any interventions that are used should be matched to the uniqueness of the client, the goals for change, and the theoretical orientation to be used, and they must take into account the effects of real-world constraints.

Matched to the Uniqueness of the Client
The chosen intervention must be appropriate for the client and his or her characteristics (Seligman, 2001). Thus, it should be well matched to the person's age, developmental level, intellectual capacity, and personality style. It should seem reasonable enough to the client to engage in and motivate him or her.

Matched to Goals
Whether the problem and eventual goals are based on presenting symptoms, symptom constellations, or inferred, underlying, etiological, and sustaining factors, the intervention ultimately chosen should be well matched to the stated goals. For example, stress management and relaxation training could be selected when the stated goal is to reduce specific symptoms of anxiety such as panic attacks, while cognitive therapy could be selected when the stated goal is to reduce the negative self-talk that is inferred to be causing a client's anxiety problems.

A Function of Theoretical Orientation
Intervention techniques should be based on the clinician's theoretical orientation in conjunction with the case conceptualization. Today, psychotherapists can come from an array of different theoretical approaches. For instance, some may adhere purely to one of the major theoretical orientations, such as client-centered, cognitive-behavioral, or psychodynamic; other clinicians integrate a preferred approach with important elements from various orientations; and some counselors use an eclectic, ad hoc mixture of techniques.

Treatment plans will give an estimate of the duration of the counseling relationship, and ultimately, this estimate will be based on the theoretical approach of the clinician and the intervention techniques chosen. Due to real-world constraints on the number of sessions available to clients, one's theoretical orientation can affect whether or not the clinician would be able to work with a particular client. For instance, a psychodynamic purist might insist on long-term counseling. Thus, this clinician would have a difficult time justifying seeing a client who is struggling with a substantial concern and who has only 15 sessions of payment from an insurance company and is unable to afford treatment by another means. On the other hand, a counselor using a behavioral approach might be able to work within a strict session limit.

Affected by Real-World Constraints
The intervention chosen must work within the real-world constraints of the counseling relationship. In general, when client motivation or ability to commit to counseling is low, or when therapeutic contacts will be very limited, more direct, active, symptom-management approaches often are selected. When client motivation and ability to commit to counseling are higher, and

BOX 10.2
Evidence-Based Treatment

How does the clinician decide which approach or combination of approaches to use? Today's clinicians look to several sources to guide their intervention planning. For counselors in training and new counselors, one important source of guidance is more experienced professionals—clinical supervisors, clinical faculty, and cotherapists or other well-trained staff. For more experienced counselors, their own previous clinical work experience—analyzing what has and has not worked well in the past with particular sorts of clients and particular sorts of concerns—provides further guidance.

In addition, today's clinicians look to the evidence: Effective counseling professionals want to know what clinical studies and other research suggest as the best courses of treatment for certain client situations and presenting concerns and which intervention approaches have been shown less effective or ineffective for certain client situations. This can be referred to as evidence-based intervention planning.

There are two types of evidential counseling research. The first type of research is used to show "absolute efficacy" (Wampold, 2001, p. 58), or the overall effectiveness of counseling and psychotherapy in general, compared with no treatment at all. As we discussed in Chapter 2, solid evidence collected over the past several decades has ended the absolute efficacy debate—research analysis tells us clearly that counseling and psychotherapy work (cf. Wampold, 2001). In fact, a review of all the evidence suggests that counseling is a "remarkably beneficial activity" (Wampold, 2001, p. 119) through which up to 80 percent of clients improve.

The second type of research is used to examine "relative efficacy" (Wampold, 2001, p. 72). Studies of relative efficacy compare different approaches—for example, psychoanalytic versus behavior treatment or cognitive therapy versus client-centered counseling—to help us understand which approaches are best for which client needs. There is a growing amount of research looking into the relative efficacy of psychotherapeutic approaches, and reports from new medical-model clinical trial studies (Henry, 1998; Wampold, 1997) and other types of studies to explain the changes derived from counseling methods (Hanna & Puhakka, 1991; Hanna & Ritchie, 1995) are published on an ongoing basis.

Therefore, counseling professionals must keep up with the research literature to be sure they are aware of the latest evidence when planning treatment.

when therapeutic contacts can be more extensive, symptom-management techniques, interventions to address inferred etiological and sustaining factors, or a combination can be used. Finally, as noted earlier, the clinician's theoretical orientation will influence the intervention used and can be a factor in deciding whether or not a specific clinician can work with a client.

BEHAVIORALLY STATED TREATMENT APPROACH When reading the treatment plan, it should be clear what will take place during the work stage of the counseling relationship, and this is accomplished by using a behavioral description of the intended intervention(s). For example, when treating a client's anger management problems using a cognitive-behavioral approach, some clearly stated interventions listed in the treatment plan might include (Peterson & Jongsma, 2003):

- During group and individual sessions, have group members and the clinician point out angry outbursts to client.
- Have client join an 8-week assertiveness-training class.

BOX 10.3

Summary of Step 2: Determining the Treatment

The clinician determines what the treatment will be, including who will be the service provider, what treatment formats will be employed, and what therapeutic approach and which interventions will be employed.

WHO WILL BE THE SERVICE PROVIDER?

- clinicians should consider the agency or counseling setting that is best suited to address the client's needs
- clinicians should refer to the mental health professional who is best equipped to address the client's needs, assigning clients to a specific clinician's caseload
- clinicians should consider whether the client's issues are better suited for referral to service providers outside the counseling arena

WHAT TREATMENT FORMATS WILL BE EMPLOYED?

- common outpatient treatment formats: individual and group counseling or psychotherapy; couples, marital, and family counseling
- emergency services or other supports for outpatients
- specialized formats such as career counseling and academic counseling
- psychological assessment, psychiatric intervention, and medication
- common inpatient treatment formats for substance abuse or mental disorders are individual, family, and group therapy; assessment; medication intervention; and milieu therapy

WHICH INTERVENTIONS WILL BE USED?

- matched to the client's unique personality, intellect, developmental level, age
- well matched to the problem and goals defined earlier in the treatment plan
- outgrowth of the clinician's theoretical and conceptual orientation
- workable within the real-world constraints of the counseling relationship

BEHAVIORALLY STATED TREATMENT APPROACH

- specific behavioral description of the intended interventions and approach

---

- Teach client, through role-playing, more effective ways of responding to irritants and self-defeating ways that client handles anger.
- Have client chart each angry outburst as well as its level of intensity. Then, have client lower the intensity and number of angry outbursts over 2 months. Chart will be examined weekly (see Boxes 10.2 and 10.3).

Step 3: Establishing How Change Will Be Measured

The completed treatment plan must specify how change will be measured and indicate the extent to which progress has been made toward realizing the stated goals. Of course, measuring change in the field of counseling and psychotherapy is a difficult task. However, keep in mind that the purpose of such measurement is not to conduct a controlled laboratory research study but to document as accurately as possible whether the client is experiencing some improvement.

Change can be assessed by a combination of subjective and objective measures (Jongsma & Peterson, 2003; Seligman, 2004). The most commonly used methods include client record and self-report, in-session observation, clinician rating and clinical estimate, and pre–post comparisons of client problem using such tools as checklist ratings and psychological testing results. Some treatment plans include measures of end goals as well as designated milestones or short-term gains; other treatment plans measure only end goals.

Client Records and Self-Report

To state the obvious, clients themselves provide one source of subjective information about the success of treatment. The treatment plan should explicitly state when client records or self-reports will be used as one measure of change.

CLIENT RECORDS Client records are written accounts documenting change. They include such items as periodic client self-reflective notes, diaries, structured logs and checklists requiring specific information at regular intervals (e.g., asking clients to record thoughts, feelings, behaviors, and physiological reactions on an hourly or daily basis), or other written records kept by the client between sessions.

CLIENT SELF-REPORT Client self-report refers to the client's self-report during the session about functioning between sessions. The counselor may use open-ended interviewing or structured questions to solicit the client's feedback about how change is being accomplished. For instance, the clinician might solicit information regarding reductions in symptoms or distress level, improvements in functioning or adjustment, and utilization of new information and behaviors learned through the counseling work.

IN-SESSION OBSERVATION Client records and self-reports mainly provide information about between-session adjustment. The client's thoughts, feelings, behaviors, and physiological reactions during individual, group, couples, or family counseling provide the clinician with direct observations about client functioning and change.

Different theoretical models may emphasize different aspects of in-session client functioning. For example, cognitive and cognitive-behavioral approaches may emphasize the client's reduction in negative self-statements over the course of counseling or the expression of fewer irrational fears. Psychodynamic approaches may emphasize improvements in the client's relationship with the therapist. For example, does the client become less dependent on the counselor to lead the session as therapy progresses? Person-centered approaches may emphasize the client's affect and self-esteem. For example, does the client make fewer negative self-attributions as counseling moves along? Regardless of theoretical approach, counseling sessions provide an opportunity to collect observational and other information about client change in the direction of stated goals, and the treatment plan should explicitly state what client changes will be observed during sessions as a measure of change.

Clinician Rating and Clinical Estimate

Along with direct observations of in-session behavior, the clinician's rating of the client's progress is often used as one measurable estimate of change. We recommend using the Global Assessment of Functioning (GAF) Scale found in the *DSM-IV-TR* (American Psychiatric Association, 2000). The GAF Scale provides one global rating of the client's overall functioning in important life roles and overall distress or psycho-emotional well-being. An advantage of the GAF is that it is widely recognized by various mental health professionals and therefore is a powerful method of communicating the clinician's estimate of how the client is doing. Using the GAF, the clinician can provide a clinical estimate of the client's functioning at some set of regular intervals, such as at the first and last session, after each session, once monthly, and so on. You can revisit Chapter 8 for a review of the GAF.

Pre–Post Comparisons

Many treatment plans rely on comparative measures to support the client's records and reports and the clinician's in-session observations and clinical estimates. One subjective outcome measure is the comparison of the client's responses to a problem checklist, or problem rating worksheet, at intake and again near the end of or soon after the termination of counseling. Comparing psychological testing results at the beginning and end of therapy provides an objective method for confirming change. Psychological testing may be used to measure global changes in functioning (e.g., with the MMPI-II) or changes in specific areas of interest (e.g., the Beck Depression Inventory, Eating Disorder Inventory, a self-esteem inventory, or career decidedness measures).

It should be stated in the treatment plan if changes in client responses to problem checklists and ratings, or in psychological testing results, will be used as a measure of counseling outcomes. We also should note that client responses to problem checklists and psychological testing results can be obtained at the end of counseling even if these measures were not used at intake; however, post-only results provide less clear information about whether counseling has had an impact on reaching the goals for change.

Milestones or Short-Term Gains

Most clinicians will not want to wait until the end of the helping relationship to find out if counseling has been effective. Therefore, today, most counselors include in their treatment plans measures of change at several points along the way. These milestones or short-term gain measurements can use any of the assessment methods previously described. When intermediate change will be measured, the timetable for these measurements should be specified in the treatment plan. For example, client behavior will be assessed weekly, after three sessions, or after each month, and so forth (see Box 10.4).

Another Look at Our Case Examples

We began this chapter by defining treatment planning and then illustrating a general treatment plan for two case examples: Sienna and Janine (Case Illustrations 10.3 and 10.4). Now that we have explained in more detail the steps involved, let's take a second look at our two case examples. Notice in these follow-up illustrations that for each case: (a) the problem now is more clearly defined and goals are more clearly stated in behavioral, operational terms; (b) treatment is clearly explained; and (c) measures of change are provided in detail.

BOX 10.4

Summary of Step 3: Establishing How Change Will Be Measured

The clinician establishes how change will be measured, including how to know whether the goals are ultimately reached by the end of the counseling relationship and what intermediate milestones or short-term gains will be indicated along the way.

CLIENT RECORDS AND SELF-REPORT
- self-reflective notes
- diaries
- structured logs and checklists
- client report of progress to clinician
- other?

IN-SESSION OBSERVATION
- clinical observation of changes
- perceptions of types of changes may be a function of theoretical orientation

CLINICAL RATING AND CLINICIAN ESTIMATE
- GAF
- other?

PRE–POST COMPARISONS
- problem checklists and ratings
- psychological testing
- post-only measurements

MILESTONES OR SHORT-TERM GAINS
- keep tabs on gains made intermittently in addition to gains made at the end of treatment
- write the timetable in treatment plan

CASE ILLUSTRATION 10.3 Revisiting Sienna's Treatment Plan

The example below illustrates a comprehensive treatment plan comprising the three steps discussed in this chapter. Step 1 is selecting achievable goals for change. Step 2 is determining the treatment. Step 3 is establishing how change will be measured. As we recall from Case Illustrations 8.1, 9.1, and 9.3, the client, Sienna, initially sought counseling for the problem of persistent, moderate depression. As we saw in Case Illustration 10.1, the counselor began to build a general treatment plan with goals to alleviate depression and decrease relationship dependence, employing primarily a humanistic treatment approach integrated with cognitive behavioral methods, and measuring change by a variety of methods. In the following illustration, the treatment plan is fully developed.

TREATMENT PLAN

Client: Sienna

Service Provider: College Counseling Center: Assigned to Staff Counselor

BEHAVIORAL DEFINITION OF PROBLEMS

1. Depression: Depressed affect, feelings of worry, sleeplessness, loss of appetite, poor concentration, lack of energy

(continued)

(continued)

2. Dependence: Inability to become self-sufficient without relying on parents, feels easily hurt by criticism and is preoccupied with pleasing others (boyfriend, mother, roommate), inability to make decisions or initiate action without excessive reassurance from others

GOALS FOR CHANGE

1. Depression:
   - Develop ability to recognize, accept, and cope with feelings of depression
   - Develop healthy cognitive patterns and beliefs about self and the world that lead to alleviation of depression symptoms
   - Alleviate depressed mood and return to previous level of effective functioning
2. Dependence:
   - Develop confidence in self so that she is capable of meeting her own needs
   - Achieve a healthy balance between healthy independence and healthy dependence
   - Decrease dependence on relationships while beginning to meet her own needs, build confidence, and practice assertiveness

THERAPEUTIC INTERVENTIONS

Short-term counseling lasting less than or up to one academic semester, integrating person-centered intervention approach with cognitive-behavioral techniques.

1. Depression:
   - Explore how depression is experienced in client's daily life
   - Encourage discussion of depressed feelings and negative thoughts to clarify them and gain insight into causes
   - Explore experiences from client's family contributing to current depression
   - Assist in developing awareness of cognitive messages that sustain hopeless and helpless feelings
   - Assist client to develop coping strategies to reduce feelings of depression (e.g., more physical exercise, less internal focus, more social involvement, more assertiveness)
   - Refer for evaluation to rule out need for medication
2. Dependence:
   - Explore client's history of psychosocial dependence beginning with unmet needs in family of origin to current boyfriend and other relationships
   - Assist client to identify the basis for fear of disappointing others
   - Assist client to identify and implement ways of increasing independence daily, and process results (e.g., speaking her mind, saying no, being assertive)
   - Assign client to psychoeducational group with the focus on support and training in assertiveness and/or time management group to increase adjustment skills

MEASURES

The development of increased healthy feelings of self-worth and accurate perceptions of self, leading to alleviation of depression symptoms and alleviation of dependence in relationships, will be measured by:

- Client weekly records of decreasing negative self-statements, increased number of positive independence/assertiveness behaviors, and decreased depression symptoms each week
- Clinician observation of increased healthy self-statements and increased mood in sessions
- Gradual increase in clinician rating of client function to GAF > 71 and rating of symptoms as no more than mild
- Increased scores on self-esteem inventory as measured pre- and posttreatment
- Decreased scores on Beck Depression Inventory as measured pre- and posttreatment

CASE ILLUSTRATION 10.4 Revisiting Janine's Treatment Plan

The example below illustrates another comprehensive treatment plan comprising the three steps discussed in this chapter. Step 1 is selecting achievable goals for change. Step 2 is determining what the treatment will be. Step 3 is establishing how change will be measured. As we recall from Case Illustrations 8.2, 9.2, and 9.4, the client, Janine, presented at a community mental health center with symptoms of a depressive mood disorder. As we saw in Case Illustration 10.2, the counselor began to build a general treatment plan with goals to alleviate depression and return Janine to her previous level of functioning, employing a cognitive approach and measuring change by a variety of methods. In the following illustration, the treatment plan is fully developed.

TREATMENT PLAN

Client: Janine

Service Provider: Community Counseling Center: Assigned to Staff Counselor

BEHAVIORAL DEFINITION OF PROBLEM

Depression: Depressed affect, suicidal thoughts, social withdrawal, feelings of hopelessness and worthlessness, diminished enjoyment of activities, loss of appetite, lack of energy, poor concentration and memory, low self-esteem

GOALS FOR CHANGE

Depression:

- Develop ability to identify and cope with feelings of depression
- Appropriately grieve job loss, poverty status, and medical diagnosis of diabetes to normalize mood and return to previous adaptive level of functioning

(continued)

(*continued*)

- Alleviate depressed mood and return to previous level of effective functioning

THERAPEUTIC INTERVENTIONS

Intermediate to longer term counseling estimated to last 12–20 sessions, using cognitive psychotherapeutic approach.

Depression:

- Explore how depression is experienced in client's day-to-day living
- Identify cognitive self-talk that is sustaining depressed mood
- Assist client to develop awareness of cognitive messages reinforcing feelings of hopelessness and helplessness
- Teach client to identify negative automatic thoughts associated with depression
- Keep a daily journal of experiences, thoughts, and feelings to clarify instances of distorted negative thinking or perceptions that precipitate depressive emotions
- Replace negative and self-defeating self-talk with verbalization of realistic and positive cognitive messages
- Monitor compliance with psychiatric referral

MEASURES

The development of healthy cognitive patterns and beliefs about self and the world, leading to the alleviation of depressive symptoms, will be measured by:

- Client weekly records of decreased negative self-statements, increased number of positive independence/assertiveness behaviors, and decreased depression symptoms each week
- Clinician observation of increased healthy self-statements and increased mood in sessions
- Improvement in Beck Depression Inventory (BDI) score from moderate depressed range at intake to minimal depressed mood range at termination
- Gradual increase in clinician rating of client function to GAF > 71 and rating of symptoms as no more than mild

Using Popular Characters to Explore Treatment Planning

A well-constructed treatment plan provides the road map for applying theory to practice during the work stage of the professional helping relationship. It does this by clearly articulating which problems will be addressed and what the goals for change will be, how treatment will proceed and what interventions will be used, and what methods will be used to measure progress toward the stated goals. As with diagnosis and case conceptualization, becoming skilled at treatment planning requires familiarity, experience, and practice. The following practice clients should give you an opportunity to begin to hone these skills.

Our Four Practice Clients

In the following section, we want to return to our four practice cases that were borrowed from popular culture (Schwitzer et al., 2005): Scarlett O'Hara, Maya Angelou's Maguerite Johnson, Hansel, and the Wicked Queen. In Chapter 9, we prepared case conceptualizations for each popular character client. In this chapter, each case demonstrates how to practice treatment planning using popular characters (Schwitzer, et al., 2005) (see Exercise 10.4).

EXERCISE 10.4 **Practicing Treatment Planning**

The characters in the following four treatment plans were introduced in Chapter 9 by four novice counselors when we were examining the case conceptualization process. For each case, if needed, first review the case conceptualization in the previous chapter. Then,

1. Develop your own treatment plan that includes a behavioral definition of the problem(s), goals for change, therapeutic interventions, and an indication of how change will be measured.
2. Meet in small groups and develop a team treatment plan.
3. Read the treatment plan given, critique it, and critique your team treatment plan and your individual treatment plans. Share your team plan in class.

SCARLETT O'HARA Drawn from the novel *Gone with the Wind* (Mitchell, 1964), Scarlett O'Hara came into the counseling center presenting stress in her marriage, grief over the death of a close friend, and feeling "out of step" with societal expectations. She reported various symptoms of stress and recurring nightmares (see Practice Client 9.1 for a review) (see Exercise 10.4).

PRACTICE CLIENT 10.1

Scarlett O'Hara

TREATMENT PLAN

Client: Scarlett O'Hara

Service Provider: Community Center for Women: Assigned to Staff Counselor

BEHAVIORAL DEFINITION OF PROBLEMS

1. Grief and Loss: Unresolved grief at death of only close friend and feelings of loss of love relationship with husband
2. Loss of Self-Confidence/Diminished Social Adjustment: Lack of satisfaction with past achievements in spite of successes, feelings misunderstood and unaccepted by peers, and lack of direction for the future

GOALS FOR CHANGE

1. Grief and Loss:
   - Begin healthy grieving process around loss of friend
   - Develop an awareness of how avoiding grief experience has negatively affected life

- Begin process of accepting and letting go of the lost friend
- Resolve loss and begin renewing old relationships and initiating new contacts with others
- Evaluate changes and perceived losses in marital relationship
- Commit to a decision to either (a) accept termination of the relationship or (b) develop the necessary skills for effective, open communication and mutually respectful and satisfying companionship within the relationship

2. Loss of Self-Confidence/Diminished Social Adjustment:
   - Increase understanding of the influence of oppressive, sexist society beliefs and practices
   - Learn to trust and act on her own experiences and intuition
   - Elevate self-esteem
   - Develop a consistent, positive self-image

THERAPEUTIC INTERVENTIONS:

Intermediate counseling with weekly sessions, lasting up to 6 months, using an existentialist-feminist approach.

1. Grief and Loss:
   - Identify the losses that have been experienced in life
   - Facilitate the identification and expression of feelings connected with the losses
   - Facilitate client understanding as to how she depended on the lost friend and intimacy of husband
   - Facilitate expression of feelings of abandonment and aloneness
   - Assist client in resolving feelings of abandonment and aloneness through expression of feelings and/or through client development of an action plan
   - Conduct a couples session to explore beginning to work on a decision to either (a) accept termination of the relationship or (b) develop the necessary skills for effective, open communication and mutually respectful and satisfying companionship within the relationship

2. Loss of Self-Confidence/Diminished Social Adjustment:
   - Explore the client's assessment of self
   - Challenge and reframe client's self-disparaging comments in social context
   - Educate the client about self in society and societal influences on women's roles, attitudes, behaviors, and experiences of self
   - Assign client to read *Women Who Run with the Wolves: Myths and Stories of the Wild Woman Archetype*
   - Discuss, emphasize, and interpret client's social experiences and how they have impacted her feelings about self
   - Assist the client to form more realistic, positive messages to self in interpreting life experiences, and reinforce these changes

MEASURES

The resolution of feelings of grief and loss, clarification regarding marital relationship, and development of increased healthy feelings of self-worth will be measured by:

- Client weekly records of increased ability to express and manage grief and loss feelings
- Clinician observation of client's increased ability to critically examine the society in which she lives

- Client report of lessened feelings of grief and alienation
- Client report of increased clarification regarding loss feelings in marriage
- Significant increase in score on the GAF Scale showing 10–15 points

---

MARGUERITE JOHNSON The main character of Angelou's (1969) autobiographical novel, *I Know Why the Caged Bird Sings*, Marguerite Johnson came into the counseling center to address feelings about abandonment by her parents and childhood sexual abuse. She reported a variety of childhood and adolescent traumas, avoids strong negative emotions, and sometimes acts on feelings in a passive-aggressive manner (see Practice Client 9.2 for a review).

PRACTICE CLIENT 10.2

Maya Angelou's Marguerite Johnson

TREATMENT PLAN

Client: Marguerite Johnson

Service Provider: Midcity Psychotherapy Center: Assigned to Staff Psychotherapist

BEHAVIORAL DEFINITION OF PROBLEMS

Adult difficulties with childhood trauma, sexual abuse, and abandonment: avoids conflict and hurt, self-blame, denial, depressed mood, feelings of numbness, inability to form close relationships, social isolation

GOALS FOR CHANGE

Adult difficulties with childhood trauma, sexual abuse, and abandonment:

- Develop an awareness of how her childhood experiences impacted and continue to impact her life
- Identify and express wide range of painful and other feelings associated with the major traumatic incidents occurring in her childhood
- Identify and express wide range of painful and other feelings associated with her mother's role in her negative childhood experiences
- Develop ability to accurately experience thoughts and feelings
- Alleviate depressed mood
- Increase client's level of trust of others, displayed by increased social interactions and increased tolerance for intimacy in relationships with others

THERAPEUTIC INTERVENTIONS:

Long-term extended psychotherapy in weekly or twice weekly sessions. The client has not addressed her reactions to her negative childhood experiences consciously, and they are therefore being managed unconsciously (in a dysfunctional manner). The corresponding therapeutic need is to bring her unconscious experiences to consciousness. Therefore, a psychodynamic approach will be used.

Adult difficulties with childhood trauma, sexual abuse, and abandonment:

- Free association: uncover repressed material locked in unconsciousness by assisting client to report and discuss feelings and thoughts immediately after censoring them
- Interpretation: explain and teach meaning of behavior
- Analyzing resistance: point out and interpret instances of resistance in therapeutic relationship at a pace tolerable to client
- Dream analysis: interpret disguised meanings in nightmares and dreams related to childhood traumas
- Interpreting transference: point out and interpret instances in which client acts out current expressions of early feelings toward childhood perpetrators of harm in the therapeutic relationship at a pace tolerable to client

MEASURES

Healthy awareness of negative childhood experiences, accurate experience of current thoughts and feelings, increased trust level and capacity for social relationships and intimacy, and alleviation of depressed mood will be measured by:

- Clinician observation of increased experience and expression of wide range of thoughts and emotions about past experiences and regarding the present
- Client record and self-report of increasing instances of forming social relationships and intimate relationships
- Gradual increase in clinician rating of client function to GAF = about 80 and rating of symptoms as no more than mild

---

HANSEL Hansel, who has a sister, Gretel, in the Grimm Brothers' fairy tale (Marshall, 1990), is a young boy brought into the counseling center by his father with symptoms of posttraumatic stress following a narrow escape from being cooked and eaten by an evil hag after being abandoned in a deep forest. The father reports that Hansel has been having recurring nightmares, avoids going into the woods to gather firewood, has difficulty concentrating on his usual games, and becomes quite agitated around gingerbread houses (see Practice Client 9.3 for a review).

Practice Client 10.3

Hansel

TREATMENT PLAN

Client: Hansel

Service Provider: Village Child Counselor: Private Practitioner

BEHAVIORAL DEFINITION OF PROBLEMS

Posttraumatic stress disorder: exposure to threatened death that resulted in an intense emotional response of fear, helplessness, and horror, with disturbing dreams associated with the traumatic event; physiological reactivity when exposed to external cues that symbolize the traumatic event; avoidance of places associated with the traumatic event; inability to recall some important aspects of the traumatic event; lack of participation in significant activities; and lack of concentration; all present for more than a month.

GOALS FOR CHANGE

Posttraumatic stress disorder:

- Reduce the negative impact the traumatic event has had on many aspects of client's life
- Recall the event without becoming overwhelmed with negative emotions
- Implement behaviors that promote healing, acceptance of past events, and ability to participate constructively in relationships with others

THERAPEUTIC INTERVENTIONS:

Eclectic child psychotherapy, including play therapy and psychodrama, three sessions weekly moving to once weekly for up to 6 months, with reevaluation at 6 months.

Posttraumatic stress disorder:

- Refer for psychiatric evaluation or psychological testing to assess presence and severity of PTSD symptoms
- Gently explore client's emotional reaction at time of trauma
- Use play therapy and psychodrama to explore client's emotions associated with traumatic event, facilitating gradual reduction in the intensity of the emotional responses
- Use art therapy to explore dream objects
- Teach imagery techniques appropriate to client's age to assist sleep transitions
- Teach developmentally appropriate cognitive and behavioral coping strategies to manage reactions
- Increase and reinforce positive beliefs about self
- Collaborate with school counseling to assist in treatment plan and assure follow-through

MEASURES

Reduced negative impact of the traumatic events on the client's life, increased ability to recall event without being overwhelmed, and increased resolution of reactions will be measured by:

- Clinician observation that the client begins to demonstrate trust in the therapeutic relationship demonstrated by sharing fears about abandonment and thoughts and feelings about trauma
- Pre–post comparison of presence and severity of PTSD symptoms assessed by psychiatric evaluation or psychological testing
- Clinician observation of increased healing and acceptance, fewer feelings of being overwhelmed, and increased interest in normal developmentally appropriate activities
- Observation and report from school counselor concerning decrease in PTSD symptoms and increase in developmentally appropriate behaviors
- Client's report and father's observations of improved sleep (sleep uninterrupted by nightmares associated with trauma), return to normal play and other activities, and observable reduction in psychoemotional distress associated with traumatic event

---

WICKED QUEEN The Wicked Queen, portrayed in the Disney movie *Snow White and the Seven Dwarfs* (Grimm, 1972; Hollis & Sibley, 1987), was referred to the counseling center for treatment of auditory and visual hallucinations in which a magic mirror began speaking to her after her husband's death. She also experiences self-absorbed narcissistic thoughts and feelings. In addition, difficulties with antisocial behaviors may be present, such as poisoning Snow White and harming others (see Practice Client 9.4 for a review).

Practice Client 10.4

The Wicked Queen

TREATMENT PLAN

Client: Wicked Queen

Service Provider: Community Services: Assigned to Doc

BEHAVIORAL DEFINITION OF PROBLEMS

1. Hallucinations: Visual and auditory perceptual disturbances
2. Traumatic Early Childhood Experiences: History of abuse and abandonment
3. Antisocial Behaviors: Refusal to follow rules, poor impulse control, failure to conform with law, suspected of repeated antisocial and criminal acts
4. Low Self-Esteem: Lack of meaningful relationships, poor self-image
5. Narcissism: Paranoia and undue preoccupation regarding physical appearance, jealousy, grandiosity, lack of acceptance of responsibility for events and actions

GOALS FOR CHANGE

1. Hallucinations: Control or eliminate active psychotic symptoms such that supervised functioning is positive
2. Traumatic Early Childhood Experiences: Develop an awareness of how childhood issues have affected and continue to affect her family life
3. Antisocial Behaviors: Become more responsible for behavior and keep behavior within the acceptable limits of the rules of society
4. Low Self-Esteem: Develop a consistent, positive self-image
5. Narcissism: Improve method of relating to world by accepting responsibility for own actions

THERAPEUTIC INTERVENTIONS AND CORRESPONDING MEASURES OF CHANGE

Eclectic solution-focused and problem-solving interventions focusing on symptom reduction and alleviation, while attempting to minimize resistance to treatment. Interventions are grouped by symptoms, and in this case, outcome measures would be a reduction of the symptoms of hallucinations, antisocial behaviors, and narcissism and an increase in self-worth and trusting behaviors as noted via clinician's observations and client self-report. In addition, intermediate significant increases on the GAF Scale and after 1 year of treatment an overall increase from a GAF score of 30 to a score of at least 60.

1. Hallucinations:
    - Accept and understand that symptoms are due to mental illness as measured by verbal statements
    - Evaluate for antipsychotic medications and monitor for adherence to taking medication by report of client and castle servants
    - Focus on the reality of the external world versus distorted fantasy as reported by client for four consecutive sessions

2. Traumatic Early Childhood Experiences:
   - Verbally describe what it was like to grow up in such an environment
   - Identify at least five feelings associated with major traumatic events
   - Increase levels of trust for others as shown by more social interactions and greater intimacy tolerance by self-report
3. Antisocial Behaviors:
   - Verbally describe history of illegal and/or unethical behavior without attempts at minimization, denial, or projection of blame
   - Develop a list of behaviors and attitudes to be modified to decrease conflict with authorities and process list with therapist
   - Make a commitment to live within the rules of society and do so for a period of at least 6 months
4. Low Self-Esteem:
   - Acknowledge feeling less competent than others
   - Increase insight into at least three historic and current sources of low self-esteem
   - Demonstrate an increased ability to identify and express personal feelings based on the use of at least four feeling statements per session
   - Form realistic, attainable goals for self in all areas of life as measured by self-report when processing with therapist
5. Narcissism:
   - Develop a list of behaviors and attitudes that must be modified to decrease her conflict with others and process list with therapist
   - Increase number of statements of accepting responsibility by at least one per session for four sessions
   - Verbally recognize own responsibility to meet the needs of others in at least five relationships

Afterthoughts about Our Practice Cases and Additional Exercises

As we discovered in Chapter 9, practice cases using popular characters can introduce important clinical issues for consideration. Exercises 10.5 and 10.6 present additional questions to ponder regarding the cases discussed and offer suggestions regarding new cases for which you can develop treatment plans.

EXERCISE 10.5 **Afterthoughts about Our Practice Cases and Treatment Planning**

For each of the following questions, first consider your own responses to the issue presented and then discuss your responses in small groups or with the class.

1. Scarlett came to the Community Center for Women for help, and this is reflected in the treatment plan, built from a feminist perspective on the relational psychology of women theoretical approach. How did her choice of counseling center affect the treatment she will receive? How might this compare with the treatment for grief and loss and loss of self-confidence that she might receive in another setting that has a behavioral or cognitive-behavioral perspective that does not include a feminist perspective?

(continued)

EXERCISE 10.5 *(continued)*

2. Scarlett's counselor conceptualized her marital concerns as part of grief and loss issues. Do you agree with this conceptualization? How would you address Scarlett's concerns about losing her attachment with her husband in your own treatment plan?

3. According to her counselor's assessment, Angelou's Marguerite Johnson's adult difficulties with childhood trauma, sexual abuse, and abandonment are present in unconscious form because the client has not consciously addressed her negative childhood experiences. Therefore, the counselor has built a psychodynamic treatment plan that brings unconscious reactions to consciousness. How does this compare with a problem-solving or solution-focused approach with direct symptom relief as the goals for change?

4. Hansel's symptoms are diagnosed as posttraumatic stress, and his counselor's treatment plan calls for child psychotherapy using humanistic, play therapy, and psychodrama interventions. How would you go about building treatment plans that are appropriate for your own clients' age and developmental level? Consider how your treatment might differ for younger children, adolescents and young adults, middle-aged adults, and geriatric clients.

5. One outcome measure in the treatment plan built for Hansel is his father's observations of change. What issues do you think might come up when relying on parents or caregivers to report on client change?

6. In Practice Client 10.4, we saw that, using the inverted pyramid method, the counselor conceptualized the Wicked Queen's difficulties using a humanistic perspective. In the conceptualization, the counselor inferred that the Wicked Queen's hallucinations, history of abuse and abandonment, antisocial behaviors, low self-esteem, and narcissism were associated with deeper concerns related to fragile self-esteem, difficulty forming relationships, and underlying undeveloped self-worth. However, the treatment plan built for the Wicked Queen uses a solution-focused, problem-solving approach focusing on direct symptom reduction and alleviation, without resolving the inferred causes of these symptoms. One rationale for this approach is that the Wicked Queen, who was court-referred to counseling, is resistant about seeking assistance and is unlikely to fully engage in the helping process.

   What do you see as the benefits and drawbacks of approaches that directly focus on symptom reduction versus approaches intended to resolve the underlying causes of symptoms? How will you decide how to match your own treatment plans to the needs, interests, and motivations of different clients?

7. The counselor's treatment plan for working with the Wicked Queen suggest that the measures of change will be the clinician's observations of the client's decrease of maladaptive behaviors for each intervention noted. What do you see as the advantages or disadvantages of this treatment plan design? For which theoretical intervention approaches is it best suited—eclectic, integrative, solution-focused and problem-solving, behavioral, cognitive or cognitive-behavioral, humanistic or existential, psychodynamic, and so on?

EXERCISE 10.6 **Additional Treatment Planning Practice Using Popular Character Clients**

Practice using popular character clients will help you develop skill and confidence using clinical tools. Select one or more popular character clients from literature or fiction writing, biography, television, movies, or another media and do the following:

1. Write a brief introduction to the character that brings out the most important elements of the person's life.

2. Write a brief case summary that presents the character as a counseling client.

3. Formulate a start-to-finish inverted pyramid method case formulation.

4. Build a start-to-finish treatment plan, including behavioral definition of problems, goals for change, therapeutic interventions, and measure of change. In class, share your efforts, discuss your work, and obtain feedback.

LEARNING TO BUILD TREATMENT PLANS: An Ongoing Process

Treatment planning requires that you apply theory to practice and answers the question: "What will the client and I *do* to bring about desired changes?" The ability to think through and write a treatment plan is essential for today's professional counselors and psychotherapists. As with diagnosis and case conceptualization, developing competence using the clinical tool of treatment planning requires advanced coursework, practice, clinical experience, and ongoing supervision (Glidewell & Livert, 1992; Loganbill, Hardy, & Delworth, 1982). You can take several steps to help with your learning, including practicing with popular character clients, becoming familiar with the work of practicing clinicians, and exploring published treatment planners.

Practice Clients

As we have demonstrated in this and the previous chapter, you don't have to wait until you have your own extensive caseload to work on treatment planning skills. Instead, start by thinking through and writing treatment plans for some of your favorite practice clients drawn from your reading, television, movies, or other popular media. Continue to use the format illustrated in this chapter: behavioral definition of problems, goals for change, therapeutic interventions, and measures. Share your work with instructors, peers, and supervisors to learn from their feedback. Eventually, you will develop your own style for building treatment plans that is based on your theoretical approach in conjunction with the real-world issues that you will face in your clinical settings (e.g., session limits).

Clinical Exposure

In this chapter, we provided a format for a generic treatment plan that is more or less transferable to any mental health setting. However, different counseling specialties, individual agency settings, and third-party reviewers often have their own unique formats for writing treatment plans. Therefore, it is a great advantage to gain exposure to the treatment planning work of as many different clinicians and settings as possible. Look for opportunities to join case conferences, case staffings, and grand rounds wherever possible. Look for opportunities to sit in at training clinics, supervising agencies, and professional development programs. During your supervised field experiences, review case files; have discussions about treatment planning with your supervisors, mentors, and additional staff; and learn how various agencies and different clinicians go about treatment planning.

Dictionaries and Published Planners

There are a variety of books to help you learn the language needed to be a good communicator when operationalizing treatment plans. For instance, dictionaries of psychological, counseling, and psychiatric terms can be a valuable reference for terms and their meanings (e.g., see Gladding, 2001). Written treatment planners may be even better resources than counseling dictionaries. Written planners provide extensive suggestions for how to define the problem, what short-term and long-term goals to set, what interventions to use, and what behavioral outcomes to expect (e.g., see Jongsma & Peterson, 2003).

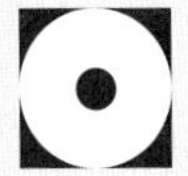

At this point, we recommend that you pause reading, turn to the DVD, and take another look at the section entitled:

Working Stage Interview.

While viewing this segment, pay particular attention to how a treatment plan is implemented.

Chapter Summary

This chapter introduced the clinical tool of treatment planning. First, we defined treatment planning and noted that it is action oriented and goal directed and helps us move from knowing what the client's concerns are to deciding what to do about them. In other words, we described treatment planning as a road map for reaching desired clinical outcomes. We highlighted the fact that treatment planning comprises three main elements: (a) selecting achievable goals, (b) determining treatment modes, and (c) documenting the attainment of goals. Next, we offered the cases of Sienna and Janine to examine how these three elements are addressed during treatment planning. We then expanded the description of treatment planning by offering a detailed description of a three-step treatment planning process based on the elements just noted.

When discussing Step 1, selecting achievable goals to be achieved, we noted that the clinician must first accurately select the problems to be addressed, determine the urgency and dysfunction of the problem(s) and make a judgment about which should be addressed first, use case conceptualization in determining appropriate goals, assess client motivation toward reaching various goals, be cognizant of real-world influences that might affect goal attainment, and use behaviorally measurable goals.

Step 2, determining the treatment, involves a number of elements. First, the clinician should determine who the service provider will be, including decisions about which setting or agency and which mental health professional or whether the client should be referred to a nonclinical service provider. The clinician should determine the treatment format, which could include such modalities as individual and group counseling or psychotherapy; couples, marital, and family counseling; emergency services or other supports for outpatients; specialized formats such as career counseling or academic counseling; psychological assessment, psychiatric intervention, and medication; or inpatient services. The clinician also should make a judgment about which interventions should be used as a function of such considerations as the client's unique personality, intellect, developmental level, and age; problems and goals as defined earlier; the clinician's theoretical and conceptual orientation; and real-world constraints affecting the helping relationship.

Finally, for Step 3, establishing how change will be measured, it was suggested that clinicians use a behaviorally stated treatment approach that involves specific behavioral descriptions of the intended interventions and approach. In measuring client gains, it was suggested that clinicians should use client records and self-report, such as self-reflective notes, diaries, structured logs and checklists, client reports of progress to clinician, and so forth; in-session observation, such as clinical observation of change (keeping in mind that this can vary as a function of the clinician's theoretical orientation); clinical ratings and estimates, such as the GAF Scale; and pre–post comparisons, such as problem checklists and ratings and psychological testing. Finally, it was suggested that many clinicians might want to keep tabs on gains made intermittently in addition to gains made at the end of treatment.

As the chapter proceeded, we expanded on the two case illustrations of treatment planning introduced earlier in this chapter. We will explore these cases again in Chapter 11 when we look at case management. Near the end of the chapter, we returned to four practice cases that were drawn from popular media. We provided illustrations of treatment plans for Scarlett O'Hara, Maya Angelou's Marguerite Johnson, the fairy-tale character Hansel, and Snow White's Wicked Queen. We suggested ways that you could practice using these and other cases drawn from popular media.

We concluded the chapter by discussing how to continue the ongoing process of learning to build and write treatment plans. We suggested that you continue to practice with fictional cases to gain skill and confidence, gain as much exposure as possible to the formats used by experienced practitioners in different settings, and use professional dictionaries and published treatment planners to sharpen your treatment planning skills.

CHAPTER 11

Case Management: Monitoring and Documenting the Professional Relationship

Along with the helping skills and clinical tools we have been discussing throughout this text, professional counselors must be competent at case management. Case management comprises all of those professional activities beyond our direct counseling skills that are needed to make the professional helping relationship successful (Sullivan, Wolk, & Hartmann, 1992; Woodside & McClam, 2003). The clinician uses case management skills to monitor and document the helping process and to keep the relationship focused on the client's well-being. Case management begins during the preinterview, is required during each of the stages of the helping relationship, and continues to be important during the postinterview phase. Whereas the natural helper has little or no understanding of most of these activities, the professional counselor realizes that case management is part of the professional context of the helping relationship (Seligman, 2004).

In this chapter, we first define and outline the components of case management. Next, we explore five key elements of case management: (a) documentation, (b) consultation, supervision, and collaboration, (c) communication with stakeholders, (d) business-related activities, and (e) caseload management. We include examples, illustrations, and practice exercises throughout the chapter to acquaint you with case management. Finally, we discuss the ongoing process of learning to become a good case manager, including why case management is so important and how good case management benefits the clinician and the client.

Defining Case Management

As in the previous two chapters, we asked our group of novice counselors how they would describe the clinical tool of case management. A few of our new counselors voiced the feelings of many clinicians when they said case management seemed to involve "paperwork! paperwork! paperwork!" and when they said case management was "much too time-consuming" and "the monotonous part" of being a counselor. Despite these protestations, and although sometimes time-consuming and tedious, case management is a powerful tool for keeping our work with clients on-track. Other novice counselors offered the following definitions:

- "Case management is the paperwork and documentation for each client on your caseload."
- "It is handling the records, files, communications, supervision, working with other staff on a case, and everything else you do in the office besides sit down with the client himself or herself."
- "Case management is documentation, recordkeeping, how you communicate about the client, and how you ethically and professionally treat your caseload."
- "Case management isn't just filing and paperwork—it's how you handle every phone call, insurance form, scheduling, information request, follow-up, time management, and giving the client good service."

We agree with our students' astute remarks. Expanding on some of them, we view case management as the following:

1. *Documentation:* recordkeeping, note taking, monitoring, and documenting all client information, including preinterview and intake materials, case notes, termination materials, and storing of records
2. *Consultation, supervision, and collaboration:* use of supervision, consultation, medical consult, referral, cotherapists, conjoint treatment, and other professional relationships when assisting clients
3. *Communication with stakeholders:* communications with interested parties who are not mental health professionals, such as the client's family and friends, courts, schools, and social services
4. *Business-related activities:* the business of counseling, including documenting contacts, billing, and interacting with third-party payers
5. *Caseload management:* managing your time and schedule and tracking and following up your caseload

In the following sections, we explore each of these areas in more detail and provide illustrations using our ongoing case examples.

Documentation

Importance and Purpose of Documentation

Accurate recordkeeping is of extreme importance for today's mental health professional (Kleinke, 1994; Reynolds, Mair, & Fischer, 1995). A complete file of the client's concerns, progress during treatment, final disposition, and other pertinent information all combine to form a client's or patient's record. Although we often refer to clinical documentation as being the client's record, notes and files actually are clinical tools used by the clinician and belong to the agency setting. Although ethical codes and laws have sometimes provided mechanisms for clients to review the records we keep about them, clinical documentation is usually the professional property of the agency that provides treatment.

Accurate recordkeeping serves two main purposes: as a clinical resource and as a mechanism for showing accountability. As an important resource, the clinician may refer to case notes and other client information during the helping relationship to keep track of presenting concerns, treatment plans, and progress toward goals. When consultations are needed, accurate records provide other professionals with a detailed summary of the client's situation. Finally, if the client seeks additional counseling at a later date, files can assist clinicians in understanding the person's counseling history.

In reference to accountability, it has often been said, "If it wasn't documented, then it didn't happen!" A complete written intake summary shows exactly what information the counselor collected and is the beginning of the treatment planning process. Clinical records show exactly what was happening during the helping relationship and can be used to show that adequate care has been taken should the clinician be challenged or sued. Termination summaries and final dispositions are often used as evaluation tools by third-party payers and administrators.

Contents of a Client Record

The exact contents of a client record vary according to the type of setting in which you work, differences in state and local requirements for recordkeeping, and according to the needs and guidelines of the specific agency in which you are employed. However, as a general rule, we can say that four components usually make up a client's record: initial contact information, diagnosis and treatment planning notes, progress notes, and termination materials.

INITIAL CONTACT INFORMATION Initial contact materials generally include information obtained prior to the first interview as well as intake materials. This often includes such items as information on record, intake data, psychological testing results, and the intake summary.

Information on Record

. . . an increasing number of people are writing and reading mental health records for an increasing number of purposes. (Reynolds et al., 1995, p. 1)

As a result of the staggering amount of information available on people, clients often enter counseling with a wealth of information that might be accessible and useful during the early stages of counseling. Depending on the setting and client needs, such information may include records from previous mental health treatment; relevant medical records; school or academic records; reports from the court, parole or probation officers, and social services; and paperwork associated with divorce, custody, financial debt, lawsuits, and the like. Frequently, clients can bring such information with them; other times, counselors may ask clients to sign a release of information so they can obtain certain records; occasionally, outside entities might send information directly to the clinician (e.g., summary notes from other professionals regarding the client, court paperwork about mandatory referrals).

Intake Data

Prior to the first interview and at the initial contact with the agency or counselor, clients generally are asked to complete quite a bit of paperwork. Usually, this includes forms that give clients a chance to explain what brought them to counseling, checklists on which clients can indicate concerns and rate distress or dysfunction, and paperwork that addresses such items as clients' family history, counseling history, and other background. Often, information from a structured interview is gathered during this time (see Chapter 6, p. 131 for an example of a structured interview format).

Psychological Testing Results

Clients sometimes are asked to complete psychological testing at the time of intake. Typical types of testing include diagnostic tests used to help form a diagnosis and are useful in treatment planning (e.g., the MMPI-II; problem-specific tests, such as the Beck Depression Inventory [BDI], which is useful in uncovering depression; and the MAST, which is an alcohol-use screening test); nondiagnostic tests used to assist clients to understand their personality dynamics (e.g., Myers-Briggs, the California Personality Inventory); and non-clinical measures of personality preferences and interests (e.g., the Strong Interest Inventory or the Self-Directed Search, which are helpful in career counseling).

Intake Summary

The intake summary is a report written by the clinician that provides a detailed snapshot of all of the basic information gathered from the client's initial contact with the agency or setting. The format of an intake summary can vary dramatically as a function of counseling settings, with some being only a few paragraphs in length and others being a full report with several subsections, such as seen in the structured interview in Chapter 6. However, a general template for a traditional intake summary includes the following sections: identifying information, presenting concerns, relevant background and family history, problem and counseling history, mental status exam, goals for counseling, and course of therapy to date.

Identifying Information. This section provides a short two- or three-sentence introduction to the client that summarizes basic demographics. Some settings simply have a basic listing of client information that includes such items as address, phone number, e-mail address, age, ethnic background, and other information (e.g., see demographic information from structured interview, Chapter 6, p. 131).

Presenting Concerns. This section provides a summary of the client's reason for seeking assistance, documents any supporting testing results, and presents the counselor's appraisal of the client's distress, dysfunction, risk for self-harm or harm or neglect of others, and imminent needs.

Background, Family, and Relevant History. This portion of the intake summary gives an encapsulated look at the client's family of origin and/or current family situation, important information about developmental history, and any other key historical data.
Problem and Counseling History. Here we find an encapsulated look at the client's history of mental health needs, counseling problems, and previous therapy, medication, or hospitalization.
Mental Status Exam. As discussed in Chapter 6, a mental status exam is an assessment of the client's appearance and behavior, emotional state, thought components, and cognitive functioning.
Goals for Counseling and Course of Counseling to Date. This section summarizes the client's goals as well as the clinician's goals for counseling at the conclusion of the intake. These may include the need for further assessment, referral, or consultation, as well as the beginnings of a detailed plan for treatment. In this section of the intake summary, the counselor also may choose to summarize whatever clinical work has already begun.

Two intake summary examples are provided using our ongoing case illustrations. Notice that the counselors supply brief summaries of information in each subheaded section of their reports. The counselors succinctly provide the information they currently have and also indicate what the next steps in assessment and treatment are expected to be (see Case Illustrations 11.1 and 11.2).

CASE ILLUSTRATION 11.1 Intake Summary: Sienna

By now, you are familiar with our client Sienna, whom we introduced in Chapter 2 and discussed again in Chapters 8, 9, and 10. Here is a sample intake summary prepared by Sienna's counselor:

Identifying Information: Sienna is a 23-year-old, second-year female African American college student at a predominantly White university. Sienna comes from an intact two-parent household, now lives on campus with an assigned roommate, and is in a romantic relationship with a male college partner.

Presenting Concern: Sienna was self-referred, coming into the counseling center presenting moderately depressed mood lasting at least several months and related depressive symptoms, including disrupted sleep, appetite, concentration, and low energy level. Sienna was very tearful during the initial meetings. She reports occasional, passing thoughts of "wanting to die" that are consistent with moderate depressed mood but denies any plan or motivation to act on these thoughts. She does not appear to be a risk for self-harm at this time.

Current stressors include ambivalence about having left home, difficulties in her currently changing relationship with her mother, confusion about her dating relationship with a culturally different White boyfriend, and conflicts with her roommate.

Sienna also describes a problematic pattern of psychoemotional and attitudinal dependence on important others, including her mother, boyfriend, and roommate. She appears to experience distress from her current reliance on important relationships for confidence, self-esteem, and decision making about important life issues.

Background, Family, and Relevant History: Sienna entered college after attending a local community college for 1 year. Her family of origin includes her mother and father and two younger brothers, both in high school.

Problem and Counseling History: Sienna reports no significant difficulties during her precollege years. She reports good academic performance, social relationships, and unremarkable dating experiences prior to her current difficulties. At the same time, she reports growing conflicts in her relationship with her mother during her high school years and says she attended a local community college for 1 year largely because she felt obligated to stay "close to my mother . . . she really needs me." Notably, she made the decision to leave home to complete a university degree at the encouragement of her high school and community college academic counselors.

Mental Status Exam: Sienna was appropriate in dress and appearance, and her eye contact seemed appropriate. She was oriented by time, place, and person. She presented with a low mood and her affect was depressed. She seemed somewhat fatigued and was a bit slow in her verbal responses. There were no apparent delusions or hallucinations. Sienna appeared to be above average intellectually and her memory was intact. Her judgment seemed good, her insight was high, and she appeared motivated for treatment. She reported occasional, passing thoughts of "wanting to die" but denies any immediate plan to act on these thoughts and does not appear to be an immediate risk for self-harm.

Goals for Counseling and Course of Counseling to Date: Sienna has been seen once for an extended intake session. Her primary goal is to reduce and eliminate her feelings of depression and return to her previous level of function. She also appears open to the goal of exploring and resolving her dependent pattern in relationships with important others.

Tentative goals are to (a) develop ability to cope with feelings of depression, develop improved cognitive patterns leading to alleviation of depression symptoms, and alleviate depressed mood and return to previous level of effective functioning and (b) resolve young adult dependence issues by developing confidence in self so that she is capable of meeting her own adult needs, forming a balance between healthy independence and dependence in changing relationship with her mother, and forming a balance between healthy independence and dependence in present relationships.

Immediate needs include referral for psychiatric evaluation for diagnosis and possible medication for a mood disorder. Additional referrals may include support or psychoeducational groups or workshops for young adult adjustment issues.

CASE ILLUSTRATION 11.2 Intake Summary: Janine

Recall our client, Janine, whom we met and discussed in Chapters 8, 9, and 10. Janine's psychotherapist prepared the following sample intake summary:

Identifying Information: Janine is a 48-year-old Anglo woman who resides in a rural area of the county. Janine currently is unemployed after losing her factory job of 15 years. She lives with her male romantic partner and appears to have limited social contact with others. Janine recently was diagnosed with diabetes.

Presenting Concern: Janine set up an initial intake appointment at the center due to feelings of depression. She was tearful with poor eye contact throughout the initial intake. She reported little desire to be around other people, loss of appetite, and diminished interest in activities that previously brought her enjoyment. She appears to have some difficulty with concentration and short-term memory. Janine reports no suicidal ideation and reports no history of self-harmful behavior.

Background, Family, and Relevant History: Janine was born the second of two children in a low-socioeconomic household in the same area of the state in which she currently resides. Her parents were never married; her mother is now deceased and she has a limited relationship with her father and a conflictual relationship with her brother.

Janine married at age 18 and had one son during the 9 years she lived with her husband. She reports that her marriage was conflictual "with problems right from the start." She moved away from her husband and raised her son alone from age 3. She reports that she has never divorced her husband, in spite of her desire to do so, because she has been unable to afford it. Her son currently lives out of state.

Problem and Counseling History: Janine described significant current distress and other symptoms of a mood disorder. She reports her symptoms began about 1 year ago, shortly following the combination of her job loss and diagnosis of diabetes. Janine reports no previous history of depressive symptoms or any other symptoms of a mental health problem and no previous history of counseling.

Mental Status Exam: Janine was appropriate in dress and appearance. During the interview, her mood appeared quite low, she appeared quite fatigued, she was tearful throughout the appointment, and eye contact was poor. She was oriented by time, place, and person. Janine appeared of average intelligence. She seemed to have some difficulty concentrating and with short-term memory recall. Her judgment seemed good, her insight was low to moderate, and she appeared motivated for treatment to relieve her symptoms. In spite of her symptoms of depression, Janine reports no suicidal ideation and denies any current or past history of self-harmful intent or behavior.

Goals for Counseling and Course of Counseling to Date: Janine has been seen twice for intake and follow-up. Her primary goal is to reduce and eliminate her feelings of depression and return to her previous level of function, including enjoyment of daily activities, desire to interact with others, and improved appetite, concentration, and memory.

Tentative goals are to (a) develop ability to identify and cope with feelings of depression; (b) appropriately adjust to job loss, poverty status, and medical diagosis of diabetes to normalize mood and return to previous level of adaptive functioning; and (c) alleviate depressed mood and return to previous level of effective functioning.

Immediate plans include further assessment: psychological testing (MMPI, BDI) and referral for psychiatric evaluation for a mood disorder. Treatment plan will include at least weekly counseling with a cognitive-behavioral focus.

DIAGNOSIS AND TREATMENT PLANNING NOTES As discussed in preceding chapters, during rapport and trust building, problem identification, and goal setting (Stages 1, 2, and 3 of the helping relationship), the clinician uses clinical tools to produce a diagnosis describing the client's concerns, uses his or her case conceptualization to understand or explain the concerns, and develops a treatment plan to determine goals for change and intervention approach. A diagnosis and treatment plan follow the preinterview and intake materials in the contents of the client record. Sometimes, a tentative diagnosis and treatment plan are described in the intake summary; however, this should always be firmed up at a later date, after the clinician has been able to gain additional information from the client and develop a deeper understanding of him or her.

CASE NOTES OR PROGRESS NOTES The clinician next must maintain a record of how counseling proceeds. Referred to either as "case notes" or "progress notes," these are always tied to the treatment plan. The notes are recorded in the client's file after each clinical contact (e.g., including individual and group counseling sessions, phone contacts, etc.). Case notes are a key part of the client's record and provide a clinical reference for professional use as well as a mechanism for showing accountability. Therefore, case notes must be written in a careful, competent, professional manner.

As with intake summaries, different types of counseling settings may use different formats for preparing case notes. However, one common template for writing case notes includes the following: **s**ubjective client report, clinician **o**bservations, current **a**ssessment, and current **p**lan, often called SOAP.

Subjective Client Report

One obvious source of information about how the treatment plan is proceeding is the client's own experience. Case notes may include a brief summary of the client's report of changes in thoughts, mood, behaviors, and physiological symptoms. Clients may report positive changes (improvements), negative changes (setbacks or deterioration), or no change. They may report on changes or experiences in different settings (at work, at home) or in various roles (marital, parenting, student).

Clinician Observations
Another source of information about how the treatment plan is progressing is the clinician's observations of the client during the clinical contact (e.g., individual, couples, family, or group counseling sessions). Case notes may include a brief summary of the counselor's observations about the client's functioning, such as apparent mood, changes in thinking, the client's appearance and behavior, and how the client interacts and relates with the therapist or others who are present during sessions.

Current Assessment
Each case note should include an assessment of the client's functioning and progress in such areas as client's overall mood, risk for harm, and general overall adjustment. Next, the clinician should include an assessment of the client's commitment and adherence to the treatment plan; follow-through on homework and outside assignments; follow-through on referrals, such as psychiatric evaluations or consultations; compliance with medication; and compliance with referrals for conjoint treatment, such as group therapy or support groups. Finally, some settings and some clinicians provide periodic updates of *DSM-IV-TR* diagnoses and Global Assessment of Functioning (GAF) scores (see Chapter 8 for more about diagnosis and GAF scores).

Current Plan
On the basis on the client's subjective report, in-session observation, and assessment, each case note should summarize what aspects of the treatment plan have been achieved, what aspects of the plan need modifying, what goals remain, and what the specific next steps in the treatment will be.

Two case note examples are provided here using our ongoing case illustrations. Notice that the counselors provide brief, clearly stated progress notes using professional, well-executed language. The counselors use the template discussed so that each case note includes one or two sentences addressing subjective client report, clinician observations, current assessment, and current plan.

CASE ILLUSTRATION 11.3 Case Note: Sienna

We have discussed our client Sienna in Chapters 2, 8, 9, and 10, and a sample intake summary was shown earlier in this chapter. Here is a sample case note prepared by Sienna's counselor. Identify how the counselor addresses each of the following: subjective client report, clinician observations, current assessment, and current plan. Also, notice that the case note is not a verbatim transcript of what was said or done in each moment of the interview; instead, the notes attempt to succinctly communicate the most important elements of the ongoing case.

Session 3 Sienna arrived on time and appeared motivated and engaged during the interview. She reports actively engaging in cognitive homework assignments since the last appointment. She reports modest improvement in sleep, appetite, and energy. Sienna describes a growing awareness of the role of family relationships in her current functioning. In the session, Sienna appeared brighter and more energetic and active than seen previously, and she reports no current thoughts of self-harm. Plan is to continue regular weekly sessions focusing on depression and dependence issues using a cognitive intervention framework. Remaining goals are to continue progress toward alleviation of remaining symptoms of depression and continue interventions to reduce dependence and improve independent adult functioning in relationships with others.

CASE ILLUSTRATION 11.4 Case Note: Janine

Our client Janine was discussed in Chapters 8, 9, and 10, and a sample intake summary was shown earlier in this chapter. Here is a sample case note prepared by Janine's counselor. Identify how the counselor addresses each of the following: subjective client report, clinician observations, current assessment, and current plan. Also, notice that the case note is not a verbatim transcript of what was said or done in each moment of the interview; instead, the notes attempt to succinctly communicate the most important elements of the ongoing case.

Session 6 Janine returned today after canceling her two previous appointments. She cited transportation problems to the missed meetings and indicates she now has resolved the problems of getting to and from the center. Agency policy regarding attendance was reviewed. Janine denied and declined to explore any psychoemotional factors potentially associated with missing recent sessions. Janine reports that in the past 3 weeks she has, on more days than not, maintained the early gains in improved mood, reduced teariness, and some improvement in sleep she experienced early in treatment. At the same time, she reports that depressed mood continues to cause distress. In the session, she appeared to have low energy and became teary at times when discussing recent stressors, especially her poor relationship with her male family members and her diagnosis of diabetes. Janine appears to continue experiencing moderate symptoms of depression, with GAF = about 52 (current) and no change in diagnosis. Plan is to monitor Janine's compliance with attending future appointments and continue with the treatment plan. Remaining goals are to consolidate progress to date and continue reducing symptoms of depression.

TERMINATION SUMMARY At the closure stage of the helping relationship, a termination summary becomes another part of the client record. The termination summary describes the overall progress made in implementing the treatment plan and achieving the goals for change. Although the specifics of these, too, can differ across settings and agencies, the basic template for a termination summary includes four components: reason for termination, treatment plan compliance, progress summary, and posttermination after-plan.

Reason for Termination

The clinician indicates the reason for termination in the termination summary. Termination may be planned as a result of reaching the stated goals for change. Termination also may be planned as a result of reaching session limitations, deciding on the need to refer the client to a more effective mode of treatment (inpatient treatment, group therapy, etc.), or deciding on the need to refer the client to another clinician.

Termination may be unplanned. Some clients leave counseling early when they begin to feel quick relief from the distress or dysfunction that brought them in but before therapeutic goals for change have been fully achieved. In this case, clients may report in a session that they have decided not to return, communicate by phone or in a written note, or simply stop showing up for appointments. Terminations also may occur prematurely due to changes in the client's life situation. For example, clients may terminate to return home at the end of a college semester, due to job relocation, due to loss of finances or insurance, or for other reasons.

Treatment Plan Compliance

The termination summary should describe the clinical work done. This should include (a) an overview of the treatment approach and interventions actually used, assignments and activities, referrals and consults, and other elements of the treatment plan that were enacted; (b) an overview of the client's ability to comply with the treatment plan, resistance and other factors encountered in the therapeutic relationship if relevant, and the client's follow-through with assignments, activities, and referrals; and (c) any important information about remaining elements of the treatment plan not yet implemented. Rather than a session-by-session recounting, this section should be a succinct summary of the overall therapeutic relationship.

Progress Summary

Based on the treatment plan, the termination summary next should describe progress achieved toward stated goals. Progress may be indicated by a combination of client report, clinician observations, pre–post comparative measures, or other methods described in our chapter on treatment planning. The progress summary should be written in clear operational language that gives a concise picture of what goals have been achieved, what unexpected changes were achieved, what setbacks or deterioration or increases in distress or dysfunction have developed, and what goals for change remain unaccomplished. Included in this section may be a final diagnostic impression, including a final estimate of global functioning using the GAF.

Posttermination After-Plan.
Finally, the clinician indicates what plans have been made for after closure. After-plans may include (a) a specified plan for the client to continue certain self-help activities to maintain positive changes made during counseling, forestall or reduce setbacks, mitigate deterioration, or continue making further progress toward unfinished or new goals; (b) specific referral to another clinician or another treatment mode to work on remaining goals, deal with setbacks or deterioration, or maintain positive changes; (c) some general suggestions for continued self-work; (d) a plan for follow-up contacts; and/or (e) a plan for no further therapeutic involvement or activities at all.

Two termination summary examples are provided using our ongoing case illustrations. Notice that the counselors write brief, clearly stated termination

CASE ILLUSTRATION 11.5 Termination Summary: Sienna

Notice that the termination is as planned. Sienna's symptoms of depression were resolved, and at termination there is no diagnosis of any mood disorder or adjustment disorder. The goals stated in the treatment plan (Chapter 9) were nearly all met, and a plan is provided for the remaining parent–child relational issues. Here is a termination summary prepared by Sienna's counselor.

Termination Summary Termination occurs as planned as a result of reaching stated goals. Sienna was seen for a total of 11 weekly sessions, using a short-term counseling treatment plan integrating a client-centered approach in session with cognitive-behavioral techniques and assignments. Sienna was on time, motivated, and compliant with the treatment plan at each scheduled appointment.

Significant progress included alleviation of depressed mood, feelings of worry, sleeplessness, poor appetite, poor concentration, and low energy nearly all day, almost every day. Sienna reports increased awareness of and use of healthy self-statements and only occasional reemergence of problematic negative self-statements. Overall remaining symptoms of depression are quite occasional and mild, with no suicidal ideation at time of termination. Significant progress also includes report of increased incidences of assertive behavior in relationships with boyfriend and roommate, subjective report of increased self-confidence, and improved awareness and understanding of influences of mother–daughter relationship dynamics on adult functioning.

Remaining goals include continuing to increase assertiveness and self-confidence and to reduce negative and guilty self-statements in relationship with mother. Posttermination after-plan is for Sienna to continue attending semistructured group counseling at the center to consolidate gains and

(*continued*)

(continued)

continue progress toward goals in relationship with her mother. Sienna will contact this therapist as needed for future support. No current plan for future individual counseling.

Diagnosis at termination:

Axis I:	V61.20 Parent–Child Relational Problem, Mild
Axis II:	No diagnosis
Axis III:	No diagnosis
Axis IV:	None
Axis V:	GAF = 80

CASE ILLUSTRATION 11.6 Termination Summary: Janine

In Janine's case the termination was due to reaching the agency's session limit. Janine made substantial progress toward her treatment goals. Here is a termination summary prepared by Janine's counselor.

Termination Summary Termination was agreed on by clinician and client. Janine was seen for a total of 16 sessions. The client rescheduled twice and no-showed one time. Janine generally appeared moderately open and motivated for change at each of the 16 interviews she attended and was moderately compliant with the treatment plan in sessions and with homework assignments between meetings.

Significant progress included client report of significantly improved mood, absence of suicidal ideation at this time, improved social interactions weekly, improved feelings of hopefulness and self-worth, and moderately good improvement in appetite, sleep, memory, and concentration. Janine also reported a decrease in negative self-statements to fewer than once daily, increased feelings of independence, and actually engaging in assertive behaviors at least weekly. In sessions, she demonstrated improvement in mood, concentration and memory, and activity and energy levels. Pre–post changes in BDI scores were positive, reflecting minimal depressed mood range at termination. Current symptoms appear mild.

Remaining goals are to continue consolidating positive changes in mood and associated features of depression. Posttermination after-plan is for client to continue independently, actively utilizing exercises to maintain realistic and positive cognitive messages to replace negative, self-defeating self-talk when it emerges. A plan for a scheduled phone contact to be initiated by client in 3 weeks was made.

Diagnosis at termination:

Axis I:	Major Depressive Disorder, Singe Episode, Mild, in Remission
Axis II:	No diagnosis
Axis III:	Diabetes
Axis IV:	Poverty, unemployment
Axis V:	GAF = 71

BOX 11.1
Summary of Documentation

Professional counselors maintain a record of all aspects of the counseling relationship.

PURPOSES OF A CLINICAL RECORD
- Documentation provides a clinical reference
- Documentation provides accountability

CONTENTS OF A CLINICAL RECORD
- Initial Contact Information
    - information on record
    - intake data
    - psychological testing results
    - intake summary
        - identifying information
        - presenting concerns
        - relevant background and family history
        - problem and counseling history
        - mental status report
        - goals for counseling
        - course of therapy to date
- Diagnosis and Treatment Planning Notes
- Case Notes or Progress Notes (SOAP)
    - subjective client report
    - clinician observations
    - current assessment
    - current plan
- Termination Materials
    - reason for termination
    - treatment plan compliance
    - progress summary
    - posttermination after-plan

STORING OF RECORDS
- security of records
- adherence to agency rules, legal statutes, ethical guidelines

summaries using just the template discussed. Each termination summary includes information about reason for termination, treatment plan compliance, progress summary, and posttermination after-plan.

Storing of Records

During the course of therapy, the client's records are securely and confidentially stored, protected, and maintained. Once the helping relationship has been closed, the termination summary has been prepared, and any postinterview follow-up has been made, the client's record and files are stored and protected according to ethical guidelines; federal, state, and local statutes; and specific agency guidelines. Final case disposition is the storing and protecting of these records. All agencies store records for a specified time period. Some settings keep the entire client file, while others destroy certain portions and retain just key information. When only selected materials are retained, ethical guidelines and legal statutes must be followed. Some sites store client materials in paper form, whereas others store records electronically. In either case, the agency and clinician must make arrangements to securely safeguard the client's information (see Box 11.1).

Consultation, Supervision, and Collaboration

Ethical codes for mental health providers (American Counseling Association [ACA], 1995; American Psychological Association [APA], 2003; National Association of Social Workers [NASW], 1999) and the various local and state statutes and regulations require that professional helpers practice within the limits of their competence. Being a professional counselor does not always mean "going it alone" when working with the client. In fact, collaboration with colleagues is a key mechanism for assuring good services that meet our clients' needs. Using and managing professional relationships with colleagues to serve clients are other aspects of case management. These professional relationships include clinical supervision; clinical, medical, and psychiatric consultation; and cotherapy and conjoint treatment.

Clinical Supervision

The use of clinical supervision is central to mental health practice. Supervision has been defined as an intensive, interpersonally focused relationship in which one person is designated to facilitate the development of therapeutic competence in one or more other persons (Loganbill, Hardy, & Delworth, 1982). Clinical supervision may focus on the use of clinical tools (diagnosis, case conceptualization, treatment planning, and case management), the clinician's counseling skills, the clinician's personal functioning as it influences his or her therapeutic work, or some combination. As a general rule, supervision tends to focus more on skill development and the content of a case earlier in training, and it moves to focus on personal functioning later in professional development. Further, although supervision can be therapeutic, it is not therapy—and if it begins to move too much in that direction, it is important that the supervisor encourage the clinician to seek personal counseling.

Students rely on supervisors to provide the intensive support and challenge and extensive expert advise they need as they begin the process of learning to be a counselor. For students, supervisors take on much of the responsibility and liability for assessment, case conceptualization, treatment planning, monitoring the implementation of the treatment plan, and managing the helping relationship through its stages.

Interns, residents for licensure, and others who are new to the field rely on supervisors to provide the moderate support, intensive challenge, and solid expert advice they need to continue building on the foundation of their early training and experiences. For interns and novice counselors, supervisors gradually shift much of the responsibility and liability for clinical skills and management of a case onto the supervisee.

Even licensed and other more experienced clinicians continue to rely on supervision for expert guidance, to learn new approaches, for assistance with specialized populations, and to address personal dynamics influencing their professional work. For example, one of the authors [Alan Schwitzer] used supervision later in his development for assistance in working with Hispanic client family dynamics, with which he was unfamiliar (a specialized population issue). He returned to supervision once again to add hypnosis skills to his clinical repertoire (to learn a new approach). Later, he used supervision to deal with problematic dreams he had while working with a client's family abuse issues (a personal dynamics issue).

Case management includes searching out and productively engaging in supervision suited to your training needs, skill and experience level, and personal-professional development needs to competently assist your clients. Use of supervision means preparing for supervision meetings by managing the necessary paperwork, reviewing cases ahead of time, bringing in audio- or videotapes as agreed on, engaging in professional dialogue about your development and your caseload, and resolving any conflicts arising in supervision that might negatively influence your work with clients.

EXERCISE 11.1 **Using Clinical Supervision**

The use of clinical supervision is central to mental health practice. Your needs as a supervisee will grow and change over your development as a clinician. To get started thinking about the use of supervision, ponder the following questions and then discuss them in small groups or in class.

1. What qualities have you found or would you like to find in your first clinical supervisors, such as those during practicum, internship, and early work?
2. What will be most important in a supervisor: An experienced clinician who can provide a lot of expert advice? Someone who will give you the freedom to make clinical decisions, right and wrong, and learn from your choices? Someone who will be emotionally supportive? Someone who is highly challenging?
3. What do you anticipate being the strengths you will bring to the supervision relationship? What are some of the roadblocks you might experience in working with a supervisor?

Clinical, Medical, and Psychiatric Consultation

Clinical supervision is an ongoing professional relationship that is defined by regular (often weekly) meetings between supervisor and supervisee. By comparison, consultation is a temporary relationship in which the clinician seeks the support, expert opinion, or advice of another professional about the needs of a specific client.

Clinical consultation occurs when the therapist engages in consultation with another mental health clinician to discuss a client's needs, explore treatment options, or gain a better understanding of the dynamics of the helping relationship. One form of clinical consultation occurs when the clinician meets with the consultant to discuss a case. Another form occurs when the clinician refers the client to meet directly with the consultant; with this form of consultation, the consultant provides input and feedback to the clinician based on his or her meeting with the client.

Medical consultation occurs when the mental health clinician refers the client to meet with a physician (or other medical practitioner, e.g., a nutritionist) for a physical exam or medical evaluation. The medical professional provides feedback about the client's physical health directly to the client and/or to the clinician.

Consultation with a psychiatrist can take the form of (a) directly discussing a case with a psychiatrist, usually with the purpose of firming up a diagnosis and/or discussing possible pharmacological alternatives, or (b) referring the client for a diagnostic or medical evaluation.

Case management includes recognizing when consultation is needed with a physician, psychiatrist, or mental health clinician and searching out an appropriate consultant. When required, it includes arranging a referral for the client to meet with the consulting professional and resolving any consultation dynamics that might negatively influence the client's counseling experience.

In many settings, case staffings, which can include any mental health or medical staff at the setting, are used to discuss client needs, provide group peer supervision and colleague consultation, and make treatment decisions. During case staffings, clinicians are asked to present a case, or cases, to assist them in case management. For the staffings, the presenting clinician must be well prepared to discuss the case(s) at hand, complete any required paperwork such as case summaries, and treat all information shared about clients ethically.

Cotherapy and Conjoint Treatment

Supervision and consultation are both characterized by relying on another professional as a "third party" in the counseling process. A different type of professional relationship used to assist clients is collaboratively working with a colleague to provide actual direct services. Colleagues either can work as cotherapists or they can provide conjoint treatment.

COTHERAPY Cotherapy occurs when two (or more) clinicians directly work together. The most common examples are group counseling in which there are two cotherapist group leaders, couples counseling in which two counselors meet together with the couple, and family counseling using two counselors working together. However, occasionally, cotherapists might work together with an individual client, such as in some inpatient settings.

Case management includes working collaboratively with a cotherapist to meet the needs of the clients involved, sorting out any relationship dynamics between cotherapists that may negatively influence the counseling process, and sharing the clinical workload.

CONJOINT TREATMENT Conjoint therapy occurs when the client is engaged in more than one mode of treatment. Perhaps the best example is the use of individual counseling plus a support group, group counseling, or group psychotherapy to meet a client's needs. A second example is individual counseling plus family counseling or couples counseling. Other examples are individual or group counseling plus specialized assistance such as career counseling, academic counseling, stress management training, anger management training, or a parenting skills class. Individual psychotherapy combined with ongoing psychiatric consultation, usually to provide and monitor medication, is another form of conjoint treatment.

Case management with conjoint treatments includes working collaboratively with other professionals involved to meet the needs of the client and being clear and specific about the goals, therapeutic activities, boundaries, and roles of each professional involved. It involves resolving any professional conflicts that arise so they do not negatively influence the client, assisting the client with scheduling and follow-through, and sharing the clinical workload (see Exercise 11.2 and Box 11.2).

EXERCISE 11.2 **Functioning in Professional Relationships**

Being a professional clinician does not always mean "going it alone." In fact, collaboration with colleagues is a key mechanism for assuring good client services. To begin preparing for the professional relationships in which you will function, respond to the following items and then discuss your responses in dyads or small groups.

1. Describe the professional and personal qualities you would hope to find in colleagues who fill the professional roles listed below. Then, write a few sentences describing your "ideal colleague."
2. Describe the professional and personal qualities you would hope to avoid in colleagues who fill the professional roles listed below. Then, write a few sentences describing the individual you believe would be the most difficult with whom to work.

Professional Roles:

1. Expert mental health consultant
2. Physician or psychiatric consultant
3. Cotherapist for individual, couples, family, and group counseling and psychotherapy

Communication with Stakeholders

The counseling relationship involves confidential communication between a client and a practicing professional. However, it is not uncommon for nonprofessionals to seek communications with the clinician about specific clients, and handling such communications is another aspect of case management. Nonprofessionals who most commonly seek to discuss client concerns with the therapist include family, friends, and other parties with an interest in an adult client's situation; the parents or legal guardians of a minor who is a client; governmental agencies, academic institutions, and other organizations; the courts; and contacts for employment checks and background investigations.

Family, Friends, and Other Interested Parties

Family, friends, supervisors and coworkers, neighbors, and others interested in an adult client's situation may seek communication with the therapist. These interested parties may seek assurance that the client is being cared for by a professional or want to volunteer information they believe is important or critical to the person's care. They may ask for an expert opinion about how to deal with the person at home, at work, or in other relationships or wish to shift the practical responsibility or emotional burden they feel toward the client onto the professional (Gallessich, 1983; Klein, 1988).

BOX 11.2
Summary of Consultation, Supervision, and Collaboration

Clinicians utilize professional relationships when needed to best serve their clients.

CLINICAL SUPERVISION
- intensive, interpersonal relationship: one person facilitates development of therapeutic competence in the other
- focus on clinical skills, clinical tools, or combination
- therapeutic, but not therapy
- those new to the field rely on supervisors to support and challenge and to build on their training and experience
- experienced clinicians rely on supervision for expert guidance, to assist in learning new approaches, and to address personal dynamics influencing their work
- case management includes review of records, audio- and videotaping, review of cases, resolving conflicts regarding clients

CLINICAL, MEDICAL, AND PSYCHIATRIC CONSULTATION
- clinical consultation: consultation with mental health clinician to discuss client needs, treatment options, or dynamics of the helping relationship
  - meet directly with consultant or
  - consultant meets with client and then clinician meets with consultant
- medical consultation: refer client to medical practitioner for physical health issues
- psychiatric consultation
  - meet with psychiatrist to firm up diagnosis and discuss medication issues
  - refer client for diagnostic and/or medical evaluation
- case management: recognizing when to consult with a physician or psychiatrist, arranging for a referral, resolving any negative consultation dynamics

COTHERAPY AND CONJOINT TREATMENT
- cotherapy involves two or more clinicians directly working together
  - examples: leading groups, couples counselors, family counselors
  - case management means working collaboratively in the client's best interests
- conjoint treatment involves two or more modes of counseling
  - examples: individual counseling plus group therapy, individual counseling plus couples or family counseling, group therapy plus stress management or anger management training
  - case management means working collabor-atively to meet the client's needs

Such interested parties may phone, e-mail, write the counselor, or even visit in person. Whether they want to discuss the client for the person's own welfare or to alleviate their own anxieties, such contacts often put quite a bit of pressure on the counselor to be responsive and helpful. Consider the mother of a college student who calls from out of town wanting to know how her son is doing with an anxiety problem, a supervisor who wants to know if it is safe to have a certain employee work with dangerous materials alone on the night shift, or a landlord who wants the counselor to "do something" about the occasional psychotic rantings of a tenant.

However, regardless of the reason for the contact and the pressure it creates for the counselor, it is the professional's responsibility to maintain confidentiality.

According to the various ethical guidelines and federal, state, and local legal statutes, as a general rule, the clinician must not discuss a client's situation with such outside parties. In fact, generally speaking, the clinician may not even acknowledge whether he or she is working with the person as a client. Exceptions are made, of course, when it is necessary to break confidentiality because the person is potentially harmful to self or another person, potentially neglectful or abusive to a child or elder, or unable to manage daily functioning. Further, communications with interested parties are allowable if specifically agreed on and consented to by the client in a written release of information.

Good case management means protecting confidentiality, while at the same time being professional and respectful when interacting with interested parties. Case management also means documenting such contacts and making a clinical decision about whether or not, and how, to discuss the contacts therapeutically with the client. When a decision to allow such communications is made, it means ensuring the client understands his or her decision and that a written consent is signed and added to the client's records and documentation of the communication itself is in the client's record.

Parents and Legal Guardians

Clients under the age of 18 years raise a different issue regarding communications and case management. As a general rule, it is the parent or legal guardian of a minor who "owns" the client's confidentiality. Generally speaking, this also may be the case with adult clients who have legal guardians, such as some adults with mental retardation or mental illnesses. Therefore, when requested by the parent or guardian, the clinician can be obligated to share any and all information about the client and his or her clinical situation.

For clients who are old enough and developmentally capable of understanding this, the clinician should clearly discuss the limits of confidentiality during the preinterview or rapport and trust building stage of the relationship. A common practice is to agree ahead of time with the parents and client as to what might be shared outside the counseling relationship and what might remain private. For example, when one of the authors [Alan Schwitzer] treated a high school student for marijuana use, it was agreed that he would share with the parents only whether or not he kept his appointments, but the content of the counseling discussion would remain private. However, it should be made clear that this is only an agreement of convenience, and the parents could change their mind once the relationship was underway. Further, not all parents and guardians are willing to accept such an agreement. Therefore, the client should be made to understand the limits of confidentiality.

Competent case management requires the clinician to disclose the minor's and parents' confidentiality rights and limitations. When requested, the clinician should communicate about the client with parents or guardians in an understandable manner, monitor and document such communications, support the welfare of the client, and document the communication in the client's record.

Government Agencies, Academic Institutions, and Other Organizations

Often, members of the local community beyond family, friends, and coworkers have a stake in a client's clinical situation. Some representatives of government agencies who might request privileged information about a client are probation and parole officers, social workers and other social services staff, public health officials, housing authorities, and similar professionals. Some representatives of academic institutions who might seek client information are K–12 school administrators, school counselors and classroom teachers, and college or university administrators, admissions staff, counselors and health staff, or individual professors. Other organizations include nonprofit and for-profit social services providers, such as staff of assisted living facilities, homeless shelters, crisis or rape response centers, and the like, who have an interest in your client's situation. Any of these entities may be interested simply in knowing whether or not the client is in treatment. They may want more detail about the person's background and current functioning. They could request detailed testing and assessment data, or they might want your professional judgment regarding current adjustment and prognosis.

As a general rule, the clinician may share information with these entities only with the client's permission, and usually, if there is no permission, they should not even acknowledge whether or not the client is in counseling. Therefore, some critical elements of case management regarding the sharing of information include (a) discussing confidentiality rights with the client and circumstances in which they might be broken, (b) assuring that a written release of information form is signed for any circumstances in which confidential information might be shared with others, and (c) assisting the client in making good decisions about when to allow the clinician to share information with outside entities and what information will be shared. Ideally, this issue is discussed during rapport and trust building; however, the topic also may come up unexpectedly later on.

Other case management tasks in relation to such information requests include maintaining good records and documentation, being knowledgeable of the statutes and laws governing this issue in your locality, seeking legal consultation when required, interacting professionally with the persons and entities seeking information, making good decisions when responding to such requests, and following through with the requests as appropriate.

Courts and Criminal Justice Mandates

An important potential exception to confidentiality is a request for communications about the client from the court or criminal justice system. Courts may demand information or communication about a client's background, current functioning, compliance with treatment, clinician's assessment of the client's situation, or other information. Court requests may come from judges (or their representatives) in civil or criminal trials, cases, and hearings; attorneys associated with court cases involving the client; judges or others responsible for making determinations about a client's safety, competence, and hospitalization; or from court officials dealing with other legal matters. The court may request written information, a verbal contact, or an appearance by the clinician. Requested information could range from general feedback about the client to specific case notes and documentation of treatment.

Except when protected by the legal right of privileged communication (see Chapter 2), generally speaking, American courts can legally require clinicians to break confidentiality. Therefore, because it involves one of the very few instances in which the counselor may be required to break confidentiality, handling court requests is an important element of case management. Clinicians may attempt to provide only limited, narrow information, resist a court request, or demand a subpoena. However, generally, there is a legal obligation to comply with the court's demand for information.

Courts also may empower other members of the criminal justice system to demand client information. For example, the court may order counseling information to be shared with probation and parole officers. Here the request for information, as we just discussed, becomes mandatory. Similarly, the courts could empower other entities such as social services and public health officials to demand client information.

Case management regarding court requests for information requires maintaining good records and documentation, being knowledgeable of the statutes and laws governing this issue in your locality, and seeking legal consultation when required. It includes interacting professionally with court personnel and making good decisions when responding to such requests. The clinician must follow through with such requests as appropriate, appear in court when demanded, discuss this issue in disclosure with the client, and document the communication in the client's record.

Employment Checks and Background Investigations

Clinicians receive requests to communicate about clients and former clients with employers in business, the government, military, law enforcement, and other settings that conduct background investigations as part of their hiring, promotion, and assignment procedures. Often, these requests come long after the helping relationship has concluded. For example, one of the authors [Alan Schwitzer] has responded to dozens of requests for background information about former college counseling clients who later sought employment in government agencies such as the CIA and FBI and entry into the U.S. military.

As with requests made from other stakeholders, the clinician may share information only with the expressed permission of the client—even if it will benefit the client. Therefore, case management first requires the clinician to obtain written permission from the client. If the client has already signed such a release for the employer seeking the information, the clinician must obtain a copy of the request from the employer. Case management in this instance requires maintaining good documentation and being knowledgeable of the statutes governing this issue. It includes seeking consultation when required, and interacting professionally with those making the request, and making good decisions when responding to such requests. The clinician should respond only to those questions asked in the request and document the communication in the client's record (see Case Illustration 11.7, Exercise 11.3, and Box 11.3).

CASE ILLUSTRATION 11.7 Communicating with a Background Investigator: Sienna

We have been working with our ongoing case illustration client Sienna. In this illustration, one year after termination, around the time of Sienna's college graduation, her counselor has been contacted by a background investigator for the FBI, who is considering Sienna's application for employment. This type of background investigation is routinely conducted for applicants. When the applicant indicates certain medical or counseling history, a request for information is sent to the provider. Notice that the counselor indicates in the letter that the client has provided consent for the communication.

In responding, the counselor writes in language that is readable and understandable to someone who is not a mental health professional. No diagnoses or psychological data are provided. Instead, Sienna's situation is explained in everyday professional language. Although the letter from the FBI is not provided here, the counselor attempts to directly answer only the specific questions provided by the investigator and only responds to questions she feels qualified to answer. She does not make any report she is unsure of, and she does not make any recommendation as to whether Sienna would be a good employee. Instead, the counselor "sticks to the facts."

Here is the counselor's letter:

John Gonzales
Special Agent, Defense Investigative Service
Washington, DC

Dear Mr. Gonzales:

I am writing in response to your Medical Information Questionnaire inquiry regarding Sienna R. with her expressed written permission as indicated by a signed Authority for Release of Information and Records.

Ms. R. was a client of the University Counseling Center for one time period during her enrollment at the university. She sought a period of brief, limited adjustment-focused services lasting for 11 weekly sessions during a single semester from February to May 2002.

Ms. R. sought support and assistance with the kinds of mood, developmental, relationship, and adjustment concerns that are not atypical of young adult college students. She appropriately sought counseling support, was a self-motivated consumer of services, made productive use of her Center contacts, and then ended counseling in mutual agreement with her counselor.

Ms. R. did not admit to the use of marijuana, prescription drugs, or excessive alcohol, and these were not a focus of her counseling. She did not report or demonstrate any bizarre, abnormal, or deviant behavior. She did not report or demonstrate any mental or nervous condition that appeared to impair her judgment or reliability. To my knowledge, she never discussed classified information in her sessions.

I would anticipate no adverse affects from sharing this information with Sienna. I hope this covers all of the information that has been requested.

Karen Hogarth
University Counselor

EXERCISE 11.3 **Communicating with Stakeholders**

The counseling relationship is generally a confidential relationship. However, nonprofessionals commonly seek communications with the clinician about specific clients. In fact, those people interested in the client's well-being often put quite a lot of pressure on counselors to discuss private information about a case. Handling communications with nonprofessionals is an important aspect of case management.

As a starting place for practicing this type of communication, complete the following role-play exercises in class. These role-plays can be completed in pairs, in triads with one learner acting as observer, or as a whole class. Complete the role play and then discuss your experience and your reactions. Rely on your course instructor as a consultant.

ROLE-PLAY 1

Stakeholder: You are an employer. Your employee mentioned that he is being seen for counseling for "mental stuff" at the local community agency and gave you his therapist's name. The employee recently had a loud, threatening verbal "blow-up" with a coworker. You call the counselor demanding to know whether this client is all right. If you can't get any straight answers from the counselor, you may suspend the employee until further notice.

Counselor: The employer calls and catches you off-guard. You do not have a signed release to discuss the client's situation. At the same time, you want to advocate for the client. How do you respond?

ROLE-PLAY 2

Stakeholder: You are a college English professor. When a student submitted a class assignment with clear suicidal themes, you referred her to the student mental health center. You call the office to be sure she made it in for her appointment, to see what is wrong with her and how she is doing, and how you should handle things when you next see her in class.

Counselor: The professor calls just as you are finishing up your intake meeting with the student, who has agreed to come in for another meeting for further assessment. You do not have a signed release

(*continued*)

EXERCISE 11.3 *(continued)*

to discuss the client's situation. At the same time, you want to be of assistance to the professor. How do you respond?

ROLE-PLAY 3

Stakeholder: You are a social services worker in public housing. Residents with drug abuse and dependence problems may be expelled from the public housing community. You have been informed that a resident is being seen at a city drug treatment center. You call the clinician for information to be used in making a determination about whether to expel the drug-using resident.

Counselor: You are, in fact, seeing the public housing resident as a client for treatment for alcohol dependence and polysubstance use. So far, the client has been resistant to treatment and has missed two of six appointments. Still, you are hopeful that with time you can make some progress. When the social services worker calls, you have in your files a signed release of information from the client. The release allows you to share any and all information with the social worker. You must decide how to proceed to be of service to the client and the caller.

ROLE-PLAY 4

Stakeholder: You are a parole officer who is working as an agent of the court. You phone a local therapist to demand that she send you a photocopy of the entire client records for one of your parolees. The information is needed in court to make a determination about whether the person has complied sufficiently with a court order to attend counseling. This determination will be used to decide (a) whether the person may retain custody of her infant, and (b) whether or not she will go back to jail to complete her sentence. Because you have the weight of the court behind you, you do not plan to take "no" for an answer.

Counselor: Your client was mandated by the court to enter counseling as a condition of parole. To date, she has been relatively compliant with the treatment plan and comes in for most of her appointments. Since she was a court referral, you already have a written release to discuss her case with the court, and you expected to do so. However, you did not expect to be asked to submit a photocopy of your entire client file, which really was not written to be read by someone who is not a mental health professional. How do you respond?

ROLE-PLAY 5

Stakeholder: You are a fifth grade teacher. You are aware that the school counselor has been seeing one of your students for group counseling once a week. The student has been acting out during the school year and has quieted down somewhat since entering group counseling. You do not know what issues the student has discussed in the group or much about the student's family background. Since the student has been doing better, you decide to approach the counselor and ask her for any suggestions regarding the student. You therefore approach the counselor, ask her to tell you a little bit about how things are going with the student, and ask for specific suggestions about how to work with the student.

Counselor: You have been working with the student for 6 months and have recently discovered that he was sexually assaulted by a "friend" about a year ago. In addition to the group counseling he is in with you, you have referred him to a private practice clinician for individual counseling. You contacted the student's parents about the assault and made a report to Child Protective Services. Counseling is going well, and the student has revealed to you that since the assault he feels "different" from everyone else in class and that is why he has taken on the persona of "class clown." It is a way for him to draw attention to his jokes so he doesn't have to feel that people see him as dirty or "gay." When the teacher approaches you, you feel good that she notices the student is doing better and want to give her some suggestions about working with the student. However, you do not want to reveal any details of the problem. How do you respond?

BOX 11.3

Summary of Communication with Stakeholders

The counseling relationship involves confidential communication between a client and a practicing professional. Some nonprofessionals will seek communications with the clinician.

FAMILY, FRIENDS, AND OTHER INTEREST PARTIES

- will try to contact you by various means (e.g., phone, e-mail, letters, directly)
- important to not acknowledge if client is in counseling and to keep confidentiality, unless you have a signed release of information form
- be respectful to stakeholders
- decide whether or not to discuss attempted contacts with clients
- document contacts

PARENTS AND LEGAL GUARDIANS

- parent or legal guardian of a minor usually "owns" the client's confidentiality
- try to agree ahead of time with parents and client as to what might be shared
- clinician can be obligated to share information about the client
- communicate about the client with parents or guardians in an understandable manner
- monitor and document such communications

GOVERNMENTAL AGENCIES, ACADEMIC INSTITUTIONS, AND OTHER ORGANIZATIONS

- these agencies may need information about the client (e.g., parole officer)
- discuss with client his or her confidentiality rights
- assure written release of information form is signed when giving out information
- assist client in making good decisions about when and what to share
- maintain good records and documentation
- be knowledgeable of the statutes and laws governing this issue
- interact professionally with the persons and entities seeking information

COURTS AND CRIMINAL JUSTICE MANDATES

- except when protected by privileged communication, generally, courts can require clinicians to break confidentiality
- therapist can attempt to provide only limited, narrow information, resist request, or demand a subpoena, but generally is obligated to comply
- maintain good records and documentation
- be knowledgeable of the statutes and laws governing this issue
- seek legal consultation when necessary
- interact professionally with court personnel and make good decisions when responding
- discuss the issue with your client and document it in the client's record

EMPLOYMENT CHECKS AND BACKGROUND INVESTIGATIONS

- may receive requests to communicate about clients and former clients regarding background investigations as part of hiring, promotion, and assignment procedures
- requests may come long after the helping relationship has concluded
- need signed release from client
- be knowledgeable of the statutes governing this issue
- make wise decisions and seek consultation when required
- interact professionally with those making the request
- respond only to questions asked
- document the communication in the client's record

Business-Related Activities

Handling the business matters of a case comprise a significant part of case management for today's professional counselors and psychotherapists (cf. Ackley, 1997). It includes such tasks as dealing with day-to-day offices issues; discussing billing procedures and collecting fees; documenting client contacts, treatment plans, and progress toward stated goals; and completing paperwork for insurance companies, HMOs, and others. It requires accuracy and business management skills regardless of the setting in which you work (see Box 11.4).

Day-to-Day Offices Issues

Although not all clinicians will have to worry about all day-to-day offices issues, every clinician will be concerned with some of them. Although it is seen by many counselors as an unfortunate side task, making sure an office runs smoothly is critical if clients are to feel safe and welcomed. Some of the many issues include assuring that the furniture and physical setting is comfortable, dealing with payments to clerical staff and, in some cases, clinical staff hiring and firing issues, paying utilities, and so forth. Although we will not cover all of these issues in detail, complete Exercise 11.4 to get a feel for some of the issues you might eventually face.

EXERCISE 11.4 **What Does a Clinical Practice Cost?**

If you are like many new counseling professionals, you might have some mixed feelings about the business matters of a case, such as client contacts, billing, and collecting payments. Certainly, the natural helper in you doesn't pay attention to money matters when offering assistance. Here is an exercise to help give you a better understanding of the "dollars and cents" of professional practice.

The following is a list (adapted from Ackley, 1997) of common office expenses for a counseling agency or independent practice. First, individually or in small groups, come up with an estimate of what you think each office practice expense might cost for a year. Second, interview an agency director or private practice clinician and find out what these items actually cost. Third, compare and discuss your findings in class.

CLINICAL PRACTICE ANNUAL EXPENSES	YOUR ESTIMATE	INTERVIEW FINDINGS
Clinical staff salaries, benefits, and/or FICA		
Office staff salaries, benefits, and FICA		
Payroll withholding taxes (federal and state)		
Unemployment insurance		
Office rent/mortgage		
Office cleaning and maintenance		
Office supplies		
Professional supplies		
Professional memberships, books, journals		
Continuing education and professional meetings		
Postage		
Telephone, Internet, fax		
Utilities		
Marketing		

Travel		
Professional liability insurance		
Medical insurance		
Income protection insurance		
Comprehensive fire, theft, office liability		
Life insurance		
Professional services (legal and accounting)		
Pension or 401K		
Depreciation on office furniture and equipment		
Miscellaneous/Other		
TOTAL	$	$

Discussing Billing Procedures and Collecting Fees

Regardless of the setting in which you work, billing issues will be a topic of discussion. Even if you are working at an agency that doesn't directly collect fees (e.g., school counselors), you often will be referring clients to settings that do, and knowing the etiquette of working with clients around "money issues" is critical.

If you are collecting fees directly, discussing fees and billing issues should occur early, during the rapport and trust building stage. Professional helpers should be clear and direct about this aspect of professional practice so that the client can make treatment decisions accordingly. Some beginning counselors experience ambivalence or personal conflict when discussing money issues with clients. However, good case management requires working through and resolving your personal concerns about the "business end" of becoming a professional helper. Not resolving these issues can result in lack of payment from clients and justified client anger when they suddenly are billed at rates or for sessions about which they were not informed. Finally, clinicians must discuss with clients exactly what, if any, information is required to be shared with third-party payers (e.g., health insurance companies, employee assistance programs). Today, it is usual for third-party payers to review diagnoses as well as treatment plans and progress toward them, and clients should be aware of this. Although federal laws now require confidentiality by insurance companies regarding this information (see HIPAA, Chapter 3), clients still should understand what, if any, information will be shared with these organizations.

Documenting Client Contacts, Treatment Plans, and Progress Toward Stated Goals

Although largely discussed in the earlier section on documentation, the business end of documentation has a somewhat different take on this important matter.

BOX 11.4
Summary of Business-Related Matters

Professional counselors manage the business aspects of their cases, which requires accuracy and business-management skills.

DAY-TO-DAY OFFICES ISSUES

- every clinician will be concerned with some of them
- assures office runs smoothly
- is critical if clients are to feel safe and welcomed
- includes comfortable furniture and environment, payments to clerical staff and, in some cases, clinical staff, hiring and firing issues, paying utilities, and much more

DISCUSSING BILLING PROCEDURES AND COLLECTING FEES

- knowledge of etiquette around "money issues" is critical
- be clear and direct and discuss fees and billing issues early, during the rapport and trust building stage
- discuss what may be required to share with third-party payers

DOCUMENTING CLIENT CONTACTS, TREATMENT PLANS, AND PROGRESS TOWARD STATED GOALS

- for accountability reasons, clinicians must assure that client contacts are documented
- have process whereby each client visit is noted and payment received is credited (e.g., ledger book, computer)
- insurance companies will want to monitor payments and number of client visits
- administrators and supervisors will want an accounting of time spent with clients

COMPLETING PAPERWORK FOR INSURANCE COMPANIES, HMOs, AND OTHERS

- forms are everywhere—a necessary burden
- assure that clinicians will be paid, funding agencies will fund, and supervisors and administrators will have a mechanism to evaluate

Often, to receive payment and for accountability reasons, clinicians must assure that each contact with a client is documented. Although documentation of progress toward stated goals is conducted through the use of progress notes, most settings also have a process whereby each client visit is noted and payment received is credited (if the client is "fee for service"). This may be completed through a business ledger book; however, in today's world, it is increasingly handled through computer programs.

Finally, many insurance companies will want to monitor payments and number of client visits, and administrators and supervisors at most settings will want an accounting of time spent with clients. Thus, clinicians must assure that this documentation is easily available to those who evaluate, supervise, and fund us. For instance, the wife of one of the authors [Ed Neukrug] is a school counselor. As a result of a state law that requires school counselors to spend 60% of their time in direct contact with students, the guidance director for the school system periodically wants all school counselors to document the number of individual, group counseling, and group guidance sessions conducted. Thus, she needs to assure that she has the proper documentation and a mechanism for periodically assessing her contact with students, and she can often be found working late at the office assuring that her paperwork is up-to-date.

Completing Paperwork for Insurance Companies, HMOs, and Others

Forms, forms, forms—they are everywhere, and increasingly, the clinician is being asked to spend a large amount of time completing them. Although a necessary burden to most, these forms assure that clinicians will be paid, that funding agencies will fund, and that supervisors and administrators will have a mechanism to evaluate. Although not the purview of this text, it should be noted that you will not get through the professional world of the counselor without having to gain some knowledge of how to complete some paperwork that you will likely call "unreasonable."

Time and Caseload Management

If you have been employed at any job, then you know the importance of time management and workload management: being on time, keeping appointments, doing your work, and so on. These basic practices become critical case management tasks for the professional counselor (see Box 11.5).

Time Management

Time management means being on time and staying as expected during assigned office hours. It requires being present, timely, and conscientious regarding all clinical duties, including individual, group, and other counseling assignments, as well as intake duty, on call and emergency staffing, phoneline responsibilities, and so on. Time management includes being present, timely, and active in all clinically related activities, such as attending supervision, consultation meetings, case staffings, and other meetings. It means allotting time for recordkeeping and documentation, professional relationships such as clinical meetings with cotherapists and group coleaders and supervision, responding to communications, and taking care of billing, reports, and other business matters. Time management means balancing regularly scheduled appointments and tasks with unexpected, emergency, or crisis needs.

Although good time management is a basic workplace skill in just about any professional setting, it takes on great importance in the professional counseling office, where appointments are scheduled in rapid succession, there is much paperwork and documentation to handle, and emergencies and crises can disrupt the daily flow of activity. Being fully available and on time for client appointments, completing reports and paperwork that serve the client's needs on time, and having a clear plan for handling unexpected client emergency needs are critical to effective treatment.

Caseload Management

Caseload management includes carefully monitoring each client's experience of the counseling relationship, his or her compliance with the treatment plan, and client progress. Clinicians must ensure that their caseload remains manageable in terms of its size, number of weekly client contacts, complexity, challenge, and psychoemotional demand.

BOX 11.5
Summary of Time and Caseload Management

Psychotherapists carefully manage their time, professional responsibilities, office practices, and carefully follow up, with a constant focus on the client's well-being.

TIME MANAGEMENT
- being present and timely for clinical duties, clinically related activities, and other assignments
- being timely and conscientious in response to recordkeeping, communications, and business matters
- balancing scheduled activities with emergency and crisis needs

CASELOAD MANAGEMENT
- monitoring client experiences, treatment, and progress
- client follow-up with missed appointments and checking in with clients between appointments
- monitoring client follow-through with referrals
- managing overall professional workload so that the focus remains on each client's well-being

Caseload management also requires the clinician to effectively follow up with clients as needed. Client follow-up can include checking in with clients (phoning, sending a note) who miss an appointment or reschedule, checking with clients at regularly scheduled intervals between appointments, if agreed on with the client, and monitoring to see that clients followed through with referrals.

Sometimes caseloads can become too large, require too many weekly contacts, demand too much therapist emotional energy, or involve too many competing workplace demands. Clinicians who find that they are no longer able to manage their caseload must consider how to reduce or change the caseload, seek the support of supervision or clinical consultation, or consult with agency management. The bottom line is that professionals must carefully manage their time, professional responsibilities, and office practices and carefully follow what is happening with each client so that the relationship stays focused at all times on the client's well-being.

Now Some Practice

In this chapter, we return once again to our four practice cases selected from popular culture to help you develop your skills using clinical tools. The characters, introduced in Chapters 9 and 10, simulate a clinical caseload. You can refer to these chapters to review the clients' basic introduction, case conceptualization, and treatment plan. In the Practice Client sections, we provide an intake case summary and diagnostic impressions for each client. Next, you are asked to develop a (simulated) case note/process note and a termination summary for each character. By practicing how to write case notes and termination summaries using popular character clients, you will have a head start when you begin your actual clinical work (see Practice Clients 11.1–11.4).

PRACTICE CLIENT 11.1

Scarlett O'Hara

Refer to Chapters 9 and 10 for the information needed to complete this exercise. Refer to the discussions of intake summaries, case notes, and termination summaries in this chapter for a guide. We provide an intake summary for the client, Scarlett O'Hara. Complete the exercise by writing (a) a case note for Session 3 and (b) a termination summary based on your understanding of the case. You can work in teams or share and discuss your work in class.

INTAKE SUMMARY

Identifying Information: Scarlett O'Hara Hamilton Kennedy Butler is a 28-year-old White woman, married to Rhett Butler, and the mother of two children. She owns and manages two successful lumber mills.

Presenting Concern: The client sought help in dealing with stress in her marriage and grief over the death of a close friend. She described herself as being "out of step" with the rest of society and said she feels restless and uncertain of what the future holds. She reports no suicidal ideation, no history of self-harm, and no history of problems with alcohol or other drug use.

Background, Family, and Relevant History: Scarlett's parents both are dead—her mother of typhoid during the war and her father in a horseback riding accident shortly after. She has two younger sisters: one is married and lives at Tara, the O'Hara family plantation; the other is a cloistered nun living in Charleston, South Carolina. Scarlett describes herself as the head of the family now.

Scarlett has been married twice previously; her first husband was a war casualty, and her second husband was killed in a raid shortly after the war. Although both marriages were brief, both produced a child, and Scarlett retains custody of the children, Wade, age 11, and Ella, age 6. She also had a child, Bonnie, with her present husband. Bonnie died in a horseback riding accident at age 5. In addition, a close friend recently passed away.

Scarlett describes her present problems as sadness and lack of direction. She reports she made her first two marriages for the sake of social convention and describes entering her current marriage for security and companionship. She reports that for many years she thought herself in love with her brother-in-law but more recently realized she feels in love with her husband. Scarlett reports that when she recently shared her feelings with him in an attempt to restore her deteriorating marriage, the husband responded by requesting a separation and reported not loving her any longer. She appears anxious to "save my marriage."

Problem and Counseling History: The client reports having stress symptoms, including nightmares, ever since leaving Atlanta to evade military attack during the war. She has never previously sought counseling.

Mental Status Exam: Scarlett was dressed in professional attire and her appearance was appropriate. At times during the interview, she appeared anxious, distressed, and saddened. She was teary at times. She was quite emotionally expressive, fully engaged, active, and maintained good eye contact. She was oriented by time, place, and person. Scarlett appeared to be above average intellectually, and her memory was intact. Her judgment seemed good, her insight was moderately high, and she appeared motivated for treatment. Scarlett reports no suicidal ideation and denies any current or past history of self-harmful intent or behavior.

Goals for Counseling and Course of Counseling to Date: Scarlett has been seen once for intake. Her primary goals are to reduce her stress symptoms and feelings of grief and loss and to resolve her marital difficulties.

Tentative goals are to (a) resolve grief at death of only close friend and feelings of loss of love relationship with husband and (b) elevate self-esteem, develop a consistent, positive self-image, and improve daily adjustment.

Diagnostic Impressions:

Axis I:	313.82 Identity Problem
	V61.10 Partner Relational Problem
	V62.82 Bereavement
Axis II:	None
Axis III:	None
Axis IV:	War survivor, marital stress, recent death of close friend
Axis V:	GAF = 60 (Current)

Case Note—Session 3:

Write your own case note using the material provided in this chapter as a guide.

Termination Summary:

Write your own termination summary using the material provided in this chapter as a guide.

PRACTICE CLIENT 11.2

Maya Angelou's Marguerite

Refer to Chapters 9 and 10 for the information needed to complete this exercise. Refer to the discussions of intake summaries, case notes, and termination summaries in this chapter for a guide. We provide an intake summary for the client, Marguerite. Complete the exercise by writing (a) a case note for Session 3 and (b) a termination summary based on your understanding of the case. You can work in teams or share and discuss your work in class.

INTAKE SUMMARY

Identifying Information: Marguerite is a 21-year-old African American female who appeared in the session to be highly intelligent and developmentally advanced for her age.

Presenting Concern: Marguerite is experiencing difficulties related to depression, a pattern of avoiding intense issues and emotions in her life, and indirectly managing strong negative emotions in a passive-aggressive manner. Marguerite appears to have never addressed and resolved issues related to her parents abandoning her to her grandmother at age 3, sexual abuse experiences in childhood and early adolescence, and other issues of family neglect. Although she appears quiet and somewhat detached interpersonally, the client appears fully cognizant. Although Marguerite appears to be experiencing significant symptoms of a mood disorder, she reports no suicidal ideation and no history of self-harm.

Background, Family, and Relevant History: Marguerite was sent by her parents to live with her maternal grandmother at age 3, lived intermittently with her mother for brief time periods, but spent most of her youth living with her grandmother. She appears to have no significant relationship with her father. The client experienced several traumas, including being stabbed once by her father's female romantic partner and being sexually assaulted at age 8 by a male romantic partner of her mother. Marguerite became selectively mute about 1 year later, when she learned that her uncle had reportedly killed the mother's boyfriend. She reports becoming pregnant during her first adolescent sexual encounter and is currently raising the baby with her mother's and stepfather's assistance.

Problem and Counseling History: The problems and problem behaviors experienced by the client throughout her youth include repressing feelings of anger, resentment, and betrayal; compensation; pregnancy; surviving sexual abuse; intense guilt; selecting to remain mute during a long period of childhood; escapism; truancy; and avoiding close interpersonal relationships. Marguerite has never received counseling or assistance.

Mental Status Exam: Marguerite was neatly dressed in dark drab clothing and her appearance was appropriate. During the interview, she generally appeared quite subdued, her mood appeared quite low, she appeared somewhat disconnected from her internal experience, was engaged but distant with the interviewer, and eye contact varied. During the interview, she mainly appeared numb and disconnected from her mood, occasionally expressing sadness, anger, and guilt. She was oriented by time, place, and person. Marguerite appeared substantially above average intellectually. Her judgment seemed good; however, her insight at this time appears minimal. Presently, she appears ambivalent about treatment. In spite of significant depression symptoms, the client reports no suicidal ideation and denies any self-harmful intent or behavior.

Goals for Counseling and Course of Counseling to Date: The client has been seen twice for intake assessment to date. The primary goals for counseling are to address and resolve adult difficulties associated with childhood trauma, sexual abuse, and abandonment. These difficulties include avoidance of conflict and hurt, self-blame, denial, depressed mood and associated symptoms of depression, feelings of numbness, inability to form close relationships, and social isolation.

Current Diagnostic Impressions:

Axis I:	296.26 Major Depressive Disorder, Single Episode, Moderate
Axis II:	V71.09 No diagnosis
Axis III:	None
Axis IV:	Problems with primary support group—disruption of family, sexual abuse
Axis V:	GAF = 50 (Lowest level observed)

Case Note — Session 3:

Write your own case note using the material provided in this chapter as a guide.

Termination Summary:

Write your own termination summary using the material provided in this chapter as a guide.

PRACTICE CLIENT 11.3

Hansel

Refer to Chapters 9 and 10 for the information needed to complete this exercise. Refer to the discussions of intake summaries, case notes, and termination summaries in this chapter for a guide. We provide an intake summary for the client, Hansel. Complete the exercise by writing (a) a case note for Session 3 and (b) a termination summary based on your understanding of the case. You can work in teams or share and discuss your work in class.

INTAKE SUMMARY

Identifying Information: Hansel is a 12-year-old White male. He lives with his father and 10-year-old sister, Gretel. His mother died when Hansel was age 5 years. His father immediately remarried. The stepmother died 5 months ago. Hansel was referred by his father for assessment and treatment.

Presenting Concern: Hansel's father sought counseling because Hansel has been experiencing a diminished interest in family activities, nightmares, and difficulty concentrating. The father reports Hansel has a desire to avoid gingerbread houses and fears going into the forest to collect firewood. Hansel's behavior changes have been ongoing for about 4 months.

About 6 months ago, Hansel and his sister had a near-death experience in the forest. The children were malnourished and lost and, as a result, stayed for a month in the cottage of an evil hag who tried to eat the children. The sister reported to the father that Hansel defended himself by pushing the evil hag into a hot oven, which resulted in her death; however, Hansel revealed that he does not fully remember these events.

Background, Family, and Relevant History: Hansel stated that his family was very close before the loss of his mother and reports feeling hurt when the father quickly remarried. Hansel reports that he is very close to his sister and father. The children currently do not attend school; however, Hansel expressed a desire to go to school in the village.

Problem and Counseling History: Hansel's concerns and behaviors have been present about 4 months. He has no previous counseling history.

Mental Status Exam: Hansel was appropriate in dress and appearance for his age and locale. During the interview, he appeared worried and anxious. He maintained good eye contact and was engaged with the interview through most of the session. He was oriented by time, place, and person; however, he was troubled by worrisome fantasies about future harm befalling him in the local forest. Hansel appeared to be of average intelligence and his memory was intact, except for difficulty recalling details of his recent trauma. His judgment, insight, and ability to engage in treatment all appeared appropriate for his age. Hansel reports no suicidal ideation and denies any self-harmful intent or behavior.

Goals for Counseling and Course of Counseling to Date: Hansel and his father have come in for one session. Current goals are to complete assessment of PTSD symptoms and initiate treatment to resolve PTSD symptoms using child psychotherapy, initiated with three sessions weekly moving to once weekly and reevaluation in 6 months.

Diagnostic Impressions:

Axis I:	309.81 Posttraumatic Stress Disorder, Chronic
Axis II:	V71.09 No diagnosis
Axis III:	None
Axis IV:	Victim of child neglect
	Victim of physical abuse as a child
	Death of mother, death of stepmother
	Exposure to trauma
Axis V:	GAF = 52 (At intake)

Case Note—Session 3:

Write your own case note using the material provided in this chapter as a guide.

Termination Summary:

Write your own termination summary using the material provided in this chapter as a guide.

PRACTICE CLIENT 11.4

Wicked Queen

Refer to Chapters 9 and 10 for the information needed to complete this exercise. Refer to the discussions of intake summaries, case notes, and termination summaries in this chapter for a guide. We provide an intake summary for the client, Wicked Queen. Complete the exercise by writing (a) a case note for Session 3 and (b) a termination summary based on your understanding of the case. You can work in teams or share and discuss your work in class.

INTAKE SUMMARY

Identifying Information: The Wicked Queen is a 30-year-old Anglo female who presently is the sole ruler of her country. She was neatly, although somewhat dramatically, dressed for the interview. Although the Wicked Queen was cooperative during the interview, she appeared to feel ill at ease and was defensive and argumentative with the interviewer.

Presenting Concern: The Wicked Queen was referred by Doc for treatment of auditory and visual hallucinations, which include seeing the image of another person's face in her "magic" mirror and hearing the face speak to her about her appearance relative to that of other females in the kingdom. Doc also shared his impression that the Wicked Queen is experiencing narcissistic and antisocial personality characteristics, and there is a concern that she may not be receptive to mental health treatment.

Background, Family, and Relevant History: The Wicked Queen currently resides in a large castle with more than 60 servants. She has been Queen since her marriage to the former King 5 years ago. She was widowed several months after her wedding, when the King died from an illness shortly after eating a stew the Wicked Queen had specially prepared for him. Her young stepdaughter, Snow White, was not prepared to assume responsibilities of the monarchy, so the Wicked Queen has ruled the country since that time.

The Wicked Queen was born into an impoverished family that lived in a hut in the forest. At age 2 years, she was abandoned by her physically abusive parents, who reportedly have a history of alcohol dependence and chronic mental illness. The Department of Social Services placed her with her paternal grandmother, an herbalist. The Wicked Queen's early developmental milestones are believed to have been normal. She was described by the grandmother as "a fussy child" who did not want to be held. The Wicked Queen reports that as a child she tortured small animals and set fires to amuse herself. She reports that her grandmother, whom she describes as overly critical, placed a great deal of emphasis on appearance, convinced that her granddaughter's beauty would provide a way out of their poverty.

Problem and Counseling History: The Wicked Queen reports that her "magic" mirror began to speak to her after the death of her husband. The Wicked Queen denies symptoms of depression and says she does not believe that her upbringing has had much of an impact on her development. She is isolated and reports no close interpersonal relationships. She appears to take great pride in both her appearance and her role as ruler of her country. She states that while her subjects do not deserve to have a queen like her, they all adore her. The Wicked Queen has a history of lying and misrepresenting herself and is alleged to have poisoned Snow White and possibly others as well, although this could not be proved.

Based on reports from Department of Social Services, it is believed that the Wicked Queen met diagnostic criteria for reactive attachment disorder of early childhood as a young child. At age 9 years, the Wicked Queen entered counseling because her grandmother was concerned about her behavior at home and her difficulty getting along with other children. At that time, her symptoms were diagnosed as oppositional defiant disorder; however, the diagnosis later was revised to conduct disorder. She appears to have been relatively unresponsive to treatment.

Mental Status Exam: The Wicked Queen was dramatically dressed and flamboyant in appearance during the interview, in a manner that would easily draw the attention of others. During the interview, she mainly appeared irritated and expressed angry mood. She was resistant to the interview and engaged the interviewer with moderate hostility. She appeared oriented to time, place, and person—with the exception that she reported the presence of specific visual and auditory hallucinations associated with a "magic talking mirror." Although she appeared above average intellectually, her insight appeared poor. Her judgment appeared uncertain and needs further assessment. She was markedly unmotivated for treatment. The Wicked Queen reported no suicidal ideation and denied any self-harmful intent or behavior. She denied any current homicidal ideation and denied any current intent to harm others. However, the credibility of the client's report is uncertain, given her resistant approach to the interview. Further evaluation is needed.

Goals for Counseling and Course of Therapy to Date: Goals for the Wicked Queen include the following: to eliminate hallucinations, to develop empathy for others, to form meaningful interpersonal relationships, to improve self-esteem, and to eliminate antisocial behavior. Immediate needs are to initiate therapy and develop client compliance with treatment plan.

Diagnostic Impressions:

Axis I:	Psychosis, NOS
Axis II:	Narcissistic Personality Disorder Antisocial Personality Disorder
Axis III:	None
Axis IV:	Problems with primary support group
Axis V:	GAF = 35 (Current)

Case Note—Session 3:

Write your own case note using the material provided in this chapter as a guide.

Termination Summary:

Write your own termination summary using the material provided in this chapter as a guide.

LEARNING TO MANAGE CASES: An Ongoing Process

It is probably accurate to say that no one chooses to become a counseling professional because of a strong desire to do case management. But don't overlook its importance! The "paperwork" in professional counseling settings can seem overwhelmingly burdensome sometimes, but good recordkeeping and documentation are essential for monitoring the progress of the counseling process. Documentation gives you a powerful tool for observing and assessing the professional helping relationship and keeping your focus on client needs.

You might be unsure or even uneasy about professional interactions and work relationships in clinical settings, but open and honest use of clinical supervision, productive use of consultation, and good use of professional relationships to provide conjoint treatment and cotherapy, when needed, are all essential to helping your clients reach their goals. You may feel unsure about the "business" aspect of clinical work, but monitoring client contacts, billing, dealing with third-party payers, and financial management are essential requirements for professional practice, whether you work as a salaried employee or as a private practitioner.

The confidential nature of the helping relationship is one of the foundational elements needed to make professional counseling work. So, it is essential that you become knowledgeable and skilled at maintaining confidentiality, communicating with nonprofessionals interested in a client's situation, and knowing when confidentiality must be broken. You must understand the differences among communications with interested family, friends, and other parties; parents and legal guardians; governmental agencies; school and university personnel; and the court and criminal justice personnel. You also must know when and how to respond to requests for client information for use in background investigations and employment checks.

Becoming good at time management, caseload management, and self-management of your own emotional energies and needs are all essential for keeping the focus clearly on the client and his or her experience and for giving the consumer good service.

All of these are elements of case management. Like counseling skills and other clinical tools, expertise at case management takes classroom instruction, practice, and, most of all, ongoing supervised field experience. We encourage you to stay cognizant of case management as you enter each new practicum placement, internship site, and professional work setting along the course of your career. The time you spend outside the clinical interview doing case management will not only benefit the client when done well, but it will also help you be a valuable asset in the competitive world of the professional helper.

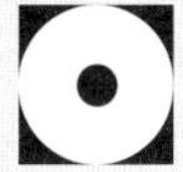

At this point, we recommend that you pause reading, turn to the DVD, and take another look at the section entitled:

Termination Interview

While viewing this segment, pay particular attention to issues related to case management.

Chapter Summary

This chapter presented the essentials of case management. We began by defining case management as the "office work" part of professional counseling—the part of being a professional that happens outside the clinical interview. We outlined five elements of this important clinical tool: documentation; consultation, supervision, and collaboration; communication with stakeholders; business-related activities; and caseload management.

Relative to documentation, we started by discussing the purposes of a clinical record, noting that it provides a clinical reference and that documentation is a mechanism for showing accountability. We then went on to discuss the contents of the clinical record. This included: the initial contact information, such as information on record, intake data, psychological test results, and intake summary (e.g., identifying information, presenting concerns, background history, counseling history, mental status report, goals, and course of therapy); diagnosis and treatment planning notes; case notes or progress notes (e.g., SOAP: **s**ubjective client report, clinician **o**bservations, current **a**ssessment, and current **p**lan); and termination materials and the storing of records.

The second aspect of case management we highlighted included consultation, supervision, and collaboration. We broke down this area into clinical supervision; clinical, medical, and psychiatric consultation; and cotherapy and conjoint treatment. We noted that clinical supervision is an intensive, interpersonal relationship that focuses on clinical skills and clinical tools. It is therapeutic, but not therapy, and it's critical to your learning process and important in addressing personal dynamics influencing your work. Supervision includes reviewing records, preparing audio- and videotaping, presenting cases, and resolving psychoemotional conflicts regarding clients. Relative to clinical, medical, and psychiatric consultation, we noted that clinical consultation occurs either when the mental health clinician meets with a consultant or has the consultant meet with a client to foster client growth. We stated that medical consultation occurs when a client is referred to a medical practitioner for physical health issues and that psychiatric consultation occurs when the psychiatrist consults regarding diagnosis and/or medication issues. Finally, we stated that cotherapy involves two or more clinicians directly working together and that conjoint treatment involves two or more modes of counseling. In all of these cases, we highlighted the fact that good case management means working collaboratively to meet the client's needs.

The third aspect of case management included communication with stakeholders. Family, friends, and other interested parties may try to contact you in many ways, and it's important not to acknowledge if a client is in counseling unless you have a release form, and to carefully consider whether or not to discuss contacts with clients. Parents and legal guardians usually "own" the client's confidentiality. You should decide early on what might be shared, and you are ultimately obligated to share and to communicate in an understandable manner. Government agencies, academic institutions, and other organizations may need information about your clients, and you should discuss confidentiality rights with your clients. When communicating with the courts and criminal justice system, except when covered by privileged communication, courts can generally require clinicians to break confidentiality. It is important to seek legal consultation when necessary and to discuss this issue with your client. Finally, you may receive requests to communicate about clients and former clients regarding background investigations as part of hiring, promotion, and assignment procedures. You should respond only after receiving a written consent to release information and only to the questions asked. In all of the above cases, we stressed the need to document any communication, to obtain a signed release form from the client, to make wise decisions, to know your ethical and legal obligations, and to maintain professional, courteous relationships with the stakeholders.

When discussing business-related issues, we highlighted four areas. First, every clinician will have to deal with some aspect of day-to-day office issues to assure that the office runs smoothly and that clients feel safe and comfortable. In the second area, billing procedures and collecting fees, it is important to know the etiquette around "money issues," to be clear and direct when addressing these issues, and to discuss fees and billing issues early. We stressed the importance of discussing with clients what information may be required to share with third-party payers. In reference to the third area—documenting client contacts, treatment plans, and progress toward stated goals—we stated that for accountability reasons, clinicians must assure that client contacts are documented and have a process whereby each client visit is noted and payment received is credited (e.g., ledger book, computer). In addition, insurance companies want to monitor payments and number of client visits, and administrators and supervisors want an accounting of time spent with clients. Finally, when completing paperwork for insurance companies, HMOs, and others, forms are everywhere, but they are a necessary burden. Completing paperwork is necessary if clinicians are to be paid, if funding agencies are to fund, and if supervisors and administrators are to have a mechanism to evaluate.

Relative to time and caseload management, we highlighted the importance of being present and timely for clinical duties, clinically related activities, and other assignments. It is important to be timely and conscientious in response to record-keeping, communications, and business matters. Clinicians must balance scheduled activities with emergency and crisis needs; monitor client experiences, treatment, and progress; conduct client follow-up with missed appointments; and check in with clients between appointments as needed. They should also monitor client follow-through with referrals, and manage the overall professional workload so that the focus remains on each client's well-being.

Near the end of the chapter, to help you get a better picture of what case management is all about, we presented two case examples, exercises and role-plays, and four practice cases using our clients drawn from popular media. Finally, we discussed how the importance of case management can be overlooked or underestimated and how critical it will be for you to pay close attention to case management in your field placements and employment settings.

Epilogue

Every person is an individual, with qualities and possibilities infinitely capable of development.

—Carl Rogers (1961; Introduction)

We have to find challenges that are sufficient to require that the individual make a really new kind of adaptation, but not so intense . . . as to force [him or her] to fall back on earlier . . . modes . . . which will serve [him or her] badly in the long run.

—Erik Erikson (1968, p. 93)

We must bring to our work as professional counselors just as much of our own selves as we possibly can, stopping, of course, at the point at which this may hamper the client's experience . . . and we must feel within ourselves that we wish to help the client as much as possible and that there is nothing at the moment more important to us.

—Alfred Benjamin (1981, p. 5)

From natural helping to professional counseling! The journey is a challenging and exciting one, and it has just begun for students using this textbook and DVD. There is much to tackle along the way: confronting our own natural styles of helping as listeners, analyzers, problem solvers, and challengers; dealing with countertransference and the imposter and white night syndromes; navigating each stage of the counseling interview, from the preinterview to rapport building to problem identification, to goal setting and treatment planning, to work, and then closure and the postinterview; mastering all of the attitudes, characteristics, foundational skills, information-gathering skills, and commonly used skills in the professional repertoire; learning to use professional tools, including diagnosis, case conceptualization, treatment planning, and case management; and learning to engage in competent and ethical clinical practice with a diverse range of clients.

Early in training, students often move back and forth between their natural style and the use of professional skills. Later, the urge to be your natural self will give way to the urge to act as a professional counselor. And finally, the natural self and professional self begin to merge so that being an effective professional clinician starts to come, well, naturally.

Fortunately, the counselor education journey provides many guides along the way: classroom instructors, practicum and internship supervisors, and mentors and supervisors for advanced growth leading up to and beyond licensure. Your education will continue to focus more on skill development and case content in your early training and probably will move on to focus more on personal functioning later in your professional development. You can rely on your instructors and supervisors to provide support, challenge, and expert advice as you engage in the process of learning to be a counselor or psychotherapist. Yet, over time, you will see the responsibility and expertise gradually shift from your educators to you.

We hope you have enjoyed and benefited from *Skill and Tools for Today's Counselors and Psychotherapists: From Natural Helping to Professional Counseling.* We would be glad if this book and DVD become important additions to your professional bookshelf.

PART FOUR

Professional Toolboxes

Professionals in every field need to have available the right tools for their jobs. Counseling professionals are no exception. Part IV of the textbook provides developing counselors with a beginning set of tools to augment the learning that takes place in the book's 11 chapters and the various segments of the DVD. You might think of the tools found in Part IV: Professional Toolboxes as a starter-kit for your own professional toolbox, which you will continue to fill during your counseling career.

The first tool you will find is listing of websites of Codes of Ethics for many of the major mental health professional associations. Earlier in the text we discussed important considerations associated with ethical and professional decision making. In Part IV, you will find website information for the ethical guidelines of the American Counseling Association (ACA), American Psychological Association (APA), National Association of Social Workers (NASW), and others.

The second tool provides specific information about counseling with diverse groups. Earlier in the textbook and in the DVD, we discussed and demonstrated important principles related to cross-cultural counseling. In Part IV, we provide more precise notes that are important to consider when providing counseling and psychotherapy for individuals of different ethnic and racial backgrounds, individuals from diverse religious backgrounds, men and women clients, gay and lesbian people, individuals who are HIV positive, homeless and poor people, older persons, the mentally ill, and individuals with disabilities.

The third tool is a sample clinical report. Part III of the textbook focused on case management and other clinical tools. The sample clinical report found in Part IV shows a start-to-finish client case write-up, such as you might be required to prepare in a counseling agency or another professional setting. The sample clinical report is based on the case of our ongoing client, Sienna, found throughout the textbook. It covers demographics, presenting problem, family background, medical and counseling history, substance use and abuse, educational-vocational history, mental status exam, assessment data, tentative diagnosis, summary and conclusion, and recommendations and treatment plan.

The fourth tool is a summary overview of Axis I and Axis II diagnoses found in the *DSM-IV-TR*. Chapter 8 of the textbook dealt with developing *DSM-IV-TR* diagnostic skills. In the toolbox, you will find as a resource a quick summary guide of all the disorders and other conditions we use on Axis I and Axis II to describe our clients' dysfunctional behaviors, distress, or foci of treatment.

Finally, the fifth tool is connected to the DVD. Here we provide samples of case conceptualization, diagnosis, case notes, and treatment planning materials—all concerning the case of Alice, whom we observe in the DVD through an intake interview, working stage interview, and closure interview. Refer to these as you watch the DVD—and later on, refer back to them as samples for case management with your own clients. This final tool provides you with a model of case conceptualization that you can use with your own clients, gives an example of how to diagnosis clients based on your case conceptualization, and demonstrates ways of developing a treatment plan.

Websites of Codes of Ethics of Select Mental Health Professional Associations

AMERICAN ASSOCIATION FOR MARRIAGE AND FAMILY THERAPY (AAMFT)
Main website: www.aamft.org
Code of ethics: www.aamft.org/resources/LRMPlan/Ethics/ethicscode2001.asp

AMERICAN ASSOCIATION OF PASTORAL COUNSELORS (AAPC)
Main website: www.aapc.org
Code of ethics: www.aapc.org/ethics.htm

AMERICAN COUNSELING ASSOCIATION (ACA)*
Main website: www.counseling.org
Code of ethics:
http://www.counseling.org/content/navigationmenu/resources/ethics/ACA_code_of_ethics.htm

AMERICAN MENTAL HEALTH COUNSELORS ASSOCIATION (AMHCA)
Main website: www.amhca.org
Code of ethics: www.amhca.org/code

AMERICAN PSYCHIATRIC ASSOCIATION (APA)
Main website: www.psych.org
Code of ethics: http://www.psych.org/psych_pract/ethics/ethics.cfm

AMERICAN PSYCHOLOGICAL ASSOCIATION (APA)
Main website: www.apa.org
Code of ethics: www.apa.org/ethics

---

* Look for revised ethical code of ACA due out in Fall of 2005.

AMERICAN SCHOOL COUNSELOR ASSOCIATION (ASCA)
Main website: www.schoolcounselor.org
Code of ethics: www.schoolcounselor.org/content.asp? contentid=173

COMMISSION ON REHABILITATION COUNSELOR CERTIFICATION (CRCC)
Main website: www.crccertification.com
Code of ethics: www.crccertification.com/code.html

NATIONAL ASSOCIATION OF SOCIAL WORKERS (NASW)
Main website: www.naswdc.org
Code of ethics: www.socialworkers.org/pubs/code/code.asp

NATIONAL ORGANIZATION OF HUMAN SERVICES (NOHS)
Main website: www.nohse.org
Ethical standards of human service professionals: www.nohse.org/ethics.html

Counseling Diverse Clients

The application of specific helping skills discussed in this text may be beneficial to some clients, but they may not be helpful, and even may be harmful, to the helping relationship when used with other clients. For instance, many Latin American clients are comfortable with less personal space than other clients and may interpret helper distance as aloofness. A Muslim may consider being touched by the left hand of a helper as obscene, because the left hand is seen as unclean and used as an aid in the process of elimination while the right hand is seen as clean and used to eat with. An African American client may be put off by eye contact from a White helper (Sue & Sue, 1990).

On a broader scale, as a function of their culture, some clients may feel defensive with the use of questions, whereas other clients may feel stonewalled because the helper uses too much empathy. Some clients may feel like they are being pushed to self-disclose—a quality viewed as weak in their culture—while other clients may feel offended that the helper has not allowed them to talk more because their culture tends to feel comfortable with the expression of feeling. Similarly, some cultures may be embarrassed with helper self-disclosure, but for others, such disclosure may bring a helper and client who are from two different cultures closer together.

Clearly, helpers need to know the cultural background of the client and understand how much a specific client's values, beliefs, and customs will play a part in the helping relationship. However, it must also be remembered that each client is unique. For instance, although many Latin American clients may be turned off by too much helper–client personal space, some will not and may indeed even feel more comfortable. Or an acculturated African American client may be offended by the intentional lack of eye contact from his or her White helper as a result of the helper's false belief that all African Americans would prefer less eye contact from White helpers.

The following sections offer some suggestions for working with select populations. Keep in mind that these are suggestions and that each client is unique.

Counseling Individuals from Different Ethnic and Racial Groups

Although cultural differences are great among African Americans, Asian Americans, Hispanic Americans, and Native Americans, there are some general suggestions for working with individuals from these and other cultures. Westwood and Ishiyama (1990), Neukrug (1994, 2004), and others note that the following should be attended to when counseling individuals from different cultures.

1. *Encourage clients to speak their own language.* A helper is not necessarily expected to be bilingual, although, no doubt, that would often be a benefit, and referral to a bilingual helper sometimes is appropriate. If a client is bilingual and you are not, make an effort to know meaningful expressions of the client's language.

2. *Do your homework and know about the cultural heritage of your clients.* Make sure that you have taken workshops or courses, gone to the library, and/or have asked your client about his or her cultural heritage.

3. *Assess the cultural identity of your clients.* Try to understand how clients view themselves as members of their culture. For example, a client who has acculturated and has little identification with his or her culture of origin is very different from a client from the same culture who is a new immigrant.

4. *Check the accuracy of your client's nonverbals.* Don't assume that nonverbal communication is consistent across cultures. Ask your client about his or her nonverbals when in doubt.

5. *Make use of alternative modes of communication.* Because of cross-cultural differences, some clients will be reticent to talk, and for others, English may be a second language. When reasonable, use other modes of communication such as acting, drawing, music, storytelling, collage making, and so forth, which may draw your client out.

6. *Encourage clients to bring in culturally significant and personally relevant items.* Have your clients bring in items that will help you understand them and their culture (e.g., book, photographs, articles of significance, culturally meaningful items, etc.).

7. *Vary the helping environment.* The helping relationship may be quite unfamiliar territory, and sitting in a small private room might create intense anxiety. Thus, it may be important to explore alternative helping environments to ease your client into the helping relationship (e.g., take a walk, have a cup of coffee at a quiet restaurant, initially meet your client at their home, etc.).

8. *Don't jump to conclusions about your client.* Don't fall into the trap of assuming your client will act in stereotypic ways. Many clients won't match your stereotype.

9. *Know yourself.* Assess your own biases and prejudices to assure they will not negatively affect your helping relationship.

10. *Know appropriate skills.* Make sure that you have taken courses and workshops and have kept up on the most recent professional literature to assure that you know the most appropriate helping skills to use and not use with your client.

Counseling Individuals from Diverse Religious Backgrounds

In working with any individual, it is important to understand his or her religious background for it may hold the key to understanding underlying values. Some pointers to keep in mind concerning religion and the helping relationship include the following:

1. *Determine the client's religious background early in the helping relationship.* As a basis for future treatment planning, know your client's religious affiliation. This can be acquired at the initial interview; however, be sensitive to any client that may initially resist such a discussion.

2. *Ask the client how important religion is in his or her life.* For some clients, religion holds little influence; for others, it is a driving force. In either case, most clients have only a rudimentary understanding of their religious tradition, and helpers should not assume that clients know much about their religion even if they present themselves as deeply religious. Assessment of the part religion plays in a client's life can assist in goal setting and treatment planning.

3. *Assess the client's level of faith development.* Low-stage faith development clients will tend to be more dualistic and concrete (Fowler, 1981). These clients work better with a fair amount of structure and setting firm goals. High-stage faith development clients see the world in complex ways and value many kinds of faith experiences. These clients likely would feel more comfortable in a helping relationship that values abstract thinking and self-reflection.

4. *Be careful not to make false assumptions about clients.* Some false assumptions are made out of a helper's stereotypic view of the client's religion. For instance, some helpers might falsely believe that all Jews keep a kosher home.

Another kind of false assumption results from the helper projecting his or her religious views onto others. For instance, some Christian helpers may assume that all faiths believe people are born with original sin, whereas this is solely a Christian belief. Most religions assume people are born holy but may require forgiveness for sins perpetrated on Earth (personal communication, Dr. John Lanci, July 22, 2003).

5. *Educate yourself concerning your client's religious beliefs*. Know about the religious affiliation of your client. Some ways you can do this are by taking a course or workshop, reading, attending a client's place of worship, and if appropriate, by asking the client.

6. *Be familiar with holidays and traditions of your client's religion*. So that you will not accidentally embarrass or offend your client, take the time to become familiar with your client's religion. For instance, learn about the more important holidays and traditions of your client's religion (e.g., a Muslim would not want to be offered food during the month of Ramadan).

7. *Understand that religion can deeply affect a client on many levels, including unconscious ones.* Some clients who deny any religious affiliation (e.g., lapsed Catholics) may still be unconsciously driven by the basic values they were originally taught. Look at clients' actions; don't only listen to their words. For instance, a lapsed Catholic may continue to feel guilty over certain issues related to the religious beliefs he or she was taught.

8. *Know yourself.* Assess your biases and prejudices to assure they will not negatively affect the helping relationship. Assess any negative or positive feelings you have toward your religious affiliation to assure these feelings do not interfere with the helping relationship.

9. *Know appropriate skills*. Make sure that you have taken courses and workshops and have kept up with the most recent professional publications to assure that you know the most appropriate helping skills to use and not use with your client.

Counseling Women

Because some mental health professionals were concerned with the ways that women were treated by helpers, the American Psychological Association developed 13 guiding principles for helpers when working with women (Fitzgerald & Nutt, 1995) (see Professional Perspectives B.1).

Feeling that the guidelines did not go far enough, some have offered a more radical approach to working with women. These individuals believe that issues brought by women to helping relationships are inextricably related to oppression against women in society (Fitzgerald & Nutt, 1995; Gladding, 1966). They suggest that the helping relationship offers women an opportunity to develop their female identity and argue that female helpers can usually be most productive in this

PROFESSIONAL PERSPECTIVES B.1
Guidelines for Working with Women

1. Be aware of the biological, psychological, and social issues that impact on women.
2. Be aware of how counseling theories and techniques help and/or hurt female clients.
3. Continually learn about special issues related to women and the helping relationship.
4. Recognize and be aware of all forms of oppression and how these interact with sexism.
5. Be knowledgeable of how verbal and nonverbal processes (particularly with regard to power in the relationship) affect women in the helping relationship.
6. Utilize skills that are particularly facilitative to women.
7. Do not have preconceived notions concerning the potential changes or goals of women.
8. Understand when it is best for a woman client to be seen by a female or male helper.
9. Use nonsexist language in counseling/therapy, supervision, teaching, and journal publication.
10. Do not engage in sexual activity with women clients under any circumstances.
11. Continually review your own values and biases and understand the effects of sex-role socialization upon your own development.
12. Be aware of how your personal functioning may influence the helping relationship with women clients. Monitor yourself through consultation, supervision, or your own therapy.
13. Support the elimination of sex bias within institutions and individuals. (Adapted from Fitzgerald & Nutt, 1995, pp. 230–252)

process (McNamara & Rickard, 1989). Downing and Roush (1985) offer one such model that includes five stages:

Stage I: Establish a relationship and demystify the helping relationship. Here helpers may downplay the "expert" role and encourage women to trust themselves. Helpers may identify with client issues and self-disclose as a way of forming a close relationship. Helpers can assist in identifying social issues related to client problem(s) and use them to set goals.

Stage II: Validate and legitimize a woman's angry feelings toward her predicament. Here helpers assist clients to understand how they have become victimized through sociopolitical forces. Helpers assist clients in combating feelings of powerlessness, helplessness, and low self-esteem. Helpers encourage participation in the examination of women's issues (books, seminars, women's groups).

Stage III: Provide a safe environment to express feelings as clients begin to form connections with other women. Here helpers validate feelings of fear and competition with other women that result from society's objectification of women. As these feelings dissipate, clients will move toward a strong and special connection to women. Helpers assist clients in understanding the difference between anger at a man and anger at a male-dominated system.

Stage IV: Help clients with conflicting feelings between traditional and new-found values. Here clients may feel torn between new-found feminist beliefs and values that do not seem congruent with those beliefs (e.g., wanting to stay home to raise the children). Helpers validate these contradictory feelings, acknowledge the confusion, and assist clients to fully explore their belief systems.

Stage V: Facilitate integration of clients' new identity. Here helpers assist clients in integrating their new-found feminist beliefs with personal beliefs, even those personal beliefs that may not seem traditionally feminist. Clients are able to feel strength in their own identity development and no longer need to rely on an external belief system.

Counseling Men

You're not allowed to have issues, you're just a male. (Kristina Williams-Neukrug)

When we were writing this section on men's issues in counseling, one of our wives made the profound statement above. You see, men in today's society are sometimes seen as not having issues because they have been in positions of power. And people in positions of power are often seen as holding a certain amount of privilege—which they do. However, helpers must be aware of the fact that there are men's issues and understand how they impact on men and on the helping relationship (Kelly & Hall, 1992; Osherson, 1986). A number of authors offer some ideas that can be incorporated into a set of guidelines when working with male clients (Osherson, 1986; Scher, 1981).

1. *Accept men where they are.* Men are particularly on guard when initially entering the helping relationship. Thus, the helper must accept men as they are in an effort to build trust. Once men feel safe, they work hard on their issues (Moore & Haverkamp, 1989; Scher, 1979).

2. *Don't push men to express what may be considered "softer feelings."* Men tend to be uncomfortable with the expression of certain feelings (e.g., deep sadness, feelings of incompetence, feelings of inadequacy, feelings of closeness) and more at ease with "thinking things through," problem solving, goal setting, and the expression of some other feelings, such as anger and pride. Push a man too quickly and you'll push him out of the helping relationship.

3. *Early in therapy, validate the man's feelings*. To protect their egos, men tend to initially blame others and society for their problems, often through the expression of anger. Men need to feel validated in these feelings if they are to continue in the helping relationship.

4. *Validate the man's view of how he has been constrained by male sex-role stereotypes.* Early in the helping relationship, it is important to note how the man is constrained by sex-role stereotypes and pressure in society (e.g., he must work particularly hard for his family). Validation of these views helps to build trust and establish the relationship.

5. *Have a plan for therapy*. Men like structure and a sense of goal directedness—even if it is changed later. Thus, the helper needs to be clear with men that he or she wants to collaborate with them on a plan for the helping relationship.

6. *Begin to discuss developmental issues.* Although each man has his own unique issues, he will likely also be struggling with common male developmental issues. The helper should be aware of and willing to discuss these issues (e.g., midlife crises) (Levinson,1986).

7. *Slowly encourage the expression of new feelings*. As trust is formed, men will begin to express what are typically considered to be more feminine feelings (e.g., tears, caring, feelings of intimacy). The helper should reinforce the expression of these new-found feelings.

8. *Explore underlying issues and reinforce new ways of understanding the world.* Expression of new feelings will lead to the emergence of underlying issues (e.g., childhood issues, feelings of inadequacy). One critical and painful issue for men is their relationship with their father: How fathers modeled emotionality and behavior, distanced themselves, and showed love become a template for men's relationships. The helper must help the male client "heal his wounded father" (Osherson, 1986).

9. *Explore behavioral change*. As men gain new insights into self, they may wish to try new ways of acting in the world. The client, in collaboration with the helper, can identify new potential behaviors and "try them out."

10. *Encourage the integration of new-found feelings, new ways of thinking about the world, and new behaviors into the man's lifestyle.* The expression of new feelings, newly gained insights, and new ways of thinking and acting will slowly take on a life of their own and be integrated into the client's way of living. Helpers can actively reinforce these new ways of being.

11. *Encourage new male relationships.* As male clients grow, new male friendships that allow the man to freely express his feelings while maintaining his "maleness" should be encouraged. Men's groups can allow men to develop more intimate relationships with other men, feel supported, and be challenged to change (Moore & Haverkamp, 1989; Williams & Myer, 1992).

12. *Say good-bye*. Although some men may want to continue in the helping relationship, many will see it as a time-limited means to a goal. Thus, the helper should be able to say good-bye and end the relationship. You have set the seeds for him to come back if he so desires.

Counseling Gay Men and Lesbian Women

Although the helper should follow the general guidelines just discussed for counseling women and men when working with gays and lesbians, the helper also should keep in mind that homosexuals have some unique concerns of their own. Thus, some authors have highlighted general guidelines for counseling gays and lesbians (Browning, Reynolds, & Dworkin, 1995; Pope, 1995; Shannon & Woods, 1995). They include the following:

1. *Adopt a nonhomophobic attitude*. Make sure that your own biases do not interfere with the helping relationship.

2. *Make few assumptions about lifestyle.* Don't assume that a gay or lesbian client is comfortable living in what the dominant culture understands as *the* gay and

lesbian lifestyle. This lifestyle, which is often portrayed in movies and on TV, in fact, usually only is found in larger metropolitan areas. The majority of lesbian and gay people in the United States inhabit a wide variety of lifestyles.

3. *Know the unique issues of lesbians and gays.* By reading professional literature and gay and lesbian literature, and by becoming involved with local lesbian and gay community groups, helpers can gain an understanding of some of the unique issues of gays and lesbians.

4. *Know community resources.* Have available community resources that might be useful to gays and lesbians.

5. *Know identity issues.* Be familiar with the identity development of gays and lesbians, especially as it relates to the coming out process (e.g., see Cass, 1979).

6. *Understand the idiosyncracies of religion toward homosexuality.* Be familiar with particular religions and spiritual concerns unique to lesbians and gays (e.g., some religions view homosexuality as abnormal).

7. *Be tuned into domestic violence issues.* Be aware that domestic violence can occur in gay and lesbian relationships as it occurs in heterosexual relationships.

8. *Know about substance abuse.* Have a firm foundation in substance abuse treatment because gays and lesbians may have a greater tendency toward the use of substances as a method of dealing with the coming out process and the inherent prejudices in society (Dyne, 1990).

9. *Be knowledgeable about AIDS.* Although AIDS is not a "gay disease," there are a disproportionate number of gay men who are HIV positive and who have AIDS.

10. *Know about sexual abuse.* Be particularly cognizant that a large percentage of lesbian women have been sexually abused before the age of 18 (38% according to Loulan, 1987).

Counseling Individuals Who Are HIV Positive

A number of challenges face the helper who works with an individual who is HIV positive or who has AIDS. Shannon and Woods (1995) and others have highlighted some points to consider when counseling the individual with HIV.

1. *Know the cultural background of the client.* HIV positive individuals are found in all cultural groups. In addition to dealing with issues unique to the HIV positive client, helpers may need to work on cross-cultural issues if the client is from a diverse background.

2. *Know about the disease and combat myths.* Individuals who are HIV positive are discriminated against and feared. Helpers need to have knowledge about the disease so they will not be fearful and will be able to effectively assist clients when they are discriminated against.

3. *Be prepared to take on uncommon helper roles*. When working with an individual who is HIV positive you may need to be an advocate, caregiver, and resource person for the client, roles with which the helper has not always been comfortable.

4. *Be prepared to deal with a number of unique treatment issues, including:*
   a. feelings about the loss of income due to the inability of the client to work and/or the high cost of medical treatment
   b. depression and feelings of hopelessness concerning declining or uncertain health and changes in the client's relationship to others
   c. the probability that the client will have friends and loved ones who are HIV positive or have died of AIDS if he or she is from a high-risk group

5. *Deal with your own feelings about mortality*. Helpers will need to be able to deal effectively with their feelings about the client's possible impending death and how those feelings may bring to the surface issues concerning the helper's own mortality.

Counseling the Homeless and the Poor

A number of unique points should be considered when counseling the homeless and the poor (Axelson & Dail, 1988; Blasi, 1990; Rossi, 1990). Some of these include the following:

1. *Focus on social issues*. When working with individuals who are struggling with basic needs, it is important for the helper to focus on social issues, such as helping a person obtain food and housing, as opposed to working on intrapsychic issues.

2. *Know the racial/ethnic/cultural background of the client*. Since a disproportionate number of homeless and the poor come from diverse racial/ethnic/cultural groups, helpers need to educate themselves about the cultural heritage of clients.

3. *Be knowledgeable about health risks*. The homeless and the poor are at greater risk of developing AIDS, tuberculosis, and other diseases. The helper should have basic knowledge of such diseases, be able to do a basic medical screening, and have referral sources available.

4. *Be prepared to deal with multiple issues*. Because as many as 50% of the homeless are struggling with mental illness and/or substance abuse, helpers often must deal with the multiple issues of homelessness, poverty, mental illness, and chemical dependence.

5. *Know about developmental delays and be prepared to refer*. Since homeless and poor children are more likely to have retarded language and social skills, be abused, and have delayed motor development, helpers should know how to identify developmental delays.

6. *Know psychological effects.* Helpers should know how to respond to the psychological and emotional response to homelessness and poverty, which can include despair, depression, and a sense of hopelessness (Blasi, 1990).

7. *Know resources.* Be aware of the vast number of resources available in your community and make referrals when appropriate.

Counseling Older Persons

Older persons have a number of problems and concerns that need to be addressed when they are counseled (Gibson & Mitchell, 1995; Schlossberg, 1995). Here are just a few of the more prevalent concerns.

1. *Adapt one's counseling style.* The helper may need to adapt the helping relationship to fit the older client's needs. For instance, use journal writing or art therapy for older persons who have difficulty hearing. For nonambulatory clients, have a session in the client's home.

2. *Build a trusting relationship.* Older persons seek counseling at lower rates than other clients (Hashimi, 1991), and those who do may be less trustful, having been raised during a time when counseling was much less common. Thus, the helper may need to spend additional time building a trusting relationship.

3. *Know potential sources of depression.* Depression can come from many sources for the older person, including the loss of loved ones, lifestyle changes, and health issues. Thus, helpers should be capable of identifying the many potential sources of depression.

4. *Know about identity issues.* Many older persons had based their identities on their career, family, or roles in the community. These individuals may need to define themselves in new ways, as they no longer find themselves in their previous roles. Helpers can assist clients in finding a new sense of who they are.

5. *Be prepared to deal with feelings that result from changes in status.* Many older persons had attained status through their life roles (e.g., in their careers, as the head of the house, etc.). However, changes in these roles can lead to feelings of depression, anxiety, or despair.

6. *Know about possible and probable health changes.* Predictable changes in health can lead to depression and concern for the future. Unpredictable changes can lead to loss of income and emotional problems. Helpers should know potential health problems, and their emotional counterparts, common to the elderly.

7. *Have empathy for changes in interpersonal relationships.* Aging brings changes in significant relationships as a result of such events as the death of a spouse, partners, and friends, changes in health status, and relocation. Helpers should know about and have empathy toward their clients concerning these changes.

8. *Know about physical and psychological causes of sexual dysfunction.* Helpers should be aware of the possible physical and psychological causes of sexual dysfunction in the elderly. Helpers also should remember that regardless of our age, we are always sexual beings.

Counseling the Mentally Ill

Helpers who work with the chronically mentally ill need to understand psychiatric disorders, psychotropic medications, and the unique needs of the chronically mentally ill such as homelessness, continual transitions, difficulty with employment, and dependent family relationships. Specific treatment issues when working with this population include the following:

1. *Help the client understand his or her mental illness.* Many clients do not have an understanding of their illness, the usual course of the illness, and the best methods of treatment. Clients should be fully informed with up-to-date knowledge about their mental illness.

2. *Help the client work through feelings concerning his or her mental illness.* Mental illness continues to be stigmatized in this society, and many clients are embarrassed about their disorder. Support groups and a nonjudgmental attitude can help to normalize the client's view of self.

3. *Help to assure attendance in counseling.* Clients may miss appointments because they are in denial about their illness, embarrassed, or simply do not care. Helpers can call clients the day before their appointment, have a relative or close friend assist the client, or work on specific strategies to help clients remember to come in for their appointments.

4. *Assure compliance with medication.* Clients may discontinue medication out of forgetfulness, denial about the illness, because they believe they won't have a relapse, or because they believe medication is not helpful. Helpers need to make sure clients continue to take their medication.

5. *Assure accurate diagnosis.* Accurate diagnosis is crucial for treatment planning and the appropriate use of medication. Helpers can assure accurate diagnosis through testing, clinical interviews, interviewing others, and through appropriate use of supervision.

6. *Reevaluate the client's treatment plan and do not give up.* The mentally ill are some of the most difficult clients, and it is easy to become discouraged. Helpers need to continue to be vigilant about their work with the mentally ill and continually reevaluate treatment plans.

7. *Involve the client's family.* Some families can offer great support to clients, and they can be a window into the client's psyche. Thus, it is important to assure adequate family involvement and to help families understand the implications of the client's diagnosis.

8. *Know resources.* The mentally ill are often involved with many other resources in the community (e.g., social security disability, housing authority, support groups). It is therefore crucial that the helper has a working knowledge of these resources.

Counseling Individuals with Disabilities

As federal laws have increasingly supported the rights to services for individuals with disabilities, the helper has taken an increasingly active role in their treatment and rehabilitation (Lombana, 1989). Some treatment issues include the following.

1. *Have knowledge of the many disabling conditions.* Obviously, a helper cannot adequately work with an individual who has a disability if he or she does not understand the emotional and physical consequences of that disability.

2. *Help the client know his or her disability.* Clients should be fully informed of their disability, the probable course of treatment, and their prognosis. Knowledge of their disability will allow them to be fully involved in any emotional healing that needs to take place.

3. *Assist the client through the grieving process.* Clients who become disabled go through stages as they grieve their loss and accept their condition. Similar to Kübler-Ross' (1997) stages of bereavement, it is usual for a client to experience denial, anger, negotiation, resignation, and acceptance. The helper can facilitate the client through these stages.

4. *Know referral resources.* Individuals with disabilities often have myriad needs. Thus, it is important that helpers are aware of community resources (e.g., physicians, social services, physical therapists, experts on pain management, vocational rehabilitation, etc.).

5. *Know the law and inform your client of the law.* By knowing the law, you can be sure the client is receiving all necessary services and not being discriminated against. Helping clients understand the law empowers them by giving them the ability to protect their rights.

6. *Be prepared to do, or refer for, career vocational counseling.* When faced with a disability, many are also faced with making a career transition. Helpers should be ready to either do career/vocational counseling or refer a client to a career/vocational helper.

7. *Include the family.* Families can offer support, assist in long-term treatment planning, and help with the emotional needs of the client. Whenever reasonable, include the family.

8. *Be an advocate.* Individuals with disabilities are faced with prejudice and discrimination. Helpers can advocate for clients by knowing the law, fighting for client rights, and assisting clients in fighting for their rights. Clients who know their rights and who advocate for themselves will feel empowered.

Clinical Report

Demographic Information

Name: Sienna Rollins
Address: Lee Residence Hall
Lower Quad, State University
Phone: 718-555-3548
E-mail: srollins@stateu.edu

Date of Birth: 07/18/82
Age: 23
Sex: Female
Ethnicity: African American
Date of Interview: 11/4/05

Intake Clinician: Karen Hogarth

Presenting Problem or Reason for Referral

Sienna was self-referred, coming into the counseling center with a moderately depressed mood (lasting at least several months) and depressive symptoms, including disrupted sleep, appetite, and concentration; and low energy level. Sienna was very tearful during initial meetings. She reports occasional, passing thoughts of "wanting to die" that are consistent with a moderately depressed mood but denies any plan or motivation to act on these thoughts. She does not appear to be a risk for self-harm at this time.

Current stressors include ambivalence about geographically leaving home, difficulties in her currently changing relationship with her mother, confusion about her dating relationship with a culturally different White boyfriend, and conflicts with her roommate.

Sienna also describes a problematic pattern of psychoemotional and attitudinal dependence on important others, including her mother, boyfriend, and roommate. She appears to experience distress from her current reliance on significant relationships for confidence, self-esteem, and decision making about important life issues.

Family Background

Sienna comes from an intact family of origin that includes her mother and father and two brothers, Sweeny, 5 years younger, and Austin, 6 years younger, both currently in high school. Socioeconomically, Sienna comes from an upper-middle-class family and grew up in a relatively affluent, predominantly African American suburb. Her father attained a master's degree and works as a civil engineer; her mother attained a bachelor's degree and works in the home. Sienna described her mother as believing her "full-time job is raising my children."

By her description, Sienna's upbringing was unremarkable. She describes home and family life as "my mother's territory," with her father deferring to mother on child-rearing, discipline, and other domestic matters. Sienna describes a fairly traditional family experience and apparently conscientious parents who attended PTA meetings, their children's little league sports and other activities, and required family attendance at AME church services. Discipline appears consistent with contemporary norms, including use of "time out," loss of privileges, and so on. Still, Sienna describes her mother as having episodes of "silence, pouting, and making me feel really guilty for going against her." It was at her mother's insistence that Sienna spent her first year of college living at home and attending a nearby community college. She says she agreed to stay "close to my mother . . . she really needs me."

Currently, Sienna is in a romantic relationship with a White male college student that has been ongoing since September. Sienna reports the couple met at a transfer student orientation picnic. She reports feeling "swept away in love" earlier on; currently, she expresses some ambivalence about the dependent role she sees herself playing in the relationship and is concerned she has been "letting him run my life too much." She also appears somewhat unresolved about being in a biracial relationship.

Significant Medical/Counseling History

Sienna reports no atypical childhood medical events. She reports that she is in good overall health, with the exception of the disruptions in sleep and appetite associated with her moderate depression. She reports no previous counseling concerns and no previous use of counseling, although she met extensively with a guidance counselor at the community college to plan her transition to a 4-year institution.

Substance Use and Abuse

Sienna states she began drinking moderately in high school in settings typical of suburban adolescents and began smoking marijuana with peers during community college. She reports currently drinking and using marijuana "just at parties" and "mostly weekends." She denies any ill effects such as missing classes and poor grades, dangerous sexual situations, or other problems as a result of her substance use. She denies use of any other prescribed or street drugs or cigarettes. She drinks coffee "every day."

Educational and Vocational History

Sienna reports having "always been an A student" during K–12. She was offered a partial scholarship to attend a 4-year college right out of high school, which she turned down to attend community college near her mother. She earned a 4.0 during her community college year and reports she is adjusting well academically to 4-year university demands, although she has some questions about choice of academic major. She did volunteer work at a local homeless shelter during high school but was not allowed to have a part-time job in order to help her mother with her two younger brothers. She says she would like to apply for on-campus work in the dining hall or student center.

Other Pertinent Information

None.

Mental Status Exam

Sienna was appropriate in dress and appearance, and her eye contact seemed appropriate. She was oriented by time, place, and person. She presented with a low mood and her affect was depressed. She seemed somewhat fatigued and was a bit slow in her verbal responses. There were no apparent delusions or hallucinations. Sienna appeared to be above average intellectually and her memory was intact. Her judgment seemed good, her insight was high, and she appeared motivated for treatment. She reported occasional, passing thoughts of "wanting to die" but denies any immediate plan to act on these thoughts and does not appear to be an immediate risk for self-harm.

Assessment

Tests used: Beck Depression Inventory (BDI), Problem Checklist.

On the Problem Checklist, Sienna endorsed as her major concerns her low mood and other moderate depression symptoms and dealing with her changing relationship with her mother. She endorsed as secondary concerns feeling dependent in, and ambivalent about, her romantic relationship and roommate conflicts.

On the BDI, Sienna obtained a score of 17, which places her in the mild to moderate range of depression.

Tentative *DSM-IV-TR* Diagnostic Impressions

Axis I:	309.0 Adjustment Disorder with Depressed Mood
	V61.20 Parent–Child Relational Problem
Axis II:	799.9 No diagnosis or condition on Axis II
Axis III:	None
Axis IV:	Problems with primary support group
Axis V:	GAF = 61 (At intake)

Summary and Conclusions

Sienna is a 23-year-old single African American female who is a second-year transfer from community college who sought counseling for relief from moderate depression symptoms and developmental concerns around autonomy from her mother. Her primary goal is to reduce and eliminate her feelings of depression and return to her previous level of function. She also appears open to the goal of exploring and resolving her dependent pattern in relationships with important others.

Tentative goals are to (a) develop her ability to cope with feelings of depression, develop improved cognitive patterns leading to alleviation of depression symptoms, and alleviate depressed mood and return to previous level of effective functioning and (b) resolve young adult dependence issues by developing confidence that she is capable of meeting her own adult needs, forming a balance between healthy independence and dependence in changing relationship with her mother, and forming a balance between healthy independence and dependence in present relationships.

Recommendations/Treatment Plan

1. Individual counseling, 1 hour weekly, limited to 12 sessions, using a combination of client-centered and cognitive approaches, to alleviate depressed mood and return to previous level of functioning, and decrease level of dependence and conflict in relationships with her mother and boyfriend.
2. Referral for psychiatric evaluation to rule out potential use of antidepressant medication and ongoing assessment in sessions.
3. Possible referral to psychoeducational group focusing on young adult autonomy as adjunct to individual counseling.

Karen Hogarth, LPC
Signature of Clinician

Overview of Axis I and Axis II of *DSM-IV-TR*

DSM-IV-TR offers a wealth of information on disorders that are used by clinicians in making sound diagnostic judgments. The following very brief overview summarizes hundreds of pages of information from Axis I and Axis II of *DSM-IV-TR*. For an in-depth review of the disorders, please see the *DSM-IV-TR* (American Psychiatric Association, 2000).

Brief Overview of Axis I Disorders

This axis includes all disorders except for those classified as personality disorders or as mental retardation (Axis II disorders). Generally, these disorders are considered treatable in some fashion and are often reimbursable by insurance companies as a function of mental health or related services. The following lists the disorders.

DISORDERS USUALLY FIRST DIAGNOSED IN INFANCY, CHILDHOOD, OR ADOLESCENCE The disorders in this section are generally found in childhood; however, at times, individuals are not diagnosed with the disorder until they are adults. Particularly important for school counselors, the disorders include learning disorders, motor skills disorders, communication disorders, pervasive developmental disorders, attention-deficit and disruptive behavior disorders, feeding and eating disorders of infancy or early childhood, tic disorders, elimination disorders, and other disorders of infancy, childhood, or adolescence.

DELIRIUM, DEMENTIA, AMNESTIC, AND OTHER COGNITIVE DISORDERS Delirium, dementia, and amnestic disorders are all cognitive disorders that represent a significant change from past cognitive functioning of the client. All of these disorders are caused by a medical condition or a substance (e.g., drug abuse, medication, allergic reaction).

MENTAL DISORDERS DUE TO A GENERAL MEDICAL CONDITION This diagnosis is made when a mental disorder is found to be the result of a medical condition and includes Axis I disorders, personality change, and mental disorder not otherwise specified. Other disorders that may at times be the result of a medical condition are listed under the following specific diagnostic categories: deliruim, dementia, amnestic disorder, psychotic disorder, mood disorder, anxiety disorder, sexual dysfunction, and sleep disorder.

SUBSTANCE-RELATED DISORDERS A substance-related disorder is a direct result of the use of a drug or alcohol, the effects of medication, or exposure to a toxin. They include alcohol, amphetamine, caffeine, cannabis, cocaine, hallucinogens, inhalants, nicotine, opioids, phencyclidine (PCP), sedatives, and hypnotics.

SCHIZOPHRENIA AND OTHER PSYCHOTIC DISORDERS All disorders classified in this section share one thing in common: psychotic symptomology as the most distinguishing feature. The disorders include schizophrenia, shizophreniform disorder, schizoaffective disorder, delusional disorder, brief psychotic disorder, shared psychotic disorder, psychotic disorder due to a general medical condition, substance-induced psychotic disorder, and psychotic disorder not otherwise specified.

MOOD DISORDERS The disorders in this category share a common feature: mood disturbances of the depressive, manic, or hypomanic type. The mood disorders are divided into four broad categories: depressive disorders, bipolar disorders, mood disorder due to a general medical condition, and substance-induced mood disorder.

ANXIETY DISORDERS There are many types of anxiety disorders, each with its own discrete characteristics. They include panic attack, agoraphobia, panic disorder with or without agoraphobia, agoraphobia without history of panic disorder, specific phobia, obsessive-compulsive disorder, posttraumatic stress disorder, acute stress disorder, generalized anxiety disorder, anxiety disorder due to a general medical condition, substance-induced anxiety disorder, anxiety disorder not otherwise specified.

SOMATOFORM DISORDERS Somatoform disorders are characterized by symptoms that would suggest a physical cause. However, no such cause can be found, and there is strong evidence that links the symptoms to psychological causes. Seven somatoform disorders include somatization disorder, undifferentiated somatoform disorder, conversion disorder, pain disorder, hypochondriasis, body dysmorphic disorder, and somatoform disorder not otherwise specified.

FACTITIOUS DISORDERS As opposed to somatoform disorders, which describe individuals who believe that their physical symptoms have a physiological etiology, factitious disorders describe individuals who intentionally feign physical or psychological symptoms to assume the sick role. Two subtypes include factitious disorder with predominantly psychological signs and symptoms and factitious disorder with predominantly physical signs and symptoms.

DISSOCIATIVE DISORDERS Dissociative disorders occur when there is a disruption of consciousness, memory, identity, or perception of the environment. Five dissociative disorders include dissociative amnesia, dissociative fugue, dissociative identity disorder (formerly called multiple personality disorder), depersonalization disorder, and dissociative disorder not otherwise specified.

SEXUAL AND GENDER IDENTITY DISORDERS This section includes disorders that focus on sexual problems or identity problems related to sexual issues. They include sexual dysfunctions, paraphilias, gender identity disorders, and sexual disorder not otherwise specified.

EATING DISORDERS These disorders focus on severe problems with the amount of food intake by the individual that can potentially cause serious health problems or death. They include anorexia nervosa, bulimia nervosa, and eating disorder not otherwise specified.

SLEEP DISORDERS These disorders have to do with severe sleep-related problems and are broken down into four subcategories: primary sleep disorders, sleep disorder related to another mental condition, sleep disorder due to a general medical condition, and substance-induced sleep disorder.

IMPULSE CONTROL DISORDERS NOT ELSEWHERE CLASSIFIED Impulse control disorders are highlighted by the individual's inability to stop exhibiting certain behaviors. They include intermittent explosive disorder, kleptomania, pyromania, pathological gambling, trichotillomania, and impulse control disorder not otherwise specified.

ADJUSTMENT DISORDERS Probably the most common disorders clinicians see in private practice, adjustment disorders are highlighted by emotional or behavioral symptoms that arise in response to psychosocial stressors. The subtypes of this diagnosis include adjustment disorders with depressed mood, with anxiety, with mixed anxiety and depressed mood, with disturbance of conduct, with mixed disturbance of emotions and conduct, and unspecified.

Brief Overview of Axis II Disorders

Axis II diagnoses tend to be long-term disorders in which treatment almost always has little or no effect on changing the presenting symptoms of the individual. The two kinds of Axis II disorders are mental retardation and personality disorders.

MENTAL RETARDATION Characterized by intellectual functioning significantly below average (below the second percentile) as well as problems with adaptive skills, mental retardation can have many different etiologies. There are four categories of mental retardation: mild mental retardation (IQ of 50–55 to approximately 70), moderate mental retardation (IQ of 35–40 to 50–55), severe mental retardation (IQ of 20–25 to 35–40), and profound mental retardation (IQ below 20 or 25).

PERSONALITY DISORDERS Individuals with a personality disorder show deeply ingrained, inflexible, and enduring patterns of relating to the world that lead to distress and impairment in a person's life. Such an individual may have difficulty understanding self and others, may be labile, have difficulty in relationships, and have problems with impulse control. Personality disorders are generally first recognized in adolescence or early adulthood and often remain throughout one's lifetime. There are three clusters of personality disorders, with each cluster representing a general way of relating to the world.

Cluster A includes paranoid, schizoid, and schizotypal personality disorder. Individuals with these disorders all experience characteristics that may be considered odd or eccentric by others.

Cluster B disorders include the antisocial, borderline, histrionic, and narcissistic personality disorders. Individuals suffering from these disorders are generally dramatic, emotional, overly sensitive, and erratic.

Cluster C includes the avoidant, dependent, and obsessive-compulsive personality disorders. Common characteristics found within this cluster are anxious and fearful traits.

In Association with the DVD, Applying Clinical Tools with Alice: Case Conceptualization, Diagnosis, Case Notes, Treatment Planning

Case Conceptualization

Applying the Inverted Pyramid Method to Alice

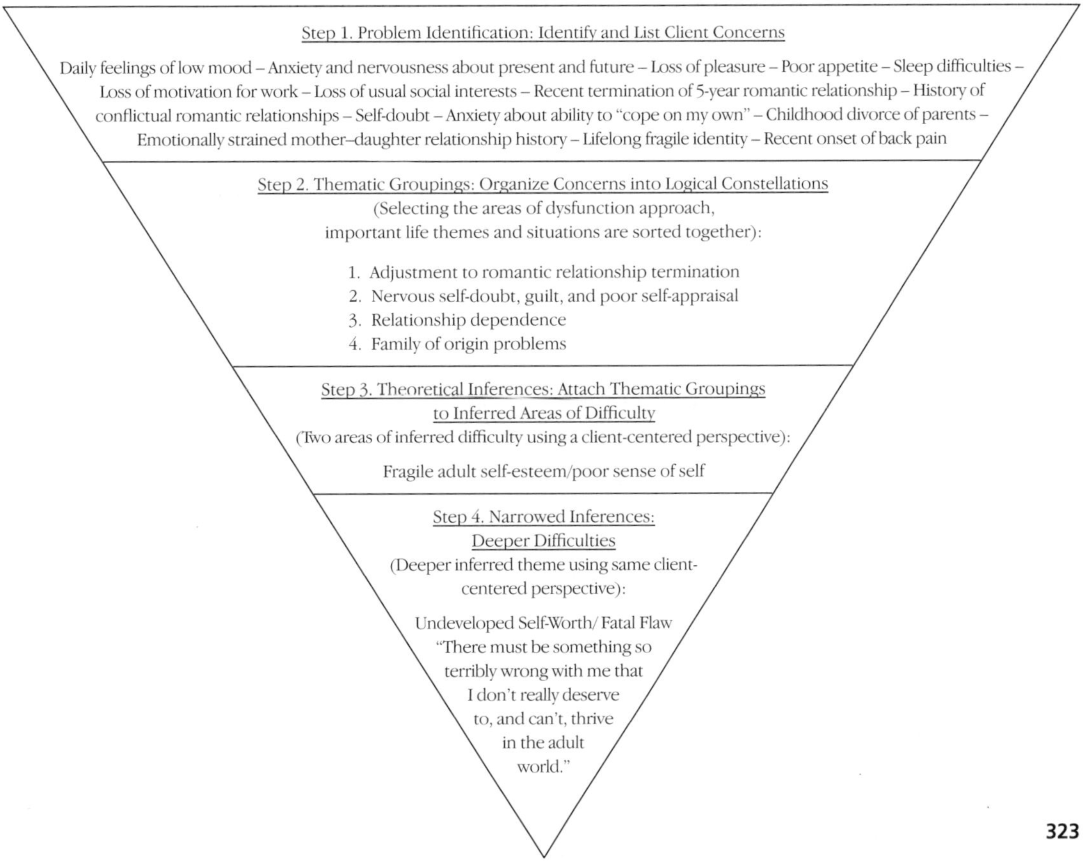

Step 1. Problem Identification: Identify and List Client Concerns

Daily feelings of low mood – Anxiety and nervousness about present and future – Loss of pleasure – Poor appetite – Sleep difficulties – Loss of motivation for work – Loss of usual social interests – Recent termination of 5-year romantic relationship – History of conflictual romantic relationships – Self-doubt – Anxiety about ability to "cope on my own" – Childhood divorce of parents – Emotionally strained mother–daughter relationship history – Lifelong fragile identity – Recent onset of back pain

Step 2. Thematic Groupings: Organize Concerns into Logical Constellations

(Selecting the areas of dysfunction approach, important life themes and situations are sorted together):

1. Adjustment to romantic relationship termination
2. Nervous self-doubt, guilt, and poor self-appraisal
3. Relationship dependence
4. Family of origin problems

Step 3. Theoretical Inferences: Attach Thematic Groupings to Inferred Areas of Difficulty

(Two areas of inferred difficulty using a client-centered perspective):

Fragile adult self-esteem/poor sense of self

Step 4. Narrowed Inferences: Deeper Difficulties

(Deeper inferred theme using same client-centered perspective):

Undeveloped Self-Worth/ Fatal Flaw "There must be something so terribly wrong with me that I don't really deserve to, and can't, thrive in the adult world."

Elements of Case Conceptualization

Element 1: Observe, assess, and measure client behaviors, thoughts, feelings, and physiological features

Alice sought counseling for feelings of moderate depression and anxiety following the end of a 5-year romantic relationship with a live-in partner. When the clinician more fully explored Alice's areas of difficulty, a number of important problems emerged:

- symptoms of moderate depression, including daily feelings of low mood and teariness; daily anxiety and nervousness about the present and future; loss of normal social interests; diminished pleasure in normal activities; disrupted sleep; poor appetite; diminished motivation to perform well at work or in other life roles.
- a history in adolescence and adulthood ("as long as I can remember") of feeling inadequate in comparison with others; feeling incompetent to manage adult work and other demands in spite of evidence to contrary; free-floating feelings of guilt, self-doubt; free-floating feelings of nervousness, anxiety
- a history of conflictual and poor romantic relationships since late adolescence/early adulthood; lifelong feelings of "needing to be in a relationship to feel ok"; emotional dependence in relationships with romantic partners, coworkers, social acquaintances, and others; deference to the decisions of others
- emotional strains in mother–daughter relationship; mother's blame for divorce on her children; feelings of inadequacy and guilt in relationship with mother
- recent chronic back pain

Element 2: Find patterns and themes by using observations, assessments, and measurements

Intuitive-logical clinical thinking is used to begin organizing symptoms according to sensible common denominators. There are four different intuitive-logical ways of clinical thinking commonly used by clinicians: (a) descriptive-diagnosis approach, which looks for diagnosable disorders; (b) clinical targets approach, which looks at thoughts, feelings, behaviors, and physiology; (c) areas of dysfunction approach, which looks for life roles and themes; and (d) intrapsychic approach, which looks for intrapersonal life themes.

The areas of dysfunction approach was used by Alice's clinician, who looked for life roles and themes:

1. Alice's daily feelings of low mood and anxiety, appetite and sleep disruptions, disruptions in motivation and pursuit of interests, and other presenting symptoms were all grouped together as symptoms associated with the end of her recent romantic relationship.

2. A theme of nervous self-doubt, guilt, and inaccurate view of self as incompetent and inadequate was formed.
3. A theme of "relationship dependence" was formed from her reports of feeling an overwhelming drive to find and stay in a romantic relationship, in spite of dissatisfaction or emotional abusiveness, deference to the decisions of others, and sense of "needing to be in a relationship."
4. A longstanding theme of "family of origin problems" was formed from her reports of early parental divorce, emotionally strained relationship with mother, and mother's fault-finding with Alice (and her sister) as a cause of divorce.

Element 3: Using the patterns and themes that are found to interpret, explain, or make clinical judgments about the person's concerns

Theoretical orientations are used to interpret, explain, or make clinical judgments about the etiological factors (underlying or root causes) and sustaining factors (features keeping the problem going) associated with the person's concerns. Major theoretical approaches such as client-centered, cognitive-behavioral, psychodynamic, solution-focused, feminist psychology of women—or an integrated or eclectic mix of these—might be used.

The client-centered, or humanistic, approach was used by Alice's clinician:

From a client-centered approach, the counselor viewed Alice's current adjustment difficulties, resulting from her recent relationship breakup, as a current situation stemming from a longer term of using relationships and dependence on others to ward off uncomfortable, deeply doubtful feelings about herself. In turn, the counselor inferred that underlying the client's current adjustment difficulties was an undue dependent need to be in relationships to feel adequate, and underlying this longstanding pattern was a fundamental fragile self-esteem, also called fragile or poor sense of self.

Next, as a still-deeper theoretical inference, the counselor believed Alice's fragile self-esteem, and the relationship problems caused by her fragile self-esteem, were linked to a core issue of undeveloped self-worth. Humanistic clinicians sometimes described this as the "fatal flaw," or the client's belief that "there must be something so terribly wrong with me that I don't really deserve to be happy, or can't really function and succeed, in the adult world." The assumption from this theoretical perspective is that a solid, firm, reliable self-worth, or sense of self, in adulthood, results from parental conditions during the "growing up years" that include parental unconditional positive regard and parental affirmation. In Alice's case, family problems with parental divorce and her mother's emotional reactions kept Alice from these necessary experiences. As a result, she developed a less-than-stable identity on which to build adult adjustment. This is the sense of being "fatally flawed" and could be selected as a focus of counseling.

These elements can be transformed into an instructive diagram using the four-step inverted pyramid method discussed in the textbook.

Notice that, as illustrated in the diagram, the clinician:

1. Casts as wide a net as possible to collect all of the relevant information about the client's needs and functioning.
2. Organizes all of the clinical information into a few logical-intuitive groupings.
3. Reduces the groupings to one or two core themes, inferred from theory, which help explain why the client's problems exist.
4. Using the same theory, reduces the themes further to their "rock-bottom" roots.

Diagnostic Impressions

Axis I:	309.28 Adjustment Disorder with Mixed Anxiety and Depressed Mood
Axis II:	V71.09 No Diagnosis or Condition on Axis II
Axis III:	Injury—Chronic Back Pain
Axis IV:	Problems with primary support group—Termination of romantic relationship
Axis V:	GAF = 55 (At intake) GAF = 75 (Highest in past year)

Case Notes

Intake Summary

IDENTIFYING INFORMATION Alice is a 41-year-old Anglo woman who resides in an urban center. Alice currently is employed as a manager in a local bank branch office. She currently lives alone, following the end of a 5-year intimate relationship with a male domestic partner. Alice experiences back pain and was recently diagnosed with a herniated disk in her lower back.

PRESENTING CONCERN Alice set up an initial intake appointment at the center due to feelings of moderate depression and anxiety following the end of a 5-year romantic relationship. She appeared to be experiencing low mood and was at times tearful during the interview. She reported diminished enjoyment in usually pleasurable activities, some difficulty remaining asleep throughout the night, some loss of appetite, loss of motivation to perform well at work or elsewhere, and loss of interest in her usual social activities and relationships. She described a sense of self-doubt, anxiety about her ability to "cope on my own," and some difficulties in concentration and focus.

BACKGROUND, FAMILY, AND RELEVANT HISTORY Alice was born the second of two children in a moderately low socioeconomic household in the same area in which she currently resides. Alice's parents divorced when she was about age 5, and subsequently, she and her sister were raised by their mother in a single-parent household. Alice expressed an impression that her mother in part faulted the presence of the two children for the parental divorce.

Alice was married briefly at age 19 while attending a public university. She described the marriage as conflictual and believes she was the victim of emotional and verbal abuse. Following divorce at age 21, Alice reports a series of romantic relationships and has not remarried.

PROBLEM AND COUNSELING HISTORY Alice describes significant current low mood and anxiety consistent with an adjustment disorder. She reports her symptoms began 4 months ago following the end of a romantic relationship. Alice reports a history of generally adequate functioning, with occasional lapses in adjustment, usually following a romantic breakup or other moderate stressor, resulting in some periods of combined moderately low mood and modest anxiety.

MENTAL STATUS EXAM Alice was appropriate in manner and appearance and maintained adequate eye contact. During the interview, her mood appeared moderately low, she appeared somewhat fatigued with low energy, she was tearful at times, and at times expressed nervousness and anxiety about her present and future. Her judgment, insight, and motivation for treatment to relieve her symptoms and perhaps address underlying symptoms all appeared good. Alice reports no suicidal ideation and denies any current or past history of self-harmful intent or behavior.

GOALS FOR COUNSELING AND COURSE OF COUNSELING TO DATE Alice has been seen twice for intake and follow-up. Her primary goal is to reduce and eliminate her feelings of moderate depression and anxiety and return to her previous level of functioning, including enjoyment of daily activities, improved appetite and mood, concentration and memory, and positive orientation toward her future. She appears open to the intermediate goal of better understanding and resolving the etiological factors affecting symptom patterns to achieve the goal of symptom reduction and elimination.

Tentative goals are: (a) identify, understand, and reduce the impact of factors causing and sustaining symptoms; and (b) appropriately adjust to ending of romantic relationship and related losses to normalize mood and return to previous level of adaptive functioning.

Treatment plan will include at least weekly contact for client-centered psychotherapy with ongoing continued assessment and reevaluation after four sessions. Possible referral for further assessment including psychological testing (MMPI, BDI) or referral for psychiatric consultation if indicated after four sessions.

Treatment Planning

A. Selecting achievable goals for change

Alice sought counseling to reduce her feelings of low mood and anxiety and related symptoms. When the counselor more fully explored all of Alice's areas of difficulty, four problem areas were conceptualized:

1. The moderate depression and anxiety symptoms of an adjustment disorder that were her presenting concerns.
2. Collateral problems of nervous self-doubt, guilt, and poor self-appraisal, which she experienced on a regular basis.
3. The collateral problem of relationship dependence, which she experienced on an ongoing basis.
4. The historical issue in her family of origin of a problematic mother–daughter relationship.

A two-part treatment plan was presented to the client, including:

1. Appropriately adjust to the current situation—that is, the ending of the romantic relationship and related losses to normalize mood and return to previous level of adaptive functioning,
2. Identify, understand, and reduce the impact of factors causing and sustaining symptoms.

With the client's agreement, a decision was made to use a client-centered approach to address not just the presenting symptoms but also the causal and sustaining factors associated with the presenting symptoms to reduce the likelihood of reemergence of similar symptoms in the future.

B. Determining treatment modes (e.g., service provider, treatment format, therapeutic approach, therapeutic interventions, and duration of counseling)

According to the case conceptualization from a client-centered perspective, Alice's themes were seen to be rooted in fragile adult self-esteem, dependence on relationships to help mitigate feelings of inability to cope alone in the adult world, and a deeper rooted underdeveloped self-worth. Correspondingly, the treatment of choice was individual counseling using client-centered interventions. Specifically, the plan would be to

a. use active client-centered listening techniques to increase the client's identification of, and understanding of, feelings and thoughts related to poor self-worth and
b. use empathy and unconditional positive regard techniques to provide a positive corrective emotional experience to

c. develop improved self-esteem and increased self-worth, which would lead to
d. alleviation of current adjustment symptoms and reduce future lapses in self-worth.

To do this, the counselor would do the following:

1. See the client 1 hour weekly for client-centered counseling.
2. Develop a positive supportive interpersonal environment in which Alice could feel open to assessing her current functioning and identifying problematic self-estimations to provide a positive corrective experience.
3. Use client-centered skills (empathy, unconditional regard, deepening reflections, etc.), with a focus on negative influences reducing her sense of self-worth, to increase client understanding.
4. Use client self-expression to organize her thoughts, feelings, and behaviors and examine their role in her adult adjustments and her role in romantic relationships.
5. Use client self-monitoring between sessions to identify and reduce influence of thoughts and feelings of fragile self-worth on mood and behavior.

C. Documenting attainment of goals

The goals of developing healthy feelings of self-worth and accurate perceptions of self that reduce the need for relationship dependence and lead to the alleviation of presenting adjustment symptoms would be measured by:

1. The client's self-reported increase in replacing feelings of poor self-esteem with positive feelings of self-worth.
2. The client's self-reported decrease in presenting adjustment symptoms over the course of counseling.
3. The client's self-reported decrease in dependence feelings and behaviors.
4. Increase in mood, decrease in anxiety, and increase in motivation and energy observed by clinician in progressive sessions.
5. Overall reduction in adjustment symptoms and increase in functioning observed by clinician reflected in positive change in GAF to at least GAF = 70 (at termination).

Case Note Session 4

Alice returned today after canceling her previous appointment. She reported a scheduling conflict with her primary care physician regarding her lower back condition and reports the conflict has been corrected for future appointments. Center policy regarding attendance was reviewed. Alice denied but appeared open to explore, if necessary, pyschoemotional factors potentially associated with missing the session.

Alice reports that in the past 3 weeks she has, on a daily basis, maintained early gains in improved mood, reduced teariness, reduced feelings of anxiety, and seen some improvement in motivation, being future oriented, and seeking out

Graphic Display Treatment Plan

GOALS FOR CHANGE	INTERVENTIONS: CLIENT-CENTERED APPROACH	OUTCOME MEASURES
1. Normalize mood and return to previously adequate level of functioning. 2. Identify, increase understanding of, and reduce the impact of factors causing and sustaining current symptoms to prevent future occurrence.	1. Use empathy and unconditional positive regard techniques to provide a positive corrective emotional experience. 2. Use active client-centered listening techniques to increase the client's identification of, and understanding of, feelings and thoughts related to poor self-worth. 3. Use client self-expression to assist client to organize her thoughts, feelings, and behaviors and examine their role in her adult adjustments and her role in romantic relationships. 4. Use client self-monitoring between sessions to identify and reduce influence of thoughts and feelings of fragile self-worth on mood and behavior.	1. Client's self-reported decrease in presenting adjustment symptoms over the course of counseling. 2. Client's self-reported increase in replacing feelings of poor self-esteem with positive feelings of self-worth. 3. Client's self-reported decrease in dependence feelings and behaviors. 4. Increase in mood, decrease in anxiety, and increase in motivation and energy observed by clinician in progressive sessions. 5. Overall reduction in adjustment symptoms and increase in functioning observed by clinician reflected in positive change in GAF to at least GAF = 70 (at termination).

pleasurable activities. At the same time, she reports that her depressed mood continues to cause distress, and low mood, anxiety, and related symptoms continue to interfere somewhat with her work performance and ability to develop new relationships, with GAF = about 61 (current) and no change in diagnosis.

Plan is to monitor Alice's continued compliance with attending future appointments and continue with treatment plan. To date, Alice has made productive use of client-centered interventions to identify, understand, and reduce the impact of etiological factors—including family of origin, identity, and relationship problems—on current functioning. Alice continues to deny any thoughts, feelings, or actions of self-harm, and referral for psychiatric evaluation is deferred at this time, pending continued monitoring at future sessions. Remaining goals are to solidify progress to date and continue reducing symptoms of adjustment disorder.

Termination Summary

Termination was agreed on by clinician and client. Alice was seen for a total of 12 sessions. The client canceled and rescheduled one time. Alice consistently was open and motivated for change at each of the 12 interviews she attended and was compliant with the treatment plan in sessions and in independent work between sessions.

Significant progress included client report of significantly improved mood, significant reduction in feelings of anxiety about present or future, improved appetite and sleep, and return to previous levels of motivation, energy, concentration, interest in pleasurable activities, and work performance. Client also reports increased understanding of, and reduction in negative impact of, influences of family of origin relationships, romantic relationship expectations, and identity on current adjustment. In sessions, client demonstrated improvement in mood, anxiety, energy, and focus. Although formal clinical assessment was not ordered, pre–post in-session comparisons are positive. Symptoms have diminished and are mild and transient when present.

Posttermination after-plan is for client to continue independently, actively using client-centered constructs to reduce and eliminate transient lapses in adjustment when they occur. No plan for future scheduled contact at this time.

Diagnosis at Termination

Axis I:	V71.09 No Diagnosis or Condition on Axis I
Axis II:	V71.09 No Diagnosis or Condition on Axis II
Axis III:	Injury–Chronic Back Pain
Axis IV:	None
Axis V:	GAF = 75

References

Ackley, D.C. (1997). *Breaking free of managed care: A step-by-step guide to regaining control of your practice.* New York: The Guilford Press.

Aiken, L. R. (2003). *Psychological testing and assessment* (11th ed.). Boston: Allyn & Bacon.

Allen, T. W. (1967). Effectiveness of counselor trainees as a function of psychological openness. *Journal of Counseling Psychology, 14*, 35–40.

American Association of Marriage and Family Therapy. (2001). *AAMFT code of ethics*. Retrieved June 1, 2001, from the World Wide Web: http://www.aamft.org/resources/lrmplan/ethics/ethicscode2001.asp

American Counseling Association. (1995). *ACA code of ethics and standards of practice*. Retrieved August 15, 2002, from the World Wide Web: http://www.counseling.org/resources/ethics.htm#ce

American Counseling Association. (1995). *Code of ethics and standards of practice* (Rev. ed.). Alexandria, VA: Author.

American Mental Health Counselors Association. (1987). *Code of ethics for mental health counselors*. Alexandria, VA: Author.

American Psychiatric Association. (1994). *Diagnostic and statistical manual of mental disorders* (4th ed.). Washington, DC: Author.

American Psychiatric Association. (2000). *Diagnostic and statistical manual of mental disorders* (4th ed., text revision). Washington, DC: Author.

American Psychiatric Association. (2001). *The principles of medical ethics with annotations especially applicable to psychiatry*. Retrieved February 12, 2004, from the World Wide Web: http://www.psych.org/psych_pract/ethics/medicalethics2001_42001.cfm

American Psychological Association. (2002). *Ethical principles of psychologists and code of conduct 2002*. Retrieved January 2, 2003 from the World Wide Web: http://www.apa.org/ethics/code2002.html

American Psychological Association. (2002). Report of the ethics committee, 2001. *American Psychologist, 57*(8), 646–653.

American Psychological Association. (2003). *Ethical principles of psychologists and code of conduct*. Retrieved June 15, 2003, from the World Wide Web: http://www.apa.org/ethics

American Psychological Association Practice Organization. (2002). *Getting ready for HIPAA: What you need to know now: A primer for psychologists,* 1–17, Washington, DC: Author.

Anderson, C. A., Lepper, M. R., & Ross, L. (1980). Perseverance of social theories: The role of explanation in the persistence of discredited information. *Journal of Personality and Social Psychology, 39,* 1037–1049.

Angelou, M. (1969). *I know why the caged bird sings*. New York: Bantam Books.

Arredondo, P. (1999). Multicultural counseling competencies as tools to address oppression and racism. *Journal of Counseling and Development, 77*(1), 102–108.

Argyle, M. (1975). *Bodily communication*. London: Methuen.

Atkinson, D. R. (1985). A meta-review of research on cross-cultural counseling and psychotherapy. *Journal of Multicultural Counseling and Development, 13,* 138–153.

Atkinson, D. R., Poston, W. C., Furlong, M. J., & Mercado, P. (1989). Ethnic group preferences for counselor characteristics. *Journal of Counseling Psychology, 36,* 68–72.

Axelson, L. J., & Dail, P. W. (1988). The changing character of homelessness in the United States. *Family Relations, 37*, 463–469.

Bachelard, G. (1960). *The Columbia world of quotations*. Retrieved January 14, 2003, from the World Wide Web: http://www.bartleby.com/66/69/5069.html

Baker, R., & Siryk, B. (1984). Measuring adjustment to college. *Journal of Counseling Psychology, 31,* 179–189.

Barry, V. C. (1982). *Moral aspects of health care.* Pacific Grove, CA: Brooks/Cole.

Baum, B. E., & Gray, J. J. (1992). Expert modeling, self-observation using videotape, and acquisition of basic therapy skills. *Professional Psychology: Research and Practice, 23*(3), 220–225.

Baumgarten, E., & Roffers, T. (2003). Implementing and expanding on Carkhuff's training technology. *Journal of Counseling and Development, 81*(3), 285–291.

Belkin, G. S. (1988). *Introduction to counseling* (3rd ed.). Dubuque, IA: William C. Brown.

Bellows-Blakely, K. F. (2000). Psychotherapists' personal psychotherapy and its perceived influence on clinical practice. *Dissertation Abstracts International, 60* (9-A), 3525. (University Microfilms International 95005-062)

Benack, S. (1984). Post-formal epistemologies and the growth of empathy. In M. Commons, F. A. Richards, & C. Armon (Eds.), *Beyond formal operations* (pp. 340–356). New York: Praeger.

Benack, S. (1988). Relativistic thought: A cognitive basis for empathy in counseling. *Counselor Education and Supervision, 27*(3), 216–232.

Benjamin, A. (1981). *The helping interview* (3rd ed.). Boston: Houghton Mifflin.

Benjamin, A. (1987). *The helping interview with case illustrations* (4th ed.). Boston: Houghton Mifflin.

Benjamin, A. (2001). *The helping interview with case illustrations* (Rev. ed.). Boston: Houghton Mifflin.

Bernard, J. M., & Goodyear, R. K. (2004). *Fundamentals of clinical supervision*. Boston: Pearson.

Beutler, L. E., Malik, M., Alimohamed, S., Harwood, T. M., Talebi, H., Noble, S., & Wong, E. (2004). Therapist variable. In M. J. Lambert (Ed.), *Bergin and Garfield's handbook of psychotherapy and behavior change* (5th ed.) (pp. 227–306). New York: Wiley.

Binswanger, L. (1962). *Existential analysis and psychotherapy.* New York: Dutton.

Binswanger, L. (1963). *Being-in-the-world. Selected papers.* New York: Basic Books.

Blasi, G. L. (1990). Social policy and social science research on homelessness. *Journal of Social Issues, 46*(4), 207–219.

Borders, L. D. (2002). School counseling in the 21st century: Personal and professional reflections. *Professional School Counseling, 5*(3), 180–185.

Bowman, J. T., & Allen, B. R. (1988). Moral development and counselor trainee empathy. *Counseling and Values, 32*(2), 144–146.

Bowman, J. T., & Reeves, T. G. (1987). Moral development and empathy in counseling. *Counselor Education and Supervision, 26*(4), 293–299.

Brammer, L. M., & MacDonald, G. (2003). *The helping relationship: Process and skills* (8th ed.). Boston: Allyn & Bacon.

Brammer, L. M., Shostrom, E. L., & Abrego, P. L. (1993). *Therapeutic psychology: Fundamentals of counseling and psychotherapy* (6th ed.). Englewood Cliffs, NJ: Prentice Hall.

Browning, C., Reynolds, A. L., & Dworkin, S. H. (1995). Affirmative psychotherapy for lesbian women. In D. R. Atkinson & G. Hackett (Eds.), *Counseling diverse populations* (pp. 289–306). Madison, WI: Brown & Benchmark.

Budman, S., & Gurman, A. (1983). The practice of brief therapy. *Professional Psychology: Research and Practice, 14,* 277–292.

Budman, S., & Gurman, A. S. (1988). *Theory and practice of brief therapy.* New York: Guilford Press.

Burlingame, G. M., & Fuhriman, A. (1987). Conceptualizing short-term treatment: A comparative review. *The Counseling Psychologist, 15,* 557–595.

Byrne, R. H. (1995). *Becoming a master counselor: Introduction to the profession.* Pacific Grove, CA: Brooks/Cole.

Carkhuff, R. (2000). *The art of helping* (8th ed.). Amherst, MA: Human Resource Development Press.

Carkhuff, R. R., & Berenson, B. G. (1977). *Beyond counseling and therapy* (2nd ed.). New York: Holt, Rinehart & Winston.

Carkhuff, R. R. (1969). *Helping and human relations* (Vol. 2). New York: Holt, Rinehart & Winston.

Cass, V. C. (1979). Homosexual identity formation: A theoretical model. *Journal of Homosexuality, 4,* 219–235.

Committee on Government Operations (fourth report). (1991). *A citizen's guide on using the freedom of information act and the privacy act of 1974 to request government records.* (House Report 102–146). Washington, DC: U.S. Government Printing Office.

Conte, H., Plutchik, R., Wild, K., & Karasu, T. (1986). Combined psychotherapy and pharmacotherapy for depressions. *Archives of General Psychiatry, 38*, 471–479.

Corey, G., & Corey, M. (2003). *Becoming a helper* (4th ed.). Pacific Grove, CA: Brooks/Cole.

Corey, G., Corey, M., & Callanan, P. (2003). *Issues and ethics in the helping professions* (6th ed.). Pacific Grove, CA: Brooks/Cole.

Corey, G. (2005). *Theory and practice of counseling and psychotherapy* (7th ed.). Pacific Grove, CA: Brooks/Cole.

Cormier, S., & Nurius, P. S. (2003). *Interviewing and change strategies for helpers: Fundamental skills and cognitive behavior interventions* (5th ed.). Pacific Grove, CA: Brooks/Cole.

Cottone, R. R. (2001). A social constructivism model of ethical decision making in counseling. *Journal of Counseling and Development, 79*(1), 39–45.

Cottone, R. R., & Claus, R. E. (2000). Ethical decision-making models: A review of the literature. *Journal of Counseling and Development, 78,* 275–283.

Council for Accreditation of Counseling and Related Educational Programs. (1994, January). *CACREP accreditation standards and procedures manual* (2nd ed.). Alexandria, VA: Author.

D'Andrea, M., & Daniels, J. (1991). Exploring the different levels of multicultural counseling training in counselor education. *Journal of Counseling and Development, 70,* 78–85.

D'Andrea, M., & Daniels, J. (1999). Exploring the psychology of white racism through naturalistic inquiry. *Journal of Counseling and Development, 77* (1), 93–101.

Daniels, J. A. (2001). Managed care, ethics, and counseling. *Journal of Counseling and Development, 79*, 119–122.

Daniels, T. (2003). A review of research on microcounseling: 1967– present. In A. Ivey and M. Ivey, *Intentional interviewing and Counseling* (5th ed.). Pacific Grove, CA: Brooks/Cole Publishing Company.

Danzinger, P. R., & Welfel, E. R. (2001). The impact of managed care on mental health counselors: A survey of perceptions, practices, and compliance with ethical standards. *Journal of Mental Health Counseling, 23,* 137–150.

Davis, J. L., & Mickelson, D. J. (1994). School counselors: Are you aware of ethical and legal aspects of counseling? *School Counselor, 42*(1), 5–13.

Davison, G. C., & Neale, J. M. (2004). *Abnormal psychology* (9th ed.). New York: Wiley.

Derlega, V. J., Lovell, R., & Chaikin, A. L. (1976). Effects of therapist disclosure and its perceived appropriateness on client self-disclosure. *Journal of Consulting and Clinical Psychology, 44,* 866.

Deutsch, C. J. (1984). Self-reported sources of stress among psychotherapists. *Professional Psychology: Research and Practice, 15*(6), 833–845.

Dinnebeil, L. A., Hale, L. M., & Rule, S. (1996). A qualitative analysis of parents' and service coordinators' descriptions of variables that influence collaborative relationships. *Topics in Early Childhood Special Education, 16*, 322–347.

Donley, R. J., Horan, J. J., & DeShong, R. L. (1990). The effect of several self-disclosure permutations on counseling process and outcome. *Journal of Counseling and Development, 67*, 408–412.

Doster, J. A., & Nesbitt, J. G. (1979). Psychotherapy and self-disclosure. In J. Chelune et al. (Eds.). *Self-disclosure: Origins, patterns, and implications of openness in interpersonal relationships* (pp. 177–242). San Francisco: Jossey-Bass.

Downing, N. E., & Roush, K. L. (1985). From passive acceptance to active commitment: A model of feminist identity development for women. *The Counseling Psychologists, 13*(4), 695–709.

Doyle, R. E. (1998). *Essential skills and strategies in the helping process* (2nd ed.). Pacific Grove, CA: Brooks/Cole.

Drum, D., & Lawler, A. (1988). *Developmental interventions: Theories, principles, and practice.* Columbus, OH: Merrill.

Drummond, R. J. (2004). *Appraisal procedures for counselors and helping professionals* (5th ed.). Columbus, OH: Merrill.

Dryden, W., & Spurling, L. (1989). *On becoming a psychotherapist.* New York: Tavistock/Routledge.

Dumont, F. (1993). Inferential heuristics in clinical problem formulation: Selective review of their strengths and weaknesses. *Professional Psychology: Research and Practice, 24,* 196–205.

Duys, D. K., & Hedstrom, S. M. 2000). Basic counselor skills training and counselor cognitive complexity. *Counselor Education and Supervision, 40*(1), 8–18.

Dyne, W. A. (1990). (Ed.). *Encyclopedia of homosexuality* (Vol. 1). New York: Garland Publishing.

Echterling, L. G., Cowan, E., Evans, W. F., Staton, A. R., Viere, G., Mckee, J. E., Presbury, J., & Stewart, A. L. (2002). *Thriving: A manual for students in the helping professions*. Upper Saddle River, NJ: Merrill.

Egan, G. (2002). *The skilled helper: A problem-management and opportunity-development approach to helping* (7th ed.). Pacific Grove, CA: Brooks/Cole.

Eisen, S. V., Clarridge, B., Stringfellow, V., Shaul, J. A., & Cleary, P. D. (2001). Toward a national report card: Measuring consumer experiences. In B. Dickey & L. I. Sederer (Eds.), *Improving mental health care: Commitment to quality* (pp. 115–134). Washington, DC: American Psychiatric Publishing.

Elliott, R., Greenberg, L. S., & Lietaer, G. (2004). Research on experiential psychotherapies. In M. J. Lambert (Ed.), *Bergin and Garfield's handbook of psychotherapy and behavior change* (5th ed., pp. 493–542). New York: Wiley.

Ellis, M. V., & Dell, D. M. (1986). Dimensionality of supervisor roles: Supervisor's perceptions of supervision. *Journal of Counseling Psychology, 33,* 282–291.

Erikson, E. (1968). *Identity, youth, and crisis.* New York: Norton.

Evans, D. R., Hearn, M. T., Uhlemann, M. R., & Ivey, A. E. (2004). *Essential interviewing* (6th ed.). Pacific Grove, CA: Brooks/Cole.

Evans, G. W., & Howard, R. B. (1973). Personal space. *Psychological Bulletin, 80,* 334–344.

Eysenck, H. J. (1952). The effects of psychotherapy: An evaluation. *Journal of Consulting Psychology, 16,* 319–324.

Fitzgerald, L. F., & Nutt, R. (1995). The division 17 principles concerning the counseling/ psychotherapy of women: Rationale and implementation. In D. R. Atkinson & G. Hackett (Eds.), *Counseling diverse populations* (pp. 229–261). Madison, WI: Brown & Benchmark.

Fong, M. L. (1995). Assessment and *DSM-IV* diagnosis of personality disorders: A primer for counselors. *Journal of Counseling Development, 73,* 635–639.

Fowler, J. (1981). *Stages of faith: The psychology of human development and the quest for meaning.* New York: Harper & Row.

Gabbard. G. O. (1995). What are boundaries in psychotherapy? *The Menninger Letter, 3*(4), 1–2.

Gallessich, J. (1983). *The profession and practice of consultation.* San Francisco: Jossey-Bass.

Garretson, D. J. (1993). Psychological misdiagnosis of African Americans. *Journal of Multicultural Counseling and Development, 21,* 119–126.

Gazda, G. M., Asbury, F. R., Balzer, F. J., Childers, W. C., Phelps, W. C., & Walters, R. P. (1999). *Human relations development: A manual for educators* (6th ed.). Boston: Allyn & Bacon.

Gelso, C., & Johnson, D. (1983). *Explorations in time-limited counseling and psychotherapy.* New York: Teachers College Press.

Gelso, C. J., & Carter, J. A. (1994). Components of the psychotherapy relationship: Their interaction and unfolding during treatment. *Journal of Counseling Psychology, 41*(3), 296–306.

George, R. L., & Cristiani, R. S. (1994). *Counseling theory and practice* (4th ed.). Boston: Allyn & Bacon.

Gibson, R. L., & Mitchell, M. H. (1995). *Introduction to counseling and guidance* (4th ed.). Englewood Cliffs, NJ: Merrill.

Gilroy, P. J., Carroll, L., & Murra, J. (2001). Does depression affect clinical practice? A survey of women psychotherapists. *Women and Therapy, 23*(4), 2001, 13–30.

Gilroy, P. J., Carroll, L., & Murra, J. (2002). A preliminary survey of counseling psychologists' personal experiences with depression and treatment. *Professional Psychology: Research and Practice, 33*(4), 402–407.

Gladding, S. (1996). *Community and agency counseling.* Upper Saddle River, NJ: Prentice Hall.

Gladding, S. (2000). *Counseling: A comprehensive profession* (4th ed.). Upper Saddle River, NJ: Merrill.

Gladding, S. T. (2001). *The counseling dictionary: Concise definitions of frequently used terms.* Upper Saddle River, NJ: Merrill/Prentice Hall.

Gladding, S., Remley, T. P., & Huber, C. H. (2001). *Ethical, legal, and professional issues in the practice of marriage and family therapy* (3rd ed.). Upper Saddle River, NJ: Merrill.

Gladstein, G. (1983). Understanding empathy: Integrating counseling, developmental, and social psychology perspectives. *Journal of Counseling Psychology, 30,* 467–482.

Glasser, W. (2000). *Reality therapy in action.* New York: HarperCollins.

Glidewell, J. C., & Livert, D. E. (1992). Confidence in the practice of clinical psychology. *Professional Psychology: Research and Practice, 23,* 151–157.

Glosoff, H. L., Herlihy, B., & Spense, B. E. (2000). Privilege communication in the counselor–client relationship. *Journal of Counseling and Development, 78*(4), 454–462.

Gompertz, K. (1960). The relation of empathy to effective communication. *Journalism Quarterly, 37*, 535–546.

Gonzales, M., Castillo-Canez, I., Tarke, H., Soriano, F., Garcia, P., & Velasquez, R. J. (1997). Promoting the culturally sensitive diagnosis of Mexican Americans: Some personal insights. *Journal of Multicultural Counseling and Development, 25*(2), 156–161.

Good, B. J. (1997). Studying mental illness in context: Local, global, or universal. *Ethos, 25*(2), 230–248.

Granello, P. F., & Witmer, M. (1998) Standards of care: Potential implications for the counseling profession. *Journal of Counseling and Development, 76,* 371–380.

Greenberg, H. R. (1993). *Screen memories: Hollywood cinema on the psychoanalytic couch.* New York: Columbia University Press.

Greenberg, L. S. (1994). What is "real" in the relationship? Comment on Gelso and Carter (1994). *Journal of Counseling Psychology, 41*(3), 307–309.

Greenberg, R. P., & Staller, J. (1981). Personal therapy for therapists. *American Journal of Psychiatry, 138*, 1461–1471.

Grimm, J. (1972). *Snow White and the seven dwarfs: A tale from the Brothers Grimm translated by Randall Jarrell.* New York: Farrar, Straus & Giroux.

Grunebaum, H. (1983). A study of therapists' choice of a therapist. *American Journal of Psychiatry, 140*, 1336–1339.

Guthmann, D. (1999). *Counseling deaf and hard of hearing persons with substance abuse and/or mental health issues: Is cross cultural counseling possible?* (ERIC Document Reproduction Service No. ED 454642). Minneapolis: The Minnesota Chemical Dependency Program for Deaf and Hard of Hearing Individuals. Also available on the World Wide Web: http://www.mncddeaf.org/articles/cross-culture_ad.htm

Hackney, H. L., & Cormier, L. S. (2005). *The professional counselor: A process guide to helping* (5th ed.). Needham Heights, MA: Allyn & Bacon.

Hanna, F. J., & Puhakka, K. (1991). When psychotherapy works: Pinpointing an element of change. *Psychotherapy, 28,* 598–607.

Hanna, F. J., & Ritchie, M. H. (1995). Seeking the active ingredients of psychotherapeutic change: Within and outside the context of therapy. *Professional Psychotherapy: Research and Practice, 26* 176–183.

Hansen, J. C., Rossberg, R. H., Cramer, S. H. (1994). *Counseling: Theory and process* (5th ed.). Boston: Allyn & Bacon.

Harvey, C., & Katz, C. (1985). *If I'm so successful, why do I feel like a fake? The imposter phenomenon*. New York: St. Martin's Press.

Harvey, V. (1997). Improving readability of psychological reports. *Professional Psychology: Research and Practice, 28,* 271–274.

Hashimi, J. (1991). Counseling older adults. In P. K. H. Kim (Ed.), *Serving the elderly: Skills for practice* (pp. 33–51). New York: McGraw-Hill.

Hayes, R. (1994). The legacy of Lawrence Kohlberg: Implications for counseling and human development. *Journal of Counseling and Development, 72*(3), 261–267.

Heibert, B., & Johnson, P. (1994). *Changes in counseling skills and cognitive structures of counselor trainees* (Report No. CG 025 436). (ERIC Document Reproduction Service No. Ed 375 335). Paper presented at the annual meeting of the American Educational Research Association in New Orleans.

Henry, W. P. (1998). Science, politics, and the politics of science: The use and misuse of empirically validated treatments. *Psychotherapy Research, 8,* 126–140.

Herr, E. (1985). *Why counseling?* (2nd ed.). Alexandria, VA: American Association for Counseling and Development.

Hersen, M., & Van Hasselt, V. B. (Eds.). (2001). *Advanced abnormal psychology* (2nd ed). New York: Plenum Press.

Hill, C. L., & Ridley, C. R. (2001). Diagnostic decision making: Do counselors delay final judgements? *Journal of Counseling and Development, 79,* 98–104

Hinkle, S. (1994a). *Psychodiagnosis for counselors: The DSM-IV* (Report No. MF01/PC01) (ERIC Document Reproduction Service No. ED 366890). Greensboro, NC: ERIC Clearinghouse on Counseling and Student Services.

Hinkle, J. S. (1994b). The *DSM-IV*: Prognosis and implications for mental health counselors. *Journal of Mental Health Counseling, 16*(2), 174–183.

Hohenshil, T. H. (1993). Teaching the *DSM-III-R* in counselor education. *Counselor Education and Supervision, 32*, 267–275.

Hohenshil, T. H. (1994). *DSM-IV:* What's new. *Journal of Counseling and Development, 73,* 105–107.

Hollis, R., & Sibley, B. (1987). *Walt Disney's Snow White and the seven dwarfs: The making of the classic film*. New York: Simon & Schuster.

Hubert, M. (1996). Confidentiality and the minor student. *The ASCA Counselor.* Alexandria, VA: Author.

Hutchins, D. E., & Cole, C. G. (1997). *Helping relationships and strategies* (3rd ed.). Pacific Grove, CA: Brooks/Cole.

Ingersoll, R. E. (2000). Teaching a psychopharmacology course to counselors: Justification, structure, and methods. *Counselor Education and Supervision, 40,* 58–69.

Ivey, A., & Ivey, M. (2003). *Intentional interviewing and counseling: Facilitating client development in multicultural society* (5th ed.). Pacific Grove, CA: Brooks/Cole.

Jaffee v. Redmond, 51F.3d 1346 (U.S. Supreme Ct., 1996).

Jaffee v. Redmond, 95–266, 116 S.C.T. 812 (U.S. Supreme Ct., 1996).

Janesick, B. J., & Goldsmith, K. L., (2000). *Managed dying*. Philadelphia: Xlibris Corporation.

Jongsma, A. E., Jr., & Peterson, L. M. (2003). *The complete adult psychotherapy treatment planner* (3rd ed). New York: Wiley.

Jourard, S. M. (1971). *The transparent self: Self disclosure and well-being* (2nd ed.). Princeton, NJ: Van Nostrand Reinhold.

Kahn, M. (1991). *Between therapist and client: The new relationship.* New York: Freeman.

Kegan, R. (1982). *The evolving self.* Cambridge, MA: Harvard University Press.

Kegan, R. (1994). *In over our heads.* Cambridge, MA: Harvard University Press.

Kelly, K. R., & Hall, A. S. (Eds.) (1992). Mental health counseling for men. [Special issue]. *Journal of Mental Health Counseling, 19*(2).

Kemp, C. G. (1962). Influence of dogmatism on the training of counselors. *Journal of Counseling Psychology, 9,* 155–157.

Kim, B. S. K., & Lyons, H. Z. (2003). Experiential activities and multicultural counseling competence training. *Journal of Counseling and Development, 81*(4), 400–408.

King, P. M. (1978). William Perry's theory of intellectual and ethical development. In L. Knetelkamp, C. Widick, & C. L. Parker (Eds.), *Applying new developmental findings* (pp. 34–51). San Francisco: Jossey-Bass.

King, P. M. (1994). Theories of college student development: Sequences and consequences. *Journal of College Student Development, 35*(6), 413–421.

Kitchener, K. S. (1984). Intuition, critical evaluation and ethical principles: The foundation for ethical decisions in counseling psychology. *The Counseling Psychologists, 12*(3), 43–45.

Kitchener, K. S. (1986). Teaching applied ethics in counselor education: An integration of psychological processes and philosophical analysis. *Journal of Counseling and Development, 64*(5), 306–311.

Klein, S. M. (1988). Psychological consultation in the college community: A psychoanalytic approach. In R. May (Ed.), *Psychoanalytic psychotherapy in a college context* (pp. 22–40). New York: Praeger.

Kleinke, C. L. (1994). *Common principles of psychotherapy*. Pacific Grove, CA: Brooks/Cole.

Kohlbery, L. (1984). *The Psychology of moral development: The nature and validity of moral stages.* San Fracisco: Harper & Row.

Kübler-Ross, E. (1997). *On death and dying.* New York: Simon & Schuster.

LaBruzza, A. L., & Mendez-Villarrubia, J. M. (1994). *Using DSM-IV: A clinician's guide to psychiatric diagnosis.* Northvale, NJ: Jason Aronson.

Ladany, N., Marotta, S., & Muse-Burke, J. L. (2001). Counselor experience related to complexity of case conceptualization and supervision preference. *Counselor Education and Supervision, 40,* 203–219.

Lambert, M. J., & Cattani-Thompson, K. (1996). Current findings regarding effectiveness of counseling: Implications for practice. *Journal of Counseling and Development, 74,* 601–608.

Lambert, M. J., & Ogles, B. (2004). The efficacy and effectiveness of psychotherapy. In M. J. Lambert (Ed.), *Bergin and Garfield's handbook of psychotherapy and behavior change* (5th ed., pp. 139–193). New York: Wiley.

Lee, W. M. L., & Mixson, R. J. (1995). Asian and Caucasian client perceptions of the effectiveness of counseling. *Journal of Multicultural Counseling and Development, 23,* 48–56.

Levinson, D. (1986). *The seasons of a man's life*. New York: Ballantine.

Locke, D. (1999). *Multicultural counseling* (Report No.EG0-CG-93-1) (ERIC Document Reproduction

Service No. ED 357316). Greensboro, NC: ERIC Clearinghouse on Counseling and Student Services.

Loewenberg, F., & Dolgoff, R. (2005). *Ethical decisions for social work practice* (7th ed.). Itasca, IL: Peacock.

Loganbill, C., Hardy, E., & Delworth, U. (1982). Supervision: A conceptual model. *The Counseling Psychologist, 10,* 3–42.

Lombana, J. H. (1989). Counseling persons with disabilities: Summary and projections. *Journal of Counseling and Development, 68*(2), 177–179.

Loulan, J. (1987). *Lesbian passion: Loving ourselves and each other*. San Francisco: Spinsters/Aunt Lute.

Lovell, C. (1999) Empathic-cognitive development in students of counseling. *Journal of Adult Development, 6*(4), 195–203.

Luborsky, L., Crits-Christoph, P., Mintz, J., & Auerbach, A. (1988). *Who will benefit from psychotherapy? Predicting therapeutic outcomes.* New York: Basic Books.

Mabe, A. R., & Rollin, S. A. (1986). The role of a code of ethical standards in counseling. *Journal of Counseling and Development, 64*(5), 294–297.

Magolda, M. B., & Porterfield, W. D. (1988). *Assessing intellectual development: The link between theory and practice.* Alexandria, VA: American College Personnel Association.

Mahalick, J. R. (1990). Systematic eclectic models. *The Counseling Psychologist, 18,* 655–679.

Mahoney, M. J. (1991). *Human change processes: The scientific foundations of psychotherapy.* New York: Basic Books.

Manderscheid, R. W., Henderson, M. J., & Brown, D. Y. (2001). Status of national efforts to improve accountability for quality. In B. Dickey & L. I. Sederer (Eds.) *Improving mental health care: Commitment to quality* (pp. 163–178). Washington, DC: American Psychiatric Publishing.

Marshall, J. (1990). *Hansel and Gretel.* New York: Dial Books.

Martin, J., Slemon, A., Hiebert, B., Halberg, E., & Cummings, A. (1989). Conceptualizations of novice and experienced counselors. *Journal of Counseling Psychology, 36,* 395–400.

Martin, W. E., Easton, C., Wilson, S., Takemoto, M., & Sullivan, S. (2004). Salience of emotional intelligence as a core characteristic of being a counselor. *Counselor Education and Supervision, 44*(1), 17–30.

May, K. M., & Sowa, C. J. (1992). The relationship between a counselor's ethical orientation and stress experienced in ethical dilemmas. *Counseling and Values, 36*(2), 150–159.

May, R. (1988). *Psychoanalytic psychotherapy in a college content.* New York: Praeger.

McAuliffe, G., Eriksen, K., & Associates (2000). *Preparing counselors and therapists: Creating constructivist and developmental programs*. Virginia Beach, VA: The Donning Company.

McAuliffe, G., & Eriksen, K. (2001). *Preparing counselors and therapists: Creating constructivist and developmental programs*. Virginia Beach, VA: The Donning Company.

McAuliffe, G., Neukrug, E., & Lovell, C. (1998). *The cognitive development of counselor trainees.* Unpublished manuscript.

McKenzie, K. (1999). Moving the misdiagnosis debate forward. *International Review of Psychiatry, 11*(2–3), 153–161.

McNamara, K., & Rickard, K. M. (1989). Feminist identity development: Implications for feminist therapy with women. *Journal of Counseling and Development, 68*, 184–189.

Mehrabian, A. (1972). *Nonverbal communication*. Chicago: Aldine-Atherton.

Mehr, J. J. (2004). *Human services: Concepts and intervention strategies* (9th ed.). Boston: Allyn & Bacon.

Mezzano, J. (1969). A note on dogmatism and counselor effectiveness. *Counselor Education and Supervision, 9*, 64–65.

Miars, R. D. (2002). Existential authenticity: A foundational value for counseling. *Counseling and Values, 46*(3), 218–225.

Midgette, T. E., & Meggert, S. S. (1991). Multicultural counseling instruction: A challenge for faculties in the 21st century. *Journal of Counseling and Development, 70*, 136–141.

Minuchin, S. (1974). *Families and family therapy.* Cambridge, MA: Harvard University Press.

Mitchell, M. (1964). *Gone with the wind.* New York: Macmillan. (Original work published 1936).

Moore, D., & Haverkamp, B. E. (1989). Measured increases in male emotional expressiveness following a structured group intervention. *Journal of Counseling and Development, 67,* 513–517.

Morrow, K. A., & Deidan, C. T. (1992). Bias in the counseling process: How to recognize and avoid it.

Journal of Counseling and Development, 70(5), 571–577.

Morse, P. S., & Ivey, A. E. (1996). *Face to face: Communication and conflict resolution in the schools.* Thousand Oaks, CA: Corwin Press.

Mowrer, O. H. (Ed.). (1967). *Morality and mental health.* Chicago: Rand McNally.

National Association of Social Workers. (1999). *Code of ethics of the National Association of Social Workers.* Retrieved May 5, 2003, from the World Wide Web: http://www.socialworkers.org/pubs/code/code.asp

National Organization of Human Service Education. (1995). *Ethical standards of human service professionals.* Fitchburg, MA: Author.

Neimeyer, G. J., Banikiotes, P. G., & Winum, P. C. (1979). Self-disclosure flexibility and counseling-related perceptions. *Journal of Counseling Psychology, 26,* 546–548.

Neimeyer, G. J., & Fong, M. L. (1983). Self-disclosure flexibility and counselor effectiveness. *Journal of Counseling Psychology, 30,* 258–261.

Neukrug, E. (1980). *The effects of supervisory style and type of praise upon counselor trainees' level of empathy and perception of supervisor.* Unpublished doctoral dissertation, University of Cincinnati, Ohio.

Neukrug, E. (1987). The brief training of paraprofessional counselors in empathic responding. *New Hampshire Journal for Counseling and Development, 15*(1), 15–19.

Neukrug, E. (1994). Understanding diversity in a pluralistic world. *The Journal of Intergroup Relations, XXI*(2), 3–12.

Neukrug, E. (1997). Support and challenge: Use of metaphor as a higher level empathic response. In H. Rosenthal (Ed.), *Favorite counseling and therapy techniques* (pp. 139–141). Bristol, PA: Accelerated Development.

Neukrug, E. (2001). Medical breakthroughs: Genetic research and genetic counseling, psychotropic medications, and the mind–body connection. In T. McClam & M. Woodside (Eds.), *Human service challenges in the 21st century* (pp. 115–132). Birmingham, AL: Ebsco Media.

Neukrug, E. (2002). *Skills and techniques for human service professionals: Counseling environment, helping skills, treatment issues.* Pacific Grove, CA: Brooks/Cole.

Neukrug, E. S. (2003a). *The world of the counselor: An introduction to the counseling profession* (2nd ed.). Pacific Grove, CA: Brooks/Cole.

Neukrug, E. S. (2003b). *The world of the counselor: A workbook for counselor educators and students* (2nd ed.). Pacific Grove, CA: Brooks/Cole.

Neukrug, E. (2004). *Theory, practice and trends in human services: An introduction to an emerging profession* (3rd ed.). Pacific Grove, CA: Brooks/Cole.

Neukrug, E., & Fawcett, R. (2006). *Essentials of testing and assessment: A practical guide for counselors, social workers, and psychotherapists.* Pacific Grove, CA: Brooks/Cole.

Neukrug, E., Lovell, C., & Parker, R. (1996). Employing ethical codes and decision-making models: A developmental process. *Counseling and Values, 40,* 98–106.

Neukrug, E., & McAuliffe, G. (1993). Cognitive development and human service education. *Human Service Education, 13*(1), 13–26.

Neukrug, E., Milliken, T., & Shoemaker, J. (2001). Counseling seeking behavior of NOHSE practitioners, educators, and trainees. *Human Service Education, 21,* 45–48.

Neukrug, E., Milliken, T., & Walden, S. (2001). Ethical practices of credentialed counselors: An updated survey of state licensing boards. *Counselor Education and Supervision, 41*(1), 57–70.

Neukrug, E., & Williams, G. (1993). Counseling counselors: A survey of values. *Counseling and Values, 38,* 51–62.

Norcross, J. C. (2000). Psychotherapist self-care: Practitioner-tested, research-informed strategies. *Professional Psychology: Research and Practice, 31*(6), 710–713.

Norcross, J. C., & Prochaska, J. O. (1982). A national survey of clinical psychologists: Affiliations and orientations. *Clinical Psychologist, 35,* 4–6.

Norcross, J. C., Strausser, D. J., & Faltus, F. J. (1988). The therapist's therapist. *American Journal of Psychotherapy, 42*(1), 53–66.

Norden, M. J. (1996). *Beyond Prozac: Brain-toxic lifestyles, natural antidotes & new generation antidepressants* (2nd ed.). New York: Regan Books.

Nwachuku, U., & Ivey, A. E. (1992). Teaching culture-specific counseling using microtraining technology. *International Journal for the Advancement of Counselling, 15,* 151–161.

Oppenheimer, M. (1998). Zen and the art of supervision. *Family Journal: Counseling and Therapy for Couples and Families, 6*(1), 61–63.

Orlinsky, D. E., & Howard, K. I. (1986). Process and outcome in psychotherapy. In S. L. Garfield & A. E. Bergin (Eds.), *Handbook of psychotherapy and behavior change* (3rd ed., pp. 311–381). New York: Wiley.

Orlinsky, D. E., Ronnestad, M. H., & Willutzki, U. (2004). Fifty years of psychotherapy process-outcome research: Continuity and change. In M. J. Lambert (Ed.), *Bergin and Garfield's handbook of psychotherapy and behavior change* (5th ed., 139–193). New York: Wiley.

Orza, J. L. (1996). Understanding the power of empathy: A qualitative study. *Dissertation Abstracts International, 56*(8-A), 3006. (University Microfilms International (95004–133)

Osherson, S. (1986). *Finding our fathers*. New York: Faucett Columbine.

Pascarella, E. T., & Terenzini, P. T. (1991). *How college affects students: Findings and insights from twenty years of research.* San Francisco: Jossey-Bass.

Patterson, C. H. (1984). Empathy, warmth, and genuineness in psychotherapy: A review of reviews. *Psychotherapy, 21,* 431–438.

Patton, M., & Robbins, S. B. (1982). Kohut's self-psychology as a model for college-student counseling. *Professional Psychology, 13,* 876–888.

Pedersen, P. B., Draguns, J. G., Lonner, W. J., & Trimble, J. E. (2002). *Counseling across cultures* (5th ed.). Thousand Oaks, CA: Sage.

Pelsma, D. M., & Borgers, S. B. (1986). Experience-based ethics: A developmental model of learning ethical reasoning. *Journal of Counseling and Development, 64*(5), 311–314.

Pennebaker, J. W., Colder, M., & Sharp, L. K. (1990). Accelerating the coping process. *Journal of Personality and Social Psychology, 58,* 528–537.

Pennebaker, J. W., & Susman, J. R. (1988). Disclosure of traumas and psychosomatic processes. *Social Science and Medicine, 26*, 327–332.

Perry, M. A., & Furukawa, M. J. (1986). Modeling methods. In F. H. Kanfer & A. P. Goldstein (Eds.), *Helping people change: A textbook of methods* (3rd ed., pp. 66–110). New York: Pergamon Press.

Persinger, M. A., Roll, W. G., Tiller, S. G., Koren, S. A., & Cook, C. M. (2002). Remote viewing with the artist Ingo Swann: Neuropsychological profile, electroencephalographic correlates, magnetic resonance imaging (MRI), and possible mechanisms. *Perceptual and Motor Skills, 94*(3, Pt. 1), 927–949.

Phelps, R. E., Taylor, J. D., & Gerard, P. A. (2001). Cultural mistrust, ethnic identity, racial identity, and self-esteem among ethnically diverse black university students. *Journal of Counseling and Development, 79*, 209–216.

Piaget, J. (1954). *The construction of reality in the child.* New York: Basic Books.

Polanski, P. J., & Hinkle, J. S. (2000). The mental status examination: Its use by professional counselors. *Journal of Counseling and Development, 78,* 357–364.

Pope, K. S., & Tabachnik, B. G. (1994). Therapists as patients: A national survey of psychologists' experiences, problems, and beliefs. *Professional Psychology: Research and Practice, 25*(3), 247–258.

Pope, M. (1995). The "salad bowl" is big enough for us all: An argument for the inclusion of lesbians and gay men in any definition of multiculturalism. *Journal of Counseling and Development, 73,* 301–303.

Pope, V. T., & Kline, W. B. (1999). The personal characteristics of effective counselors: What 10 experts think. *Psychological Reports, 84*(3, Pt. 2), 1339–1344.

Poston, W. S. C., Craine, M., & Atkinson, D. R. (1991). Counselor dissimilarity, confrontation, client cultural mistrust, and willingness to self-disclose. *Journal of Multicultural Counseling and Development, 19*, 65–73.

Prochaska, J. O., & Norcross, J. C. (1983). Contemporary psychotherapists: A national survey of characteristics, practices, orientations, and attitudes. *Psychotherapy: Theory, Research and Practice, 20*(2), 161–173.

Public Citizen (2002). The Freedom of Information Act: A user's guide. Retrieved January 16, 2005 from the World Wide Web:http://www.citizen.org/litigation/free_info/articles.cfm?ID=5208

Purkey, W. W., & Schmidt, J. J. (1996). *Invitational counseling: A self-concept approach to professional practice.* Pacific Grove, CA: Brooks/Cole.

Reeves, T. G., Bowman, J. T., & Cooley, S. L. (1989). Relationship between the client's moral development level and empathy of the counseling student. *Counselor Education and Supervision, 28*(4), 299–305.

Remen, N., May, R., Young, D., & Berland, W. (1985). The wounded healer. *Saybrook Review, 5,* 84–93.

Remley, R. P., Herlihy, B., & Herlihy, S. B. (1997). The U.S. Supreme Court decision in *Jaffe v. Redmond:* Implications for counselors. *Journal of Counseling and Development, 75,* 213–218.

Rest, J. R. (1984). Research on moral development: Implications for training counseling psychologists. *The Counseling Psychologist, 12,* 19–29.

Reynolds, J. F., Mair, D. C., & Fischer, P. C. (1995). *Writing and reading mental health records: Issues and analysis* (2nd ed.). Mahwah, NJ: Erlbaum.

Ridgway, I. R., & Sharpley, C. F. (1990). Empathic interactional sequences and counsellor trainee effectiveness. *Counselling Psychology Quarterly, 3*(3), 257–265.

Robbins, S. B., & Zinni, V. R. (1988). Implementing a time-limited treatment model: Issues and solutions. *Professional Psychology: Research and Practice, 19,* 53–57.

Robertiello, R. C., & Schoenewolf, G. (1987). *101 Common therapeutic blunders: Countertransference and counterresistance in psychotherapy.* Northvale, NJ: Jason Aronson.

Rogers, C. (1989a). A client-centered/person-centered approach to therapy. In H. Kirschenbaum (Ed.), *The Carl Rogers reader* (pp. 135–152). Boston: Houghton Mifflin. (Original work published 1986).

Rogers, C. (1989b). Reinhold Niebuhr's The self and the dramas of history: Review by Carl Rogers. In H. Kirschenbaum (Ed.), *Carl Rogers: Dialogues* (pp. 208–211). Boston: Houghton Mifflin. (Original work published 1956)

Rogers, C. R. (1942). *Counseling and psychotherapy: New concepts in practice*. Boston: Houghton Mifflin.

Rogers, C. R. (1957). The necessary and sufficient conditions of therapeutic personality change. *Journal of Counseling Psychology, 21*(2), 95–103.

Rogers, C. R. (1959). A theory of therapy, personality and interpersonal relationships as developed in the client-centered framework. In S. Koch (Ed.), *Psychology: A study of science: Vol. 3. Formulations of the person and the social context* (pp. 184–256). New York: McGraw-Hill.

Rogers, C. R. (1961). *On becoming a person.* Boston: Houghton Mifflin.

Rokeach, M. (1960). *The open and closed mind.* New York: Basic Books.

Rossi, P. H. (1990). The old homeless and the new homelessness in historical perspective. *American Psychologist, 45*(8), 954–959.

Russo, J. R., Kelz, J. W., & Hudon, G. R. (1964). Are good counselors open-minded? *Counselor Education and Supervision, 3,* 74–77

Safran, J. D., & Muran, J. C. (2000). *Negotiating the therapeutic alliance: A relational treatment guide.* New York: Guilford Press.

Sarwer-Foner, G. J. (1993). The relationship between psychotherapy and pharmacotherapy: An introduction. *American Journal of Psychotherapy, 47,* 387–392.

Schatzberg, A. F., & Nemeroff, C. B. (2001). *Textbook of psychopharmacology* (3rd ed.). Washington, DC: American Psychiatric Press.

Scher, M. (1979). On counseling men. *Personnel and Guidance Journal, 57,* 252–254.

Scher, M. (1981). Men in hiding. *Personnel and Guidance Journal, 60,* 199–202.

Schinka, J. A. (2003). *Mental status checklist–adult.* Lutz, FL: Psychological Assessment Resources.

Schlossberg, N. K. (1995). *Counseling adults in transition* (2nd ed.). New York: Springer.

Schwitzer, A. M., Boyce, D., Cody, P., Holman, A., & Stein, J. (2005). *Counselor training using clients from literature, popular fiction, and entertainment media.* Manuscript submitted for publication.

Schwitzer, A. M., & Everett, A. (1997). Reintroducing the *DSM-IV*: Responses to ten counselor reservations about diagnosis. *The Virginia Counselors Journal, 25,* 54–64.

Schwitzer, A. M. (1996). Using the inverted pyramid heuristic in counselor education and supervision. *Counselor Education and Supervision, 35,* 258–267.

Schwitzer, A. M. (1997). The inverted pyramid framework applying self psychology constructs to conceptualizing college student psychotherapy. *Journal of College Student Psychotherapy 11,* 29–48.

Scissons, E. D. (1993). *Counseling for results*. Pacific Grove, CA: Brooks/Cole.

Seligman, L. (1993). Teaching treatment planning. *Counselor Education and Supervision, 33,* 287–297.

Seligman, L. (1996). *Diagnosis, and treatment planning in counseling* (2nd ed.) NY: Plenum Press.

Seligman, L. (1998) *Selecting effective treatments: A comprehensive, systematic guide to treating mental disorders* (Rev. ed.). San Francisco: Jossey-Bass.

Seligman, L. (2001). *Systems, strategies, and skills of counseling and psychotherapy.* Upper Saddle River, NJ: Merrill/Prentice Hall.

Seligman, L. (2004). *Diagnosis and treatment planning in counseling* (3rd ed.). New York: Plenum Press.

Sexton, T. (1993). A review of the counseling outcome research. In G. R. Walz & J. C. Bleuer (Eds.), *Counselor efficacy: Assessing and using counseling outcomes research* (Report No. ISBN-1-56109-056-5) (ERIC Document Reproduction Service No. Ed 362 821). Ann Arbor, MI: ERIC Clearinghouse on Counseling and Personnel Services.

Sexton, T. L. (1999). *Evidence-based counseling: Implications for counseling practice, preparation, and professionalism* (No. ED435948) (ERIC Document Reproduction Service No. ED99CO0014). Greensboro, NC: ERIC Clearinghouse on Counseling and Student Services.

Sexton, T., & Whiston, S. C. (1991). A review of the empirical basis for counseling: Implications for practice and training. *Counselor Education and Supervision, 30,* 330–354.

Sexton, T., & Whiston, S. C. (1994). The status of the counseling relationship: An empirical review, theoretical implications, and research directions. *The Counseling Psychologist, 22,* 6–78.

Sexton, T. L., Whiston, S. C., Bleuer, J. C., & Walz, G. R. (1997). *Integrating outcome research into counseling practice and training.* Alexandria, VA: American Counseling Association.

Shannon, J. W., & Woods, W. J. (1995). Affirmative psychotherapy for gay men. In D. R. Atkinson & G. Hackett (Eds.), *Counseling diverse populations* (pp. 307–324). Madison, WI: Brown & Benchmark.

Sharpley, C. F., & Sagris, A. (1995). When does counsellor forward lean influence client-perceived rapport? *British Journal of Guidance and Counselling, 23,* 387–394.

Sherman, J. B. (2000). Required psychotherapy for psychology graduate students: Psychotherapists' evaluations of process. *Dissertation Abstracts International: Section B: The Sciences and Engineering, 60(9-B)*, 4910. (University Microfilms International 95006–122).

Sieber, J. E. (1992). *Planning ethically responsible research.* Newbury Park, CA: Sage.

Smith, D. S. (1982). Trends in counseling and psychotherapy. *American Psychologist, 37,* 802–809.

Smith, H. B. (1999). Managed care: A survey of counselor educators and counselor practitioners. *Journal of Mental Counseling, 21,* 270–284.

Snarey, J. (1985). Cross-cultural universality of social-moral development. *Psychological Bulletin, 97*(2), 202–232.

Sodowsky, G. R., & Taffe, R. C. (1991). Counselor trainees' analysis of multicultural counseling videotapes. *Journal of Multicultural Counseling and Development, 19,* 115–129.

Solomon, A. (1992). Clinical diagnosis among diverse populations: A multicultural perspective. *The Journal of Contemporary Human Services, 73*(6), 371–377.

Speight, S. L., Myers, J., Cox, C. I., & Highlen, P. S. (1991). A redefinition of multicultural counseling. *Journal of Counseling and Development, 70,* 29–36.

Sue, D. W., Arredondo, P., & McDavis, R. J. (1992). Multicultural counseling competencies and standards: A call to the profession. *Journal of Counseling and Development, 70*(4), 477–486.

Sue, D. W., & Sue, D. (1990). *Counseling the culturally different: Theory and practice* (2nd ed.). New York: Wiley.

Sue, D. W., & Sue, D. (2002). *Counseling the culturally different: Theory and practice* (4th ed.). New York: Wiley.

Sullivan, W., Wolk, J., & Hartmann, D. (1992). Case management in alcohol and drug treatment: Improving client outcome. *Families in Society: The Journal of Contemporary Human Services, 73,* 195–204.

Swenson, L. C. (1997). Psychology and law for the helping professions (2nd ed.). Pacific Grove, CA: Brooks/Cole.

Tafoya, T. (1996, June). *New heights in human services: Multiculturalism.* Keynote address at National Organization of Human Services Annual Conference. St. Louis, MO.

Tamase, K., & Arake, M. (1993). Questions sequence and intimacy of open and closed questions. *Bulletin of Nara University of Education, 29,* 181–189.

Tamase, K., Baker, S., & Ivey, A. (1999). *Differences in effects of open and closed questions and types of open questions.* Unpublished manuscript, Nara Unviersity of Education, Nara, Japan.

Tennyson, W. W., & Strom, S. M. (1986). Beyond professional standards: Developing irresponsibleness. *Journal of Counseling and Development, 64*(5), 298–302.

Thompson, J. J. (1973). *Beyond words: Nonverbal communication in the classroom*. New York: Citation Press.

Thompson, R. (2002). *Counseling techniques: Improving relationships with others, ourselves, our families and our environment* (2nd ed.). Washington, DC: Accelerated Development.

Tosi, D. J. (1970). Dogmatism within the counselor–client dyad. *Journal of Counseling Psychology, 17,* 284–288.

Toth, P. L., & Erwin, W. J. (1998). Applying skill-based curriculum to teach feedback in groups: An evaluation study. *Journal of Counseling and Development, 76*(3), 294–301.

Truax, C. B., & Mitchell, K. M. (1971). Research on certain therapist interpersonal skills in relation to process and outcome. In A. E. Bergin & S. L. Garfield (Eds.), *Handbook of psychotherapy and behavior change: An empirical analysis* (pp. 299–344). New York: Wiley.

U.S. Department of Health and Human Services. (2003). *HIPAA*. Retrieved August 7, 2003, from the World Wide Web: http://www.hhs.gov/ocr/hipaa/

Van Hoose, W. H. (1980). Ethics and counseling. *Counseling and Human Development, 13,* 1–12.

Van Hoose, W. H., & Paradise, L. V. (1979). *Ethics in counseling and psychotherapy.* Cranston, RI: Carroll Press.

Van Zandt, C. D. (1990). Professionalism: A matter of personal initiatives. *Journal of Counseling and Development, 68,* 243–245.

Wampold, B. E. (2001). *The great psychotherapy debate: Models, methods, and findings.* Mahwah, NJ: Erlbaum.

Watzlawick, P. (1967). *Pragmatics of human communication*. New York: Norton.

Weaver, K. M. (2000). The use of the California Psychological Inventory in identifying personal characteristics of effective beginning counselors. *Dissertation Abstracts International, 60*(12-A), 4334. (University Microfilms International 95011–031).

Welfel, E. R., & Lipsitz, N. E. (1983). Ethical orientation of counselors: Its relationship to moral reasoning and level of training. *Counselor Education and Supervision, 23*(1), 33–45.

Welfel, E. R. (2002). *Ethics in counseling and psychotherapy: Standards, research, and emerging issues* (2nd ed.). Pacific Grove, CA: Brooks/Cole.

Westwood, M. J., & Ishiyama, F. I. (1990). The communication process as a critical intervention for client change in cross-cultural counseling. *Journal of Multicultural Counseling and Development, 18,* 163–171.

Wheeler, S. (1991). Personal therapy: An essential aspect of counsellor training, or a distraction from focusing on the client? *Journal for the Advancement of Counselling, 14,* 193–202.

White, P. E., & Franzoni, J. B. (1990). A multidimensional analysis of the mental health graduate counselors in training. *Counselor Education and Training, 29*(4), 258–267.

Whitson, S. C., & Coker, J. K. (2000). Reconstructing clinical training: Implications from research. *Counselor Education and Supervision, 39*, 228–253.

Widick, C. (1977). The Perry scheme: A foundation for developmental practice. *The Counseling Psychologist, 6*(4), 35–38.

Williams, R. C., & Myer, R. A. (1992). The men's movement: An adjunct to traditional counseling approaches. *Journal of Mental Health Counseling, 14,* 393–404.

Williams, S. C. (1999). Counselor trainee effectiveness: An examination of the relationship between personality characteristics, family of origin functioning, and trainee effectiveness. *Dissertation Abstracts International: Section B: The Sciences and Engineering, 59*(8-B), 4494. (University Microfilms International 95004–227)

Wilson, L. L., & Stith, L. L. (1991). Culturally sensitive therapy with Black clients. *Journal of Multicultural Counseling and Development, 19,* 32–43.

Wolfgang, A. (1985). The function and importance of nonverbal behavior in intercultural counseling. In P. B. Pedersen (Ed.), *Handbook of cross-cultural counseling and therapy*. (pp. 99–115) Westport, CT: Greenwood Press.

Woodside, M., & McClam, T. (2003). *Generalist case management: A method of human service delivery* (2nd ed.). Pacific Grove, CA: Brooks/Cole.

Wright, W. (1975). Counselor dogmatism, willingness to disclose, and clients' empathy ratings. *Journal of Counseling Psychology, 22,* 390–394.

Wylie, M. S. (1995, September/October). The new visionaries. *The Family Therapy Networker*, pp. 20–29, 32–35.

Yeh, C. J., & Hwang, M. Y. (2002). Interdependence in ethnic identity and self: Implications for theory and practice. *Journal of Counseling and Development, (78)*4, 420–429.

Young, M. E. (1992). *Counseling methods and techniques: An eclectic approach.* New York: Macmillan.

Young, M., & Long, L. (1998). *Counseling and therapy for couples.* Pacific Grove, CA: Brooks Cole.

Yutrzenka, B. A. (1995). Making a case for training in ethnic and cultural diversity in increasing treatment efficacy. *Journal of Consulting and Clinical Psychology, 63*(2), 197–296.

Zuckerman, E. (2003). *The paper office: Forms, guidelines, and resources to make your practice work ethically, legally, and profitably* (3rd ed.). New York: Guilford Press.

Index

Note: Page numbers with a (t) are tables